Hepatitis: Management and Treatment

Hepatitis: Management and Treatment

Editor: Terry May

AMERICAN
MEDICAL PUBLISHERS
www.americanmedicalpublishers.com

AMERICAN
MEDICAL PUBLISHERS
www.americanmedicalpublishers.com

Cataloging-in-Publication Data

Hepatitis : management and treatment / edited by Terry May.
p. cm.
Includes bibliographical references and index.
ISBN 978-1-63927-192-4
1. Hepatitis. 2. Hepatitis--Management. 3. Liver--Diseases. 4. Liver--Diseases--Treatment. I. May, Terry.
RC848.H42 H47 2022
610.285--dc23

American Medical Publishers,
41 Flatbush Avenue,
1st Floor, New York,
NY 11217, USA

ISBN 978-1-63927-192-4 (Hardback)

Contents

Preface

Hepatitis refers to an inflammatory condition of the liver. Some of the symptoms of hepatitis include yellow discoloration of the skin, whites of the eyes, vomiting, tiredness, abdominal pain, poor appetite and diarrhea. Viruses commonly cause hepatitis. It can be classified into hepatitis A, B, C, D and E. Heavy alcohol use, toxins, autoimmune diseases and non-alcoholic steatohepatitis can give rise to the disease. Contaminated water and food cause hepatitis A and E. Hepatitis B is transmitted sexually. It can also be transmitted from mother to baby during pregnancy. Hepatitis C is spread through infected blood and needle sharing. Hepatitis can be diagnosed on the basis of symptoms, medical history, blood tests, imaging and liver biopsy. Hepatitis A, B and D can be prevented with immunization. Certain medications, physical activity, a healthy diet and weight loss programs are recommended for its treatment. The topics included in this book on hepatitis are of utmost significance and bound to provide incredible insights to readers. Its objective is to give a general view of hepatitis and its management and treatment. Those in search of information to further their knowledge will be greatly assisted by this book.

The researches compiled throughout the book are authentic and of high quality, combining several disciplines and from very diverse regions from around the world. Drawing on the contributions of many researchers from diverse countries, the book's objective is to provide the readers with the latest achievements in the area of research. This book will surely be a source of knowledge to all interested and researching the field.

In the end, I would like to express my deep sense of gratitude to all the authors for meeting the set deadlines in completing and submitting their research chapters. I would also like to thank the publisher for the support offered to us throughout the course of the book. Finally, I extend my sincere thanks to my family for being a constant source of inspiration and encouragement.

Editor

1

The prevalence of functional dyspepsia using Rome III questionnaire among chronic hepatitis C patients

Hala I. Mohamed*, Hamdy A. Mokarib, Zienab M. Saad and Wael M. Abd El Ghany

Abstract

Background: Hepatitis C virus (HCV) is a common chronic infection that is widely associated with symptoms of fatigue and abdominal pain. The aim of the present study was to determine the prevalence of functional dyspepsia (FD) among patients with hepatitis C.

Methods: This study included 252 patients with chronic hepatitis C and 150 healthy volunteers. Clinical and laboratory data were recorded for every patient. All patients and controls were administered a questionnaire of FD according to Rome III criteria.

Results: The percentage of patients with FD was significantly higher in patients with chronic HCV than normal controls (65.9 % vs 28.7 %, respectively). In chronic HCV patients, post prandial distention syndrome (PDS) subtype was the predominant type (86.1 %). The percentage of patients with a high fibrosis score (F2–3) and raised ALT were significantly higher in patients with FD than in patients without FD ($P < 0.001$; $P < 0.04$; respectively). A multivariate regression analysis revealed a significant association between fibrosis score, BMI and FD

Conclusion: FD is more prevalent in patients with chronic hepatitis C. Obese chronic HCV and those with higher fibrosis scores are more likely to have FD.

Keyword: FD, Hepatitis C, PDS, Rome III

Background

FD is a clinical syndrome defined by unexplained chronic or recurrent upper abdominal symptoms [1]. Symptoms are frequently related to meals and include epigastric pain, early satiety, fullness or bloating, belching, nausea and vomiting. In previous report abdominal pain, nausea, bloating, and early satiety were found to occur more frequently in patients with chronic liver disease compared to healthy controls [2]. According to another study, dyspeptic symptoms without any apparent organic cause were reported by 28/62 patients with cirrhosis [3].

The most widely applied criteria used in previous studies were Rome I and Rome II criteria. Due to the strict criteria in Rome II; new Rome III criteria was introduced. In Rome III criteria two subtypes of FD were identified epigastric pain syndrome (EPS) and post prandial distress syndrome (PDS) [4]. little is known about these subtypes especially in our Egyptian community.

Functional dyspepsia have been studied in patients with hepatitis C [5], but no published data are yet available about the possible association between FD and chronic HCV infection. The aim of this study was to investigate the possible association between chronic hepatitis C and FD.

Methods

This study was under taken at the Virology and Hepatology clinic of Minia University Hospital, Minia, Egypt. The study was approved by the institutional review board of the Minia Faculty of Medicine, Minya University, Egypt. Written, informed consent was obtained from every participant (for both participation in the study and publication of the data). In total, 252 consecutive patients with chronic hepatitis C genotype 4, diagnosed by HCV-RNA

* Correspondence: halaibrahem@mu.edu.eg
Faculty of Medicine, Gastroenterology and Endemic Medicine Department, Minya University, Minya, Egypt

and liver biopsy using the Metavir score, were enrolled in the study. One hundred and fifty controls were randomly selected from healthy volunteer (medical officer, nurses, medical staff and medical students. They were matched in age and sex to the patients. All patients and controls were requested to fill out a self-report questionnaire. The questionnaires were dispensed to patients and controls by the researchers. They were requested to consult the doctor if they did not understand a question in the questionnaire. A researcher assisted those with literacy difficulties.

The validated Rome III diagnostic questionnaire for FD was designed by the Rome committee. The FBDs module was downloaded from the Rome Foundation website (http://www.romecriteria.org/questionnaires/).

FD patients were classified into two subtypes PDS and EPS. PDS must include all of the following: Bothersome postprandial fullness, occurring after ordinary sized meals, at least several times per week. Early satiation that prevents finishing a regular meal, at least several times per week. EPS must include all of the following: 1) Pain or burning localized to the epigastrium, of at least moderate severity at least once per week, 2) The pain is intermittent, 3) Not generalized or localized to other abdominal or chest regions, 4) Not relieved by defecation or passage of flatus, 5) Not fulfilling criteria for biliary pain, 6) Criteria fulfilled for the last 3 months with symptom onset at least 6 months prior to diagnosis..

The alarm (or red flags symptoms) are also included in the questionnaire. The presence of alarm symptoms as melena, hematemesis, loss of weight, history of gastric cancer potentially indicative of organic diseases that warrant further investigations and necessitates for further evaluation.

In addition to that the psychological alarm questionnaire which help to detect associated psychological problems related to FD. The questions include anxiety, depressive symptoms, suicidal ideation, severity of pain, physical impairment and abuse behavior. Patients who fulfilled the criteria for FD based on Romi III questionnaire were referred to endoscopy to rule out the organic cause.

Statistical analysis

Statistical analysis was applied using Graph pad prism software with curve fitting version 4 and SPSS computer program (version 13 windows). Contingency tables used (chi square and Fisher's tests) for binomial variables and T test and AVOVA tests for the other variables. Multivariate regression analysis was done. P value equal to or less than 0.05 was considered significant. Results were expressed as mean ± SD unless otherwise stated.

Results

Total of 272 HCV patients and 150 normal controls patients were studied. Twenty one patients were non responders as they did not complete the questionnaire (10 patients) and refusing endoscopy (11 patients). Of the 251 HCV infected patients were included in the study; 187 fulfilled the criteria of functional dyspepsia and underwent upper endoscopy. One hundred sixty six had normal endoscopy and were diagnosed as having functional dyspepsia, 5 subjects had lower esophagitis, 8 patients had gastro esophageal reflux disease, 6 subjects had antral gastritis and duodenal ulcer recorded in 2 patients

There was significant difference in the demographics between the control groups and the HCV group with regard to age, sex, smoking and BMI ($P < 0.001$; $P < 0.0001$; $P < 0.0001$; $P < 0.003$, respectively),other socio-demographics character of the precipitants was shown in (Table 1).

The percentage of patients with FD diagnosed according to Rome III criteria were significantly higher in patients with chronic HCV infection than normal controls (65.9 %, 28.7 %; respectively; $P < 0.0001$) Fig. 1. Regarding to functional dyspepsia subtypes, the PDS subtype was significantly predominant than The EPS one in both patients and controls ($P < 0.005$, $P < 0.03$) (Table 2).

To study the possible risk factors of FD in patients with chronic HCV, we compared patients with FD to those without. It was found that ALT level and fibrosis stages were significantly higher in patients with FD than

Table 1 Socio-demographic and clinical criteria of the patients and controls

Parameter	HCV patients 252	Normal control 150	*P*-value
Age (mean ± SD)	45.5 ± 8.08	33.6 ± 12.09	<0.001*
Sex			<0.0001*
Male	161 (63.9 %)	53 (35.3 %)	
Female	91 (36.1 %)	97 (64.7 %)	
Residence			<0.9
Urban	156 (61.9 %)	93 (62 %)	
Rural	96 (38.1 %)	57 (38 %)	
Years of education (Mean ± SD)	9.70 ± 2.9	10.4 ± 1.8	<0.13
Smoking			<0.0001*
Yes	138 (54.8 %)	13 (8.7 %)	
No	114 (45.2 %)	137 (91.3 %)	
BMI (kg/m^2)	29.4 ± 3.9	23.9 ± 3.5	<0.003*
Red flag symptoms			<0.09
Yes	10 (4 %)	2 (1.3 %)	
No	242 (96 %)	148 (98.7 %)	
Psycho-social symptoms			<0.2
Yes	9 (3.6 %)	12 (8 %)	
No	243 (96.4 %)	138 (92 %)	

HCV hepatitis C virus, *BMI* body mass index, *FD* functional dyspepsia
*Statistically significant

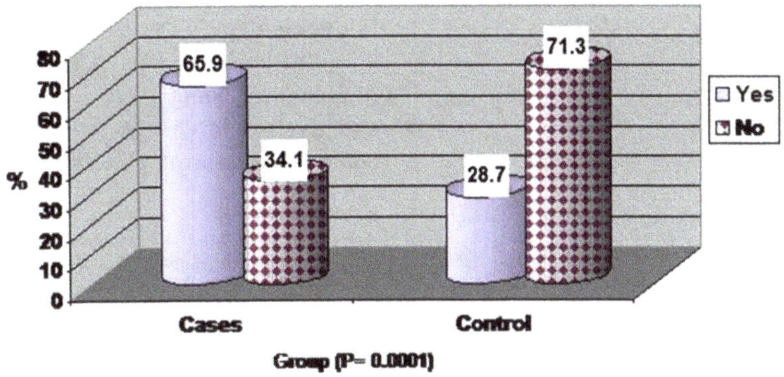

Fig. 1 Prevalence of Functional dyspepsia in patients with chronic hepatitis C. Percentage of patients with FD diagnosed according to Rome III criteria was significantly higher in patients with chronic hepatitis C virus (65.9 %) than in controls (28.7 %)

in patients without ($P < 0.04$, $P < 0.0001$), there was no significant difference in HCV viral load in patients with FD than in patients without ($P < 0.2$) (Table 3).

Multivariate regression analysis was done to clarify the association between patient's risk factors and functional dyspepsia. The most important predictors of FD in HCV patients were BMI ($P < 0.01$) and fibrosis stage ($P < 0.001$). There was no significant association between age, sex, smoking, ALT, HCV viraemia and FD (Table 4).

Discussion

Patients with Chronic hepatitis C usually have different abdominal complaints. Abdominal pain or discomfort is frequently seen in clinical practice in patients with chronic HCV without organic lesion, the functional origin of abdominal complaints is claimed in many patients [6].

We have seen this association frequently in clinical practice, but this is the first designed study to investigate the possible association between FD and chronic hepatitis C.

In this study, the prevalence of FD was significantly high in HCV patients than healthy controls (65.9 % vs 28.7 %). It was found that the majority of the HCV infected patients in this study had symptoms of PDS which constituted about 86.1 % of them while 13.9 % of patients had EPS.

This finding was similar to most studies performed as a population based research. Aro et al. [7] in Sweden who found that PDS was more prevalent than EPS.

Table 2 Prevalence of functional dyspepsia subtypes among HCV patients and controls

Parameter	HCV positive patients n = 166	Normal controls n = 43
Patients with PDS	153 (86.1 %)	28 (65.1 %)
Patients with EPS	13 (13.9 %)	15 (34.9 %)
P value	<0.005**	<0.03**

HCV Hepatitis C virus; *PDS* Post prandial distress syndrome; *EPS* Epigastric pain syndrome
**Statistically significant

These findings indicate that patients with liver disease have meal-related symptoms that may be under recognized. Further investigational studies of gastric neuromuscular function, such as gastric emptying studies and electrogastrogram testing, are warranted. Intestinal motility disorders have been described in cirrhosis but not previously reported or studied in chronic hepatitis [8].

Alternative explanations for these postprandial symptoms might include meal-related increases to portal blood flow and volume changes. Duplex ultrasound and MRI have shown that patients with chronic hepatitis C have a greater volume change to the left lobe of the liver with a relatively smaller change in portal blood flow than do controls [9].

Theoretically, portal flow and volume changes in patients with inflammatory conditions of the liver may result in more congestion and subsequent stretch of Glisson's capsule, in turn leading to more stimulation of hepatic vagal afferent activity with resultant symptoms of postprandial pain, nausea, and fullness [10].

Grassi et al., reported FD in 28.8 % of patients with chronic liver diseases and 71.2 % had organic cause of

Table 3 Biochemical, serological and pathological characteristics of HCV patients with functional dyspepsia

Parameter	Patients with FD 166	Patients without FD 86	*P*-Value
Serum ALT			
Normal	9 (45 %)	11 (55 %)	<0.04*
Elevated	157 (67.7 %)	75 (32.3 %)	
Fibrosis score			<0.0001*
F0-F1	13 (37.1 %)	22 (62.9 %)	
F2-F3	153 (70.5 %)	64 (29.5 %)	
HCV RNA (PCR)			<0.2
Median	147,160	180,603	
Range	(1000–2 220 000)	(800–4 080 000)	

ALT alanine transaminase; *FD* functional dyspepsia; *PCR* Polymerase chain reaction
*Statistically significant

Table 4 Multivariate regression analysis of factors associated with FD In HCV patients

Parameter	Adjusted odds ratio (95 % CI)	P-value
Age > 40	1.4 (0.96–1.04)	<0.8
Male Sex	0.74 (0.37–1.46)	<0.3
BMI >25 kg/m^2	1.61 (1.35–3.16)	<0.01*
Smoking	1.77 (0.87–3.58)	<0.1
High serum ALT	1.2 (0.98–0.01)	<0.8
High viraemia (PCR)	1 (1–1)	<0.2
Fibrosis score (F3-F4)	3.8 (1.76–8.52)	<0.001*

ALT alanine transaminase, *FD* functional dyspepsia, *PCR* Polymerase chain reaction; *CI* confidence interval
*statistically significant

dyspepsia as gastroesophageal reflux disease, congestive gastropathy, gastric or duodenal ulcer and gallbladder stones. Severity of dyspeptic symptoms was similar in both organic and functional forms; symptoms tend to occur with moderate intensity, worsening in parallel with the aggravation of liver disease. The predominance of functional forms in liver diseases is practically the same as that reported in the general population [11].

By multivariate analysis, the most important factors that predicts FD were BMI and fibrosis scores. While gender, age, residence, smoking and viral load were not significantly associated. Aro et al. demonstrated that obesity (BMI > 30 kg/m^2) was predictive for uninvestigated FD but no significant association between obesity and FD [7].

A higher fibrosis scores in HCV patients with FD can indicate a prolonged duration of HCV infection and associated motor or inflammatory changes in the bowel mucosa. Previous studies indicated that patients with cirrhosis were found to have increased severity of gastrointestinal symptoms correlating with the severity but not the etiology of the liver disease [12]. This means that increasing grade of fibrosis is associated with increase occurrence of FD this may occur as a result of immunological changes that occur with advanced liver diseases.

Gastrointestinal sensorimotor disturbances have previously been reported in patients with cirrhosis and might be involved in the pathogenesis of gastrointestinal symptoms in these patients.

In summary FD is a prevalent finding in HCV patients and its pattern is not different from that of the general population.

Conclusion

FD is more prevalent in patients with chronic hepatitis C. Obese, chronic HCV patients and those with higher fibrosis scores are more likely to have FD. Further studies are needed to determine why. Is infectious pathogenesis, motor dysfunction, or psychological disturbance?.

Limitation of the study: as this study employed questionnaire method for data collection it might lead to recall bias and language bias. Also some subjects in this study had actually being treated for their dyspeptic symptoms and this would change the course of the symptoms and could affect the true prevalence of FD.

Abbreviations

HCV: hepatitis C virus; FD: functional dyspepsia; PDS: post prandial distention syndrome; EPS: epigastric pain syndrome; ALT: alanine aminotransferase; BMI: Body Mass Index; 95 % CI: 95 % confidence interval; OR: odds ratio.

Competing interests

The authors declare that they have no competing interests

Authors' contributions

H.I. participated in the design of the study and application of questionnaire; Z.M. participated in acquisition of data and analysis of the data ; H.M. performed the statistical analysis, and drafted the manuscript; WA conceived of the study, and participated in its design. All authors read and approved the final manuscript.

Acknowledgements

The author would like to express sincere appreciation to Dr. Madeha Makhlouf for her valuable advice and guidance. My sincere thanks also goes to Dr. Yasser Mahrous for giving us the access to the research facilities. Finally we are indebted to all patient health workers who agreed to participate in the present study.
All author declare that there was no fund provided to this research regarding to study design; in the collection, analysis, and interpretation of data; in the writing of the manuscript.

References

1. Talley NJ, Stanghellini V, Heading RC, Koch KL, Malagelada JR, Tytgat GN. Functional gastroduodenal disorders. Gut. 1999;45 Suppl 2:37–42.
2. Galati JS, Monsour HP, Dyer CH, Seagren S, Quigley EMM. A survey of the frequency of gastrointestinal complaints in patients with chronic liver disease. Gastroenterology. 1995;108:A1068.
3. Dumitrascu DL, Pascu O, Draghici A, Pop S, Dumitrascu D, Iacob G. Functional dyspepsia in liver cirrhosis. Rom J Intern Med. 1996;34:91–6.
4. Dumitrascu DL, Drossman DA. New standard for functional gastrointestinal disorder. J of Gastrointestin Liver Dis. 2006;15(3):237–41.
5. Riley T, Chinchilli V, Shoemaker M, Koch K. Is nausea associated with chronic hepatitis C infection? Am J Gastroenterol. 2001;96:3356–60.
6. Lehman EM, Wilson ML. Epidemic hepatitis C virus infection in Egypt: estimates of past incidence and future morbidity and mortality. J Viral Hepat. 2009;16:650–8.
7. Aro P, Talley NJ, Ronkainen J, Storkrubb T, Virth M, Johannson E, Strernvald E, Agreus L. Anexiety is associated with uninvestigated and functional dyspepsia (Rome criteria) in a Sewedish population- based study. Gastroenterology. 2009;137:94–100.
8. Madrid AM, Cumsille F, Defillippi C. Altered small bowel motility in patients with liver cirrhosis depends on severity of liver disease. Dig Dis Sci. 1997;42:738–42.
9. Barbaro B, Manfredi R, Bombardieri G. Correlation of MRI liver volume and Doppler sonographic portal hemodynamics with histologic findings in patients with chronic hepatitis C. J Clin Ultrasound. 2000;28:461–68.
10. Rathgaber S, Rex DK. Right upper quadrant abdominal pain (Diagnosis in patients without evident gallstones). Postgrad Med. 1993;94:153–61.
11. Grassi M, Albiani B, De Matteis A, Fontana M, Lucchetta MC, Raffa S. Prevalence of dyspepsia in liver cirrhosis: a clinical and epidemiological investigation. Minerva Med. 2001;92(1):7–12.
12. Fouad YM, Makhlouf MM, Khalaf H, Mostafa Z, Raheem EA, Meneasi W. Is irritable bowel syndrome associated with chronic hepatitis C? J Gastroenterol Hepatol. 2010;25:1285–8.

2

Long-term outcomes of liver transplantation in patients with hepatitis C infection are not affected by HCV positivity of a donor

Maria Stepanova[1,2], Mehmet Sayiner[1], Leyla de Avila[1], Zahra Younoszai[1], Andrei Racila[1] and Zobair M. Younossi[1,3*]

Abstract

Background: The use of HCV-positive livers for HCV-positive recipients is becoming more common. Our aim is to evaluate long-term outcomes in liver transplant recipients transplanted with HCV antibody-positive organs.

Methods: From the Scientific Registry of Transplant Recipients (1995–2013), we selected all adult liver transplant recipients with HCV, and cross-sectionally compared long-term graft loss and mortality rates between those who were transplanted from HCV antibody-positive (HCV+) vs. HCV antibody-negative donors.

Results: We included 33,668 HCV+ liver transplant recipients (54.0 ± 7.7 years old, 74.1% male, 71.0% white, 23.6% with liver malignancy). Of those, 5.7% ($N = 1930$) were transplanted from HCV+ donors; the proportion gradually increased from 2.9% in 1995 to 9.4% in 2013. Patients who were transplanted from HCV+ positive donors were more likely to be discharged alive after transplantation (95.4% vs. 93.9%, $p = 0.006$), but this difference was completely accounted for by a greater proportion of HCV+ donors in more recent study years ($p = 0.10$ after adjustment for the transplant year). After transplantation, both mortality in HCV patients transplanted from HCV+ donors (12.5% in 1 year, 24.2% in 3 years, 33.0% in 5 years) and the graft loss rate (2.2% in 1 year, 4.8% in 3 years, 7.5% in 5 years) were similar to those in HCV patients transplanted from HCV-negative donors (all $p > 0.05$).

Conclusions: Over the past two decades, the use of HCV+ organs for liver transplantation has tripled. Despite this, the long-term outcomes of HCV+ liver transplant recipients transplanted from HCV+ donors were not different from those who were transplanted with HCV-negative organs.

Keywords: Liver transplant, HCV, Extended criteria donor

Background

Chronic hepatitis C infection is currently the most common indication for liver transplantation in the U.S. [1]. After the disease progresses to its most advanced stages which include hepatocellular carcinoma and liver failure, the only alternative to liver-related death is receiving a liver transplant. Since the progression rate increases with age [2], and given that the highest prevalence of HCV infection in the U.S. has been reported in the baby boomer population [3] who are currently between 50 and 70 years of age, the need for liver transplantation in HCV-infected patients is likely to remain high in the coming years. It is unclear whether the recently approved direct-acting antiviral (DAA) regimens for HCV, for which their high efficacy and minimal contraindications are at this point counter-balanced by access-related barriers [4–6], are able to reverse this trend at the national level any time soon.

Due to the shortage of organs, the use of HCV-infected grafts has long been considered as a potentially viable alternative for patients who are already infected with HCV. Although concerns about the presence of

* Correspondence: zobair.younossi@inova.org
[1]Betty and Guy Beatty Center for Integrated Research, Inova Health System, Claude Moore Health Education and Research Building 3300 Gallows Road, Falls Church, VA 22042, USA
[3]Center for Liver Diseases, Department of Medicine, Inova Fairfax Hospital, Falls Church, VA, USA
Full list of author information is available at the end of the article

HCV-related damage to the graft and about viral transmission initially seemed plausible, in the last two decades, an increasing number of centers have adopted the practice of extending their criteria to include HCV-positive donors for using in HCV-positive recipients. As of now, the results reported from both single-center and multi-center studies have been largely consistent about the lack of an additional risk to a recipient associated with the presence of HCV infection in a graft, given that both a recipient and a donor meet other selection criteria [7–11]. It is important to note that most of these studies had a relatively short follow-up. On the other hand, the results reported from other multi-center studies have suggested that the use of HCV-positive donors is not truly risk-free and may, in fact, result in an additional clinical burden which includes an increased risk of developing advanced post-transplant fibrosis and more rapid recurrence of hepatitis in the graft [12, 13]. It is unclear whether this burden could eventually translate into compromised long-term outcomes with long enough follow-up.

The aim of this study is to report post-transplant outcomes in HCV-positive recipients transplanted from HCV-positive donors, and to evaluate the risk for mortality and graft loss associated with the use of HCV-positive donors, using the most recent long-term follow-up data from a nationwide registry of liver transplant recipients.

Methods

Study cohort

This study used data from the Scientific Registry of Transplant Recipients (SRTR). The SRTR data system includes data on all donor, wait-listed candidates, and transplant recipients in the U.S., submitted by the members of the Organ Procurement and Transplantation Network (OPTN), and has been described elsewhere. The Health Resources and Services Administration (HRSA), U.S. Department of Health and Human Services provides oversight to the activities of the OPTN and SRTR contractors.

In this study, we included all liver transplant recipients with HCV of at least 18 years of age and older who underwent liver transplantation between 1995 and 2013 in the U.S. In both recipients and donors, their anti-HCV serology status was used to define those with and without HCV (HCV+ and HCV-, respectively). No HCV RNA testing was reported in SRTR.

The length of hospital stay for patients following liver transplantation was calculated in days from the date of transplant to the date of discharge. Inpatient mortality and history of acute rejection during inpatient stay were recorded. We also collected information on organ donors that included high risk donors classified by the CDC criteria, basic demographics and clinical history (diabetes, cancer), and recorded procurement from a non-heart beating donor.

The primary outcomes included in this study were inpatient mortality, post-transplant mortality (calculated by matching with the Social Security Death Master File, provided by SRTR), and post-transplant graft failure (defined as a documented re-transplant or a graft loss-related cause of death). Patients undergoing re-transplantation were included in the mortality analysis with their most recent transplants only.

Liver transplant recipients discharged alive were followed at 6 and 12 months post-transplant, and then annually until death, re-transplantation, or loss to follow-up. Patients with no documented date of death were presumed alive as of September 1, 2015. The time to events for survival analysis was calculated from the date of transplant.

Statistical analysis

The clinico-demographic parameters and outcomes of liver transplant recipients with HCV+ were compared between those transplanted from HCV+ and HCV- donors using a Kruskall-Wallis non-parametric test and a chi-square test for homogeneity. The association of a donor's HCV positivity with time to post-transplant mortality and graft failure was evaluated by a Cox proportional hazard model with adjustment for clinical and demographic parameters of both donors' and recipients' and for immunosuppressant medications used in follow-up. *P*-values of 0.05 or lower were considered statistically significant. All analyses were run in SAS 9.3 (SAS Institute, Cary, NC).

For this study, a data use agreement with SRTR was signed, and a permission to publish the manuscript was obtained. The study was granted a non-human subject research exemption by Inova Institutional Review Board.

Results

There were 106,427 liver transplants conducted between 1995 and 2013 included in SRTR. Of those, 95,710 were in individuals of at least 18 years of age, and in 75,469 of those the HCV status of a recipient, the HCV status of a donor, and a recipient's mortality status were available. Of this subpopulation, 33,668 (44.6%) liver transplant recipients were HCV+.

There was a substantial increase in the proportion of HCV+ recipients being transplanted from HCV+ donors during the study years. Indeed, the increase in less than 20 years was more than three-fold, from less than 3% in 1995 to more than 9% in 2013. The greatest change in the trend happened in 2010 which resulted in a nearly 50% increase in the proportion of HCV+ donors used for transplantation in the following 3 years, by at least 10% annually (Fig. 1).

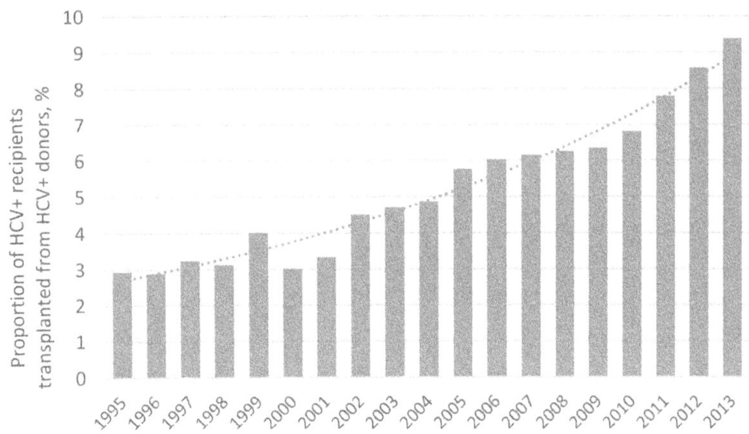

Fig. 1 The proportion of HCV+ donors used for transplantation in HCV+ recipients by year

Comparison of clinico-demographic parameters of HCV+ liver transplant recipients transplanted from HCV+ and HCV- donors is included in Table 1. There was a greater proportion of African-American patients receiving HCV+ transplants, as well as more patients with pre-transplant type 2 diabetes, liver cancer, and a greater proportion of re-transplants (all $p < 0.05$) (Table 1). Despite this, patients transplanted with HCV+ organs had lower MELD scores both with and without adjustment for the presence of liver cancer (both $p < 0.0001$).

The HCV+ donors were, on average, older, less frequently non-heart-beating at the time of procurement, and were substantially more frequently classified as high risk (all $p < 0.0001$). There was no difference in donors' gender and history of diabetes or cancer (all $p > 0.05$) (Table 1).

The short-term outcomes of HCV+ liver transplant recipients were more favorable in those transplanted from HCV+ donors, including a lower rate of inpatient acute rejection events and inpatient mortality, and a shorter inpatient stay (all $p < 0.007$) (Table 1). However, when adjusted for the year of transplant, no difference in any of those outcomes was found (all $p > 0.10$).

Long-term outcomes were similar in patients transplanted from HCV+ and HCV- donors (Table 1, Fig. 2). Indeed, a borderline significant difference was observed for 1 and 2 years post-transplant mortality (1 year: 12.5% in patients transplanted from HCV+ donors vs. 14.1% in patients with HCV- donors, $p = 0.059$; 2 years: 18.4% vs. 20.2%, $p = 0.054$) which was again completely explained out by the bias in the year of transplant (both $p > 0.21$ after adjustment for year). At the same time, the following years after transplantation revealed nearly identical mortality rates (all $p > 0.5$).

Similarly, the graft loss rates were insignificantly lower in patients transplanted from HCV+ donors up to 3 years post-transplant (2.2% vs. 2.8% at 1 year, $p = 0.15$; 3.6% vs. 4.5% at 2 years, $p = 0.090$; 4.8% vs. 5.9% at 3 years, $p = 0.089$) due the yearly distribution of HCV+ donors (all $p > 0.13$ after adjustment for year).

In a Cox proportional hazard model, after adjustment for the year of transplant, recipient's age, gender, race, elements of medical history, MELD score, donor's age and medical history, and the use of immunosuppressant medications, the association of a donor's HCV+ status with post-transplant graft loss and mortality in HCV+ liver transplant recipients was highly insignificant: adjusted hazard ratio (aHR) (95% CI) = 1.045 (0.954–1.145) for time to post-transplant mortality, aHR = 0.922 (0.727–1.169) for time to graft loss (both $p > 0.33$) (all mortality and graft loss predictors tested in the Cox proportional hazard models are included in Additional file 1: Table Table S1). Furthermore, the lack of association of donors' HCV positivity with the studied outcomes was also confirmed in a separate round of case–control analysis where the outcomes of patients transplanted from HCV+ donors were compared to those of propensity score-matched controls (all $p > 0.15$) (Additional file 2: Table S2). In contrast, a more recent year of transplant was a major predictor of both lower mortality rate (aHR = 0.963 (0.956–0.971) per year) and lower graft failure rate (aHR = 0.950 (0.934–0.967) per year) (both $p < 0.0001$) even after adjustment for the type of immunosuppressants used in follow-up (Additional file 2: Table S2).

Discussion

In this study, we reported post-transplant outcomes in patients with HCV transplanted from HCV antibody-positive donors and compared these outcomes to those of HCV patients transplanted from HCV-negative donors using 20 years of data from the nationwide transplant registry. Our study shows that there are no differences in

Table 1 Comparison of HCV+ liver transplant recipients, donors and outcomes in transplantations from HCV+ and HCV-donors

	HCV+ donor	HCV- donor	*P*
N	1930	31,738	
Recipients:			
Age, years	55.1 ± 7.2	53.9 ± 7.7	<0.0001
Male gender	1448 (75.0%)	23,508 (74.1%)	0.35
Race/ethnicity: Caucasian	1346 (69.7%)	22,575 (71.1%)	0.19
Race/ethnicity: African-American	267 (13.8%)	3249 (10.2%)	<0.0001
Race/ethnicity: Hispanic	254 (13.2%)	4664 (14.7%)	0.06
Co-infected with HBV (HBV sAg+)	51 (2.7%)	959 (3.1%)	0.32
Pre-transplant history of type 2 diabetes	236 (13.3%)	3335 (11.7%)	0.0441
Liver cancer	544 (28.2%)	7414 (23.4%)	<0.0001
Liver re-transplant	3 (0.2%)	6 (0.0%)	0.0004
MELD score	18.2 ± 8.3	20.3 ± 9.7	<0.0001
MELD score excl. liver cancer	19.9 ± 8.3	22.4 ± 9.5	<0.0001
Donors:			
Age, years	42.0 ± 11.8	39.6 ± 16.4	<0.0001
Male gender	1196 (62.0%)	19,513 (61.5%)	0.67
Non-heart-beating	31 (1.6%)	1138 (3.6%)	<0.0001
History of diabetes	167 (8.7%)	2491 (7.9%)	0.19
History of cancer	39 (2.0%)	834 (2.6%)	0.11
History of high risk behavior	808 (42.4%)	2044 (6.5%)	<0.0001
Heterotopic transplant	2 (0.1%)	35 (0.1%)	0.95
Outcomes:			
Acute rejection episodes before discharge	36 (2.4%)	809 (4.1%)	0.0020
Discharged alive	1842 (95.4%)	29,808 (93.9%)	0.0063
Length of inpatient stay, days	15.7 ± 20.3	16.4 ± 21.9	0.0013
Mortality: 1 year	242 (12.5%)	4467 (14.1%)	0.059
Mortality: 3 years	399 (24.2%)	7190 (24.8%)	0.58
Mortality: 5 years	424 (33.0%)	8028 (32.5%)	0.68
Mortality: 10 years	281 (47.5%)	7019 (48.6%)	0.59
Graft failure: 1 year	38 (2.2%)	782 (2.8%)	0.15
Graft failure: 3 years	63 (4.8%)	1375 (5.9%)	0.09
Graft failure: 5 years	70 (7.5%)	1465 (8.1%)	0.56
Graft failure: 10 years	50 (13.9%)	1160 (13.5%)	0.86

both short- and long-term outcomes between patients who were transplanted from HCV-positive and HCV-negative donors. This is largely consistent with prior reports of similar findings reported from smaller studies with shorter follow-up.

This finding provides an additional support to the practice of using HCV-positive donors for HCV-positive recipients which has become nearly universal in multiple transplant centers. Indeed, we have shown that the use of HCV-positive organs has tripled over less than two decades. Nevertheless, our data confirm that the medium-term outcomes of patients with HCV are similar regardless of HCV positivity of the organs. Furthermore, the short-term outcomes, including being discharged alive from the hospital, having a rejection episode before discharge, and 1 year mortality, all seem to be lower in HCV-positive organ recipients. This superior short-term survival, in addition to the impact of a greater proportion of patients receiving HCV-positive organs in the most recent study years, may also be related to less advanced liver disease in these patients suggesting a cautious use of HCV-positive organs. Indeed, patients receiving HCV-positive organs had lower MELD scores which remained true even after excluding those

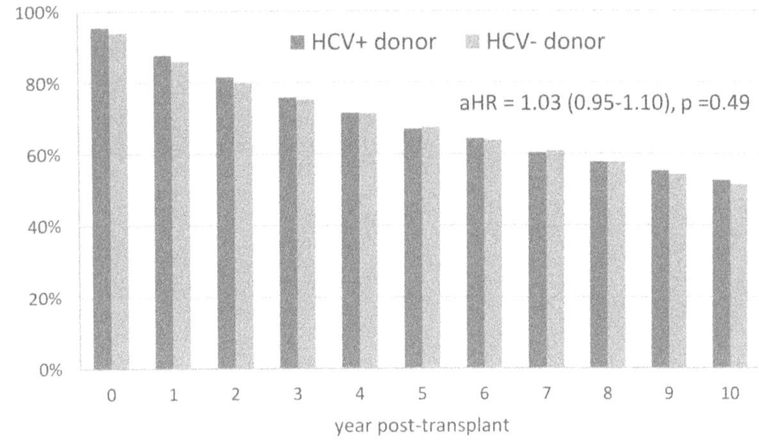

Fig. 2 Post-transplant survival in HCV+ liver transplant recipients transplanted from HCV+ and HCV- donors. $P > 0.05$ at all time points. aHR – adjusted hazard ratio. Mortality at the zero time point represents inpatient mortality at transplant

who received MELD exclusion for hepatocellular carcinoma (HCC).

While there seems to be no evidence supporting the presence of an increased risk of post-transplant mortality and allograft losses arisen solely from the HCV-positivity of a donor, this finding should be interpreted with caution. In particular, it is necessary to understand that hepatocytes in an HCV-positive graft might still have been injured by chronic inflammation, so a careful selection of both grafts and recipients will be important [13]. Nevertheless, it is interesting to note that in our study, we have failed to find any evidence of an increased risk of adverse post-transplant outcomes associated with being HCV-positive in the group of donors age 45 or older or in the donors with history of type 2 diabetes (all $p > 0.05$).

With the new DAAs becoming more widely available, the utility of HCV-seropositive organs becomes even more important. Indeed, we suggest that the use of HCV-positive organs in HCV-positive recipients who can be safely and effectively treated post-transplant will become increasingly a viable option. However, it is important to note that although preliminary studies have shown notable benefits of treating post-transplant HCV patients with DAAs [14, 15], long-term data is still not available.

The study did have a limitation related to the lack of HCV RNA results for the donors, so the impact of active viremia in both donors and recipients could not be evaluated, while it is reasonable to believe that such impact may exist. We also did not have access to histology data for the grafts so the risk associated with the presence and/or degree of hepatic steatosis and fibrosis in an allograft could not be studied. The outcomes were limited to mortality and graft loss only, while other clinical outcomes, such as developing hepatic inflammation and fibrosis, could also significantly affect patients' well-being in the post-transplant period.

Conclusions

In this study which used the most recent nationwide registry of liver transplant recipients, we have found no evidence of an increased risk for adverse post-transplant outcomes that could be associated with HCV positivity of a donor. Therefore, we postulate that while we, as a society, are working on decreasing wait-list mortality in liver transplant candidates, HCV-positive allografts could be a reasonably safe option for patients with chronic HCV infection who are in need of a liver transplant. It is important to note that our data cannot be used in support of indiscriminate use of HCV-positive donors, especially those who are HCV RNA-positive, given previously reported unfavorable histologic outcomes which could not be ruled out in this study. Further studies are needed to establish evidence-based selection criteria for HCV-positive donors which could provide patients with the best possible risk-to-benefit ratio.

Abbreviations

aHR: Adjusted hazard ratio; BMI: Body mass index; COPD: Chronic obstructive pulmonary disease; CVD: Cardiovascular disease; DAA: Direct-acting antiviral; HBV: Hepatitis B virus; HCC: Hepatocellular carcinoma; HCV: Hepatitis C virus; ICU: Intensive care unit; MELD: The model for end-stage liver disease; SRTR: The Scientific Registry of Transplant Recipients

Acknowledgements

The data reported here have been supplied by the Minneapolis Medical Research Foundation (MMRF) as the contractor for the Scientific Registry of Transplant Recipients (SRTR). The interpretation and reporting of these data are the responsibility of the authors and in no way should be seen as an official policy of or interpretation by the SRTR or the U.S. Government.

Funding
This study was supported by the Beatty Liver and Obesity Research Fund and Liver Outcomes Research Fund, Inova Health System, Falls Church, VA.

Authors' contributions
MaS - study concept and design, analysis and interpretation of data; drafting of the manuscript. MeS, LdA, ZaY, AR - critical revision of the manuscript for important intellectual content. ZoY - study concept and design; critical revision of the manuscript for important intellectual content; obtained funding; study supervision. All authors read and approved the final manuscript.

Competing interests
Maria Stepanova is an active Associate Editor for BMC Gastroenterology. Other coauthors have no conflict of interest related to this manuscript to disclose.

Consent for publication
Not applicable.

Ethics approval and consent to participate
Per Data Use Agreement (DUA) with SRTR, the authors were required to use the data solely for bona fide research/analysis described in a pre-approved research plan, and were specifically required not use the data for any commercial purpose which could have a negative impact on patient welfare, such as offering, denying, or allocating insurance; and adverse selection (e.g., identifying patients with high risk diagnoses). The text of the manuscript was reviewed by SRTR to ensure compliance with the terms of the DUA regarding confidentiality, and approved for publication. The study was granted a non-human subject research status by Inova Institutional Review Board.

Author details
[1]Betty and Guy Beatty Center for Integrated Research, Inova Health System, Claude Moore Health Education and Research Building 3300 Gallows Road, Falls Church, VA 22042, USA. [2]Center for Outcomes Research in Liver Diseases, Washington, DC, USA. [3]Center for Liver Diseases, Department of Medicine, Inova Fairfax Hospital, Falls Church, VA, USA.

References
1. Stepanova M, Wai H, Saab S, Mishra A, Venkatesan C, Younossi ZM. The portrait of an adult liver transplant recipient in the United States from 1987 to 2013. JAMA Intern Med. 2014;174(8):1407–9.
2. Westbrook RH, Dusheiko G. Natural history of hepatitis C. J Hepatol. 2014; 61(1 Suppl):S58–68.
3. Coilly A, Roche B, Duclos-Vallée JC, Samuel D. News and challenges in the treatment of hepatitis C in liver transplantation. Liver Int. 2016;36 Suppl 1: 34–42. doi:10.1111/liv.13017. Review.
4. Stepanova M, Younossi ZM. Interferon-free regimens for chronic hepatitis C: barriers due to treatment candidacy and insurance coverage. Dig Dis Sci. 2015;60(11):3248–51.
5. Adinolfi LE, Guerrera B. All-oral interferon-free treatments: the end of hepatitis C virus story, the dream and the reality. World J Hepatol. 2015; 7(22):2363–8.
6. Do A, Mittal Y, Liapakis A, Cohen E, Chau H, Bertuccio C, Sapir D, Wright J, Eggers C, Drozd K, Ciarleglio M, Deng Y, Lim JK. Drug authorization for sofosbuvir/ledipasvir (Harvoni) for chronic HCV infection in a real-world cohort: a new barrier in the HCV care cascade. PLoS One. 2015;10(8), e0135645.
7. Plotkin JS, Ridge L, Kuo PC, Lim J, Njoku MJ, Johnson LB. Extending the boundaries of acceptable organ donors: a means of expanding the donor pool for liver transplantation. Transplant Proc. 1997;29(8):3288.
8. Marroquin CE, Marino G, Kuo PC, Plotkin JS, Rustgi VK, Lu AD, Edwards E, Taranto S, Johnson LB. Transplantation of hepatitis C-positive livers in hepatitis C-positive patients is equivalent to transplanting hepatitis C-negative livers. Liver Transpl. 2001;7(9):762–8.
9. Burr AT, Li Y, Tseng JF, Saidi RF, Bozorgzadeh A, Shah SA. Survival after liver transplantation using hepatitis C virus-positive donor allografts: case-controlled analysis of the UNOS database. World J Surg. 2011;35(7):1590–5.
10. Álvaro E, Abradelo M, Fuertes A, Manrique A, Colina F, Alegre C, Calvo J, García M, García-Sesma A, Cambra F, Sanabria R, Moreno E, Jimenez C. Liver transplantation from anti-hepatitis C virus-positive donors: our experience. Transplant Proc. 2012;44(6):1475–8.
11. Northup PG, Argo CK, Nguyen DT, McBride MA, Kumer SC, Schmitt TM, Pruett TL. Liver allografts from hepatitis C positive donors can offer good outcomes in hepatitis C positive recipients: a US National Transplant Registry analysis. Transpl Int. 2010;23(10):1038–44.
12. Ballarin R, Cucchetti A, Spaggiari M, Montalti R, Di Benedetto F, Nadalin S, Troisi RI, Valmasoni M, Longo C, De Ruvo N, Cautero N, Cillo U, Pinna AD, Burra P, Gerunda GE. Long-term follow-up and outcome of liver transplantation from anti-hepatitis C virus-positive donors: a European multicentric case–control study. Transplantation. 2011;91(11):1265–72.
13. Lai JC, O'Leary JG, Trotter JF, Verna EC, Brown Jr RS, Stravitz RT, Duman JD, Forman LM, Terrault NA, Consortium to Study Health Outcomes in HCV Liver Transplant Recipients (CRUSH-C). Risk of advanced fibrosis with grafts from hepatitis C antibody-positive donors: a multicenter cohort study. Liver Transpl. 2012;18(5):532–8.
14. Saab S, Greenberg A, Li E, Bau SN, Durazo F, El-Kabany M, Han S, Busuttil RW. Sofosbuvir and simeprevir is effective for recurrent hepatitis C in liver transplant recipients. Liver Int. 2015;35(11):2442–7.
15. Brown RS Jr, O'Leary JG, Reddy KR, Kuo A, Morelli GJ, Burton JR Jr, Stravitz RT, Durand C, Di Bisceglie AM, Kwo P, Frenette CT, Stewart TG, Nelson DR, Fried MW, Terrault NA; HCV-TARGET Study Group. Interferon-free therapy for genotype 1 hepatitis C in liver transplant recipients: real world experience from HCV-TARGET. Liver Transpl. 2015. doi: 10.1002/lt.24366

3

Efficacy, safety and pharmacokinetics of simeprevir and TMC647055/ritonavir with or without ribavirin and JNJ-56914845 in HCV genotype 1 infection

Stefan Bourgeois[1*], Hans Van Vlierberghe[2], Christophe Moreno[3], Hans Orlent[4], Frederik Nevens[5], Keikawus Arastéh[6], Yves Horsmans[7], Jörn M. Schattenberg[8], Peter Buggisch[9], Sven Francque[10], Leen Vijgen[11], Thomas N. Kakuda[12], Eva Hoeben[13], Donghan Luo[14], An Vandebosch[13], Bert Jacquemyn[11], Pieter Van Remoortere[14] and René Verloes[13]

Abstract

Background: A Phase 2a, open-label study (NCT01724086) was conducted to assess the efficacy and safety of a once-daily, 2-direct-acting-antiviral-agent (2-DAA) combination of simeprevir + TMC647055/ritonavir ± ribavirin and of the 3-DAA combination of simeprevir + TMC647055/ritonavir + JNJ-56914845 in chronic hepatitis C virus genotype (GT)1-infected treatment-naïve and prior-relapse patients.

Methods: The study comprised four 12-week treatment panels: Panel 1 ($n = 10$; GT1a) and Panel 2-Arm 1 ($n = 12$; GT1b): simeprevir 75 mg once daily + TMC647055 450 mg once daily/ritonavir 30 mg once daily + ribavirin 1000–1200 mg/day; Panel 2-Arm 2 ($n = 9$; GT1b): simeprevir 75 mg + TMC647055 450 mg/ritonavir 30 mg without ribavirin; Panel 3: simeprevir 75 mg + TMC647055 600 mg/ritonavir 50 mg with (Arm 1: GT1a; $n = 7$) or without (Arm 2: GT1b; $n = 8$) ribavirin; Panel 4: simeprevir 75 mg + TMC647055 450 mg/ritonavir 30 mg + JNJ-56914845 30 mg once daily (Arm 1: $n = 22$; GT1a/GT1b) or 60 mg once daily (Arm 2: $n = 22$; GT1a/GT1b). Primary endpoint was sustained virologic response 12 weeks after end of treatment (12 weeks of combination treatment; SVR12).

Results: In Panel 1 and Panel 2-Arm 1, 5/10 and 6/12 (50%) GT1a/GT1b + ribavirin patients achieved SVR12, versus 3/9 (33%) GT1b without ribavirin patients in Panel 2-Arm 2. In Panel 3-Arm 1 and Panel 3-Arm 2, 6/7 (86%) GT1a + ribavirin and 4/8 (50%) GT1b without ribavirin patients, respectively, achieved SVR12. In Panel 4, 10/14 (71%) and 14/15 (93%) GT1a patients in Arms 1 and 2 achieved SVR12 compared with 8/8 and 7/7 (100%) GT1b patients in each arm, respectively. No deaths, serious adverse events (AEs), Grade 4 AEs or AEs leading to treatment discontinuation occurred.

Conclusions: The 2- and 3-DAA combinations were well tolerated. High SVR rates of 93% and 100% in GT1a- and GT1b-infected patients, respectively, were achieved in this study by combining simeprevir with JNJ-56914845 60 mg and TMC647055/ritonavir.

Keywords: Simeprevir, TMC647055/ritonavir, JNJ-56914845, Ribavirin, Direct-acting antiviral agents, Hepatitis C virus, genotype 1, Efficacy, Safety

* Correspondence: stefan.bourgeois@zna.be
[1]Department of Gastroenterology & Hepatology, ZNA Antwerp, Antwerpen, Belgium

Background

Interferon (IFN)-free regimens comprising direct-acting antivirals (DAA) with different mechanisms of action can result in high sustained virologic response (SVR) rates in patients chronically infected with hepatitis C virus (HCV). Combination regimens comprising an HCV NS3/4A protease inhibitor (PI), a non-nucleoside inhibitor (NNI) of the HCV NS5B polymerase and/or an HCV NS5A replication complex inhibitor with/without ribavirin have been shown to be successful in the treatment of chronic HCV infection [1]. For example, the combination of the PI paritaprevir, the NNI dasabuvir and the NS5A inhibitor ombitasvir, with ritonavir included as a pharmacologic booster for paritaprevir, is approved for the treatment of chronic HCV genotype (GT) 1 infection. In the PEARL-III (HCV GT1b) and PEARL-IV (HCV GT1a) Phase 3 studies, treatment of previously untreated patients with paritaprevir/ritonavir, dasabuvir and ombitasvir for 12 weeks resulted in SVR 12 weeks after end of treatment (SVR12) rates of 99.5% and 97.0% in the presence of ribavirin, and 99.0% and 90.2% in the absence of ribavirin, respectively [2].

Simeprevir is a once-daily, HCV NS3/4A PI approved as part of an IFN-free combination with sofosbuvir for HCV GT1 infection. In addition, simeprevir with sofosbuvir is approved for HCV GT4 infection and HCV/human immunodeficiency virus (HIV) co-infection in the European Union (EU). Simeprevir is also approved in combination with pegylated IFN (pegIFN)/ribavirin for chronic HCV GT1 and GT4 infection in the United States and EU [3]. Simeprevir is a cytochrome P450 (CYP) 3A substrate and mild inhibitor (intestinal only). Simeprevir also inhibits organic anion transporting polypeptide (OATP) 1B1/3 and P-glycoprotein [4].

TMC647055 is an NNI of the HCV NS5B polymerase, binding in the NNI-1 pocket on the polymerase. TMC647055 has in vitro antiviral activity against HCV GT1, 3, 4, 5 and 6 [5]. In a Phase 1 study (NCT01202825), TMC647055 1000 mg twice daily in combination with simeprevir 150 mg once daily for 10 days demonstrated good antiviral activity and was well tolerated in HCV GT1a- and GT1b-infected patients [6]. However, the systemic exposure to both compounds decreased during treatment to levels potentially lower than required for complete viral suppression. Co-administering TMC647055 with the potent CYP3A4 inhibitor ritonavir was expected to increase exposure by overcoming CYP3A4 induction [5].

JNJ-56914845 (previously known as GSK-2336805) is a potent HCV NS5A replication complex inhibitor, with in vitro antiviral activity against HCV GT1, 4, 5 and 6a/6b [7, 8]. It is a CYP3A and P-glycoprotein substrate and, in vitro, it inhibits P-glycoprotein, OATP1B1/3 and breast cancer resistance protein (data on file).

This Phase 2a, open-label study (NCT01724086) assessed the efficacy, pharmacokinetics, safety and tolerability of the 2-DAA combination of simeprevir with TMC647055 and a low dose of ritonavir with or without ribavirin for 12 weeks in chronic HCV GT1-infected treatment-naïve and prior-relapse patients. The study also included the addition of a third DAA, JNJ-56914845, to the simeprevir and TMC647055 combination to assess the potential of further increasing the efficacy of the regimen by combining three DAAs with different mechanisms of action. Results from the final analysis, when all patients in all panels had completed the study, are presented here.

Methods

Patients and study design

This was a Phase 2a, open-label study, conducted between 12 September 2012 and 16 December 2014 at 12 sites in Belgium and Germany. The study was approved by the Institutional Review Board or Independent Ethics Committee at each participating centre, and met the ethical principles of the Declaration of Helsinki and Good Clinical Practice guidelines. All patients provided written, informed consent.

Adults (18–70 years of age) with chronic HCV GT1a/GT1b infection and screening plasma HCV RNA >10,000 IU/mL who were treatment-naïve or had relapsed following previous treatment with pegIFN/ribavirin were eligible for inclusion. Patients had to have a documented liver biopsy within 3 years of the screening visit, or have an elastography prior to first dosing.

Exclusion criteria included liver cirrhosis, hepatic decompensation, liver disease of non-HCV aetiology, infection/co-infection with non-GT1a/GT1b HCV, hepatitis A or B, or HIV-1/-2, and significant laboratory abnormalities, including total bilirubin ≥1.5 x upper limit of normal and platelet count <90,000/mm^3. Patients who had received prior HCV-specific DAA treatment or a liver transplant were also excluded.

The study comprised four 12-week treatment panels (Fig. 1). Panels 1 and 2, which ran in parallel, comprised the first part of the study and were sequentially followed by Panels 3 and 4. Panels 1–3 evaluated simeprevir in combination with TMC647055/ritonavir (at two different doses of TMC647055) with ribavirin in GT1a-infected patients and with or without ribavirin in GT1b-infected patients. Panel 4 evaluated the triple combination of simeprevir with TMC647055/ritonavir plus the NS5A inhibitor JNJ-56914845 at a low and high dose in GT1a/b-infected patients.

More specifically, patients in Panels 1 and 2 received simeprevir 75 mg once daily, TMC647055 450 mg once daily, ritonavir 30 mg once daily and ribavirin 1000–1200 mg (patients in Panel 2-Arm 2 did not receive ribavirin). Patients in Panel 3 received simeprevir 75 mg

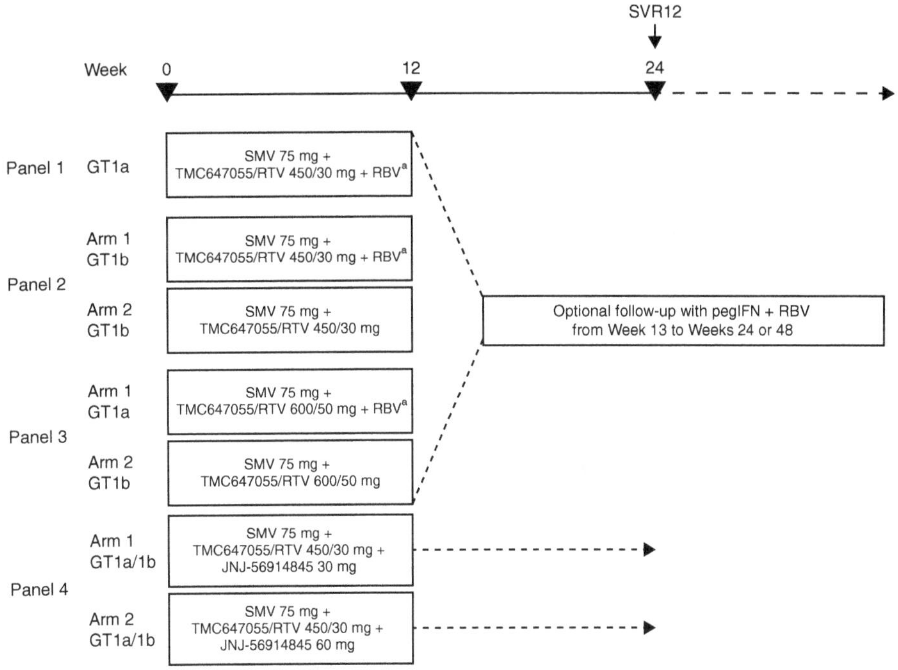

Fig. 1 Study design. [a]Ribavirin given twice daily at a dose of 1000–1200 mg. Follow-up therapy with pegIFN/RBV was based on on-treatment response and was initiated only if: Week 4 HCV RNA ≥25 IU/mL (Panels 1–3: 36 weeks of follow-up therapy); Week 4 HCV RNA <25 IU/mL detectable or HCV RNA confirmed detectable between Week 4 and Week 11 (Panels 1–2: 12 weeks of follow-up therapy). *GT* genotype, *HCV* hepatitis C virus, *pegIFN* pegylated interferon α-2a, *RBV* ribavirin, *RTV* ritonavir, *SMV* simeprevir, *SVR12* sustained virologic response 12 weeks after end of treatment

once daily, TMC647055 at a higher dose of 600 mg once daily, ritonavir 50 mg once daily and ribavirin 1000–1200 mg (patients in Panel 3-Arm 2 did not receive ribavirin). Patients in Panel 4 received simeprevir 75 mg once daily, TMC647055 450 mg once daily, ritonavir 30 mg once daily and JNJ-56914845 30 (Arm 1) or 60 mg (Arm 2) once daily. Simeprevir was dosed at 75 mg once daily (rather than the 150 mg dose approved) to account for CYP3A inhibition by ritonavir, which is not a part of the approved regimen for simeprevir. Further details on the dosing rationale are provided in Additional file 1. For ethical reasons, patients in Panels 1–3 received follow-up treatment with pegIFN/ribavirin for an additional 12 or 36 weeks if their Week-4 HCV RNA levels did not comply with predefined criteria (Fig. 1). For patients in Panel 4 receiving the 3-DAA regimen, no follow-up treatment was planned.

Central randomisation was implemented in Panel 2, with patients randomly assigned 1:1 to Arm 1 or Arm 2 based on a computer-generated schedule prepared before the study, balanced by using randomly permuted blocks, and stratified by *IL28B* genotype (CC and non-CC). Patients in Panel 3 were not randomised as their treatment was dependent on their HCV geno/subtype (1a or 1b) (Fig. 1). In Panel 4, patients were randomised in a 1:1 ratio between Arm 1 or Arm 2, stratified by HCV geno/subtype.

To avoid unnecessary drug exposure, the following virologic stopping rules were adopted: all study drugs were discontinued for patients with viral breakthrough (confirmed on-treatment increase of >1 log_{10} IU/mL in HCV RNA from the lowest level reached, or confirmed HCV RNA >100 IU/mL in patients whose HCV RNA had previously been <25 IU/mL), or with inadequate virologic response (confirmed HCV RNA >100 IU/mL at Week 4 or afterwards until Week 11).

Details on protocol deviations are provided in Additional file 1.

Outcomes

The primary efficacy endpoint was SVR12. Patients achieved SVR12 if they received no pegIFN/ribavirin follow-up treatment after 12 weeks of combination treatment (Panels 1–3 only) and achieved HCV RNA <25 IU/mL undetectable/detectable 12 weeks after actual end of treatment (Panels 1–4). Patients in Panels 1–3 who received follow-up therapy and had HCV RNA <25 IU/mL at 12 weeks after end of treatment were also classed as having achieved SVR12; however, they were considered as failures with regards to the primary endpoint of the study, which focused on the 12-week DAA therapy. The primary safety endpoints included the proportion of patients with adverse events (AEs), serious AEs (SAEs) or abnormal changes in safety-related laboratory values. Secondary endpoints included: the proportion of patients with SVR 24 weeks after end of treatment (SVR24); Week-4 pharmacokinetics of the study drugs; on-treatment virologic failure, including patients with viral breakthrough (defined in the previous section); viral relapse (defined as HCV RNA <25 IU/mL undetectable at the actual end of treatment and confirmed HCV RNA ≥25 IU/mL during post-treatment follow-up); and the presence of HCV NS3/4A, NS5A and/or NS5B variants at baseline and at time of failure in patients not achieving SVR.

Assessments

Blood samples for HCV RNA level determination were collected at screening and at predefined time points throughout the treatment phase and follow-up period. HCV RNA was measured using the COBAS® TaqMan® HCV Test version 2.0 (Roche Molecular Diagnostics, Pleasanton, CA, USA) for use with the High Pure System assay (lower limit of quantification: 25 IU/mL; limit of detection: 10–15 IU/mL).

HCV geno/subtypes were determined pre-treatment based on sequencing of a part of the NS5B gene (at baseline) when available or by the VERSANT® HCV Genotype 2.0 assay (LiPA) or Trugene HCV Genotyping assay (at screening) (Siemens Healthcare Diagnostics, Erlangen, Germany).

Standard population-based sequencing of the HCV NS3/4A and NS5B regions in Panels 1–3 and of the NS3/4A, NS5A and NS5B regions in Panel 4 was performed at baseline for all patients and post-baseline for patients not achieving SVR12 based on the HCV RNA changes observed in each individual patient and the limits of the sequencing assay.

Plasma pharmacokinetic samples for simeprevir, TMC647055, ritonavir and JNJ-56914845 were collected over 24 h (pre-dose, 1, 2, 3, 4, 5, 6, 8, 10, 12 and 24 h post-dose) at Week 4 from all patients and assayed using validated liquid chromatography-tandem mass spectrometry methods with lower limits of quantification for simeprevir, TMC647055, ritonavir and JNJ-56914845 of 5.0, 5.0, 2.0 and 1.0 ng/mL, respectively (data on file) [9]. Pharmacokinetic parameters including maximum plasma concentration (C_{max}) and area under the plasma concentration–time curve over 24 h (AUC_{0-24h}) were calculated using non-compartmental analysis (Phoenix WinNonlin® 6.2.1; Certara, Princeton, NJ, USA).

AEs were monitored throughout the treatment phase and follow-up period and up to 24 weeks after actual end of treatment. AEs were coded using the Medical Dictionary for Regulatory Activities (version 16.0 for Panels 1 and 2 and version 17.0 for Panels 3 and 4).

Statistical analyses

Statistical analyses were performed using SAS® version 9.1 or higher (SAS Institute Inc, Cary, NC, USA).

No formal sample size calculations were performed as this was a proof-of-concept study. For each efficacy endpoint, the proportion of patients was summarised descriptively together with a 95% confidence interval by treatment group and population. The change in $\log_{10}$ HCV RNA from baseline at all time points was calculated using descriptive statistics. Pharmacokinetic parameters were calculated using non-compartmental analysis (Phoenix WinNonlin® 6.2.1). All safety and tolerability data were summarised descriptively.

All analyses were conducted using data from the intent-to-treat population, which comprised all patients who received at least one dose of study drug.

Results

Patient disposition and baseline characteristics

In total, 125 patients were screened, and 90 (n = 10, 21, 15 and 44 in Panels 1, 2, 3 and 4, respectively) were treated (intent-to-treat population) (Fig. 2). Four (3%) patients discontinued the study prematurely (lost to follow-up, n = 3 [Panels 2 and 3]; withdrawal of consent, n = 1 [Panel 4]).

In Panel 1, 5/10 (50%) patients completed their treatment regimen. In Panel 2, the majority of patients completed treatment (GT1b/with ribavirin group: 11/12 [92%]; GT1b/without ribavirin group, 8/9 [89%]). Most patients also completed treatment in Panel 3 (GT1a/with ribavirin, 7/7 [100%]; GT1b/without ribavirin, 7/8 [88%]) and Panel 4 (30-mg group, 22/22 [100%]; 60-mg group, 21/22 [96%]). All treatment discontinuations were due to viral breakthrough, as detailed in the next section.

Baseline demographics and disease characteristics are shown in Table 1.

Virologic response

Figure 3 shows the treatment outcome in each of the four panels. In Panel 1, 5/10 (50%) patients achieved SVR12. In Panel 2, SVR12 was achieved in 6/12 (50%) and 3/9 (33%) patients in the GT1b/with ribavirin and GT1b/without ribavirin groups, respectively. In Panel 3, 6/7 (86%) and 4/8 (50%) patients in the GT1a/with ribavirin and GT1b/without ribavirin groups, respectively, achieved SVR12. In Panel 4, SVR12 was achieved in 18/22 (82%) and 21/22 (95%) patients in the JNJ-56914845 30- and 60-mg groups, respectively. In the 30-mg group, SVR12 was achieved in 10/14 (71%) GT1a/other-infected patients and in all (8/8; 100%) GT1b-infected patients. In the 60-mg group, SVR12 was achieved in 14/15 (93%) GT1a/other-infected patients and in all (7/7; 100%) GT1b-infected patients.

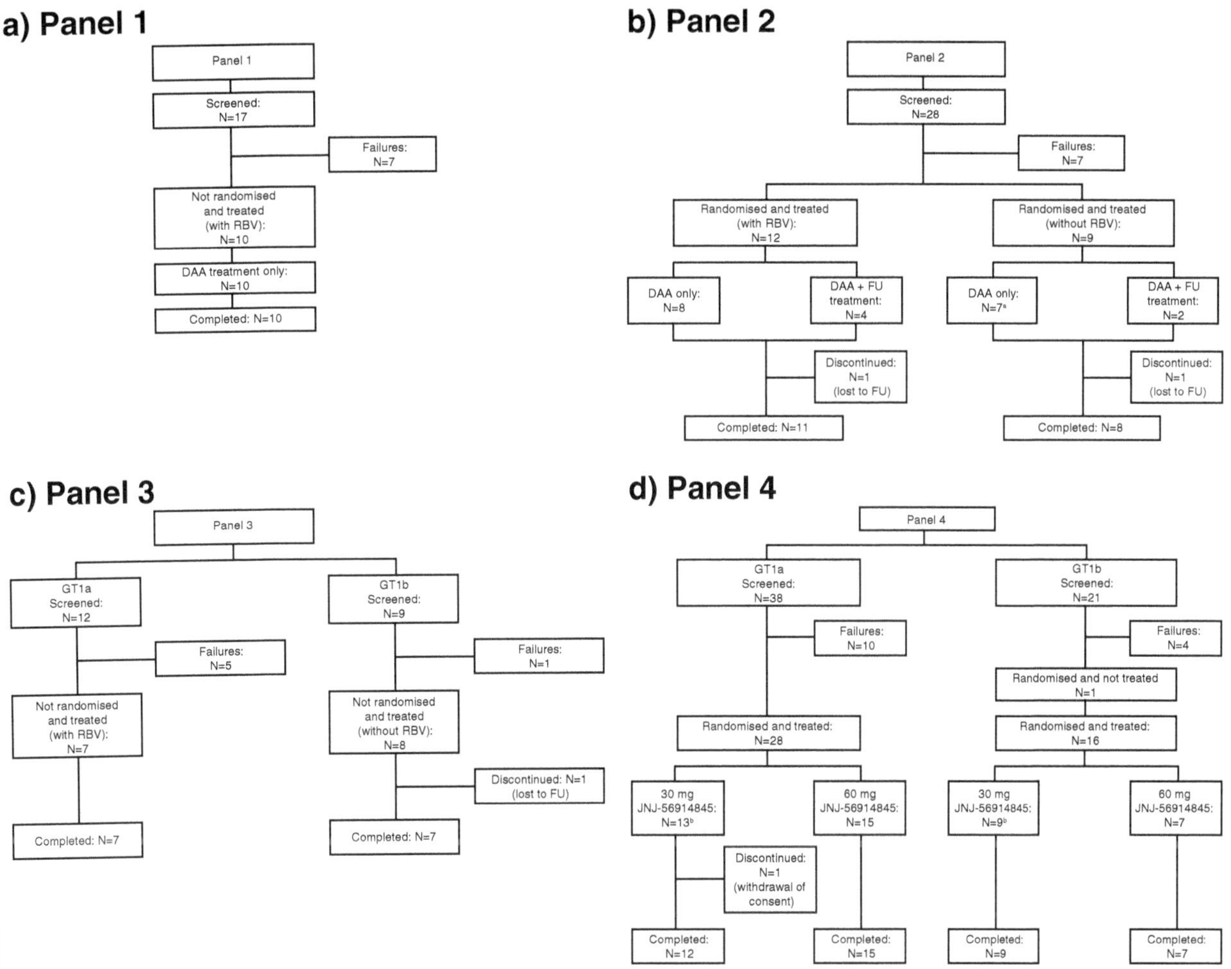

Fig. 2 Patient disposition. [a]In Panel 2, one patient in the GT1b/without RBV group had <25 IU/mL detectable HCV RNA at Week 4 and, therefore, met the criterion for a 12-week follow-up treatment with pegIFN/RBV. This patient refused to receive follow-up treatment. [b]In Panel 4, the results of the Trugene or LiPA test performed at screening were used to randomise the patients to the 30-mg or 60-mg dose of JNJ-56914845. For analyses purposes, NS5B sequencing was used to determine the HCV geno/subtype. Based on this method, the geno/subtype for two patients in the 30-mg group was found to be non-1a, non-1b (1c, $n = 1$; 1l, $n = 1$) based on geno/subtyping using NS5B sequencing. These two patients were analysed together with the GT1a-infected patients in the category 'GT1a/other'. *DAA* direct-acting antiviral agent, *FU* follow-up, *GT* genotype, *HCV* hepatitis C virus, *pegIFN* pegylated interferon α-2a, *RBV* ribavirin

All patients who achieved SVR12 also went on to achieve SVR24, with the exception of one patient in Panel 1 and one patient in the GT1b/without ribavirin group in Panel 3 who had HCV RNA ≥25 IU/mL 24 weeks after end of treatment (1,830,000 IU/mL and 2770 IU/mL, respectively).

An overview of treatment outcome, including reasons for not achieving SVR12, is shown in Fig. 3. A total of 5/10 (50%), 1/12 (8%) and 1/9 (11%) patients in Panel 1 and in the GT1b/with ribavirin and GT1b/without ribavirin groups of Panel 2, respectively, experienced viral breakthrough. In Panel 3, 1/8 (13%) patients in the GT1b/without ribavirin group had viral breakthrough compared with 1/22 (5%) patients in the 60-mg group of Panel 4 (Fig. 3). Among the patients with undetectable HCV RNA at end of treatment and with at least one post-treatment follow-up HCV RNA measurement available, 2/6 patients (33%) in each of the Panel 2 and Panel 3 GT1b/without ribavirin groups and 4/14 (18%) GT1a-infected patients in the Panel 4 30-mg group experienced viral relapse. At the time of the final analysis, one patient in Panel 1 and one patient in the Panel 3 GT1b/without ribavirin group achieved SVR12 but had HCV RNA ≥25 IU/mL 24 weeks after end of treatment.

Virologic resistance testing

At baseline, the NS3 Q80K polymorphism was observed in 2/10 (20%) GT1a-infected patients in Panel 1 and in 2/13 (15%) GT1a-infected patients in the 30-mg group

Table 1 Baseline patient demographics and disease characteristics (intent-to-treat population)

	Simeprevir 75 mg + TMC647055/ ritonavir 450/30 mg			Simeprevir 75 mg + TMC647055/ritonavir 600/50 mg		Simeprevir 75 mg + TMC647055/ ritonavir 450/30 mg + JNJ-56914845 30 mg	Simeprevir 75 mg + TMC647055/ritonavir 450/30 mg + JNJ-56914845 60 mg
	Panel 1	Panel 2		Panel 3		Panel 4	
	GT1a/with ribavirin ($n = 10$)	GT1b/with ribavirin ($n = 12$)	GT1b/without ribavirin ($n = 9$)	GT1a/with ribavirin ($n = 7$)	GT1b/without ribavirin ($n = 8$)	GT1a/b/other ($n = 22$)[a]	GT1a/b/other ($n = 22$)[b]
Caucasian, n (%)	10 (100)	12 (100)	8 (89)	7 (100)	6 (75)	20 (91)	21 (96)
Male, n (%)	8 (80)	4 (33)	7 (78)	7 (100)	3 (38)	16 (73)	17 (77)
Treatment-naïve, n (%)	10 (100)	8 (67)	8 (89)	7 (100)	4 (50)	20 (91)	19 (86)
Prior relapser, n (%)	0 (0)	4 (33)	1 (11)	0 (0)	4 (50)	2 (9)	3 (14)
Age, median, years (range)	46.5 (38–52)	47.5 (29–62)	37.0 (18–64)	44.0 (28–58)	48.5 (43–66)	50.5 (24–70)	48.0 (27–58)
HCV RNA, median, $\log_{10}$ IU/mL (range)	6.52 (4.4–7.2)	6.69 (5.8–7.5)	5.98 (5.3–7.1)	6.32 (6.0–7.4)	6.76 (6.1–7.0)	6.78 (5.5–7.4)	6.62 (5.2–7.1)
METAVIR score, n (%)							
F0–F2	5 (50)	6 (50)	6 (67)	4 (29)	3 (38)	7 (32)	5 (23)
F3	1 (10)	1 (8)	1 (11)	1 (14)	0	2 (9)	4 (18)
Missing	4 (40)	5 (42)	2 (22)	2 (29)	5 (63)	13 (59)	13 (59)
IL28B genotype, n (%)							
CC	5 (50)	4 (33)	2 (22)	0 (0)	2 (25)	9 (41)	6 (27)
CT	4 (40)	6 (50)	6 (67)	6 (86)	5 (63)	8 (36)	11 (50)
TT	1 (10)	2 (17)	1 (11)	1 (14)	1 (13)	5 (23)	5 (23)

GT genotype, *HCV* hepatitis C virus

[a]GT1a/other, $n = 14$; GT1b, $n = 8$. GT1a/other includes one patient with HCV GT1c and one patient with GT1l, as determined by NS5B sequencing

[b]GT1a/other, $n = 15$; GT1b, $n = 7$

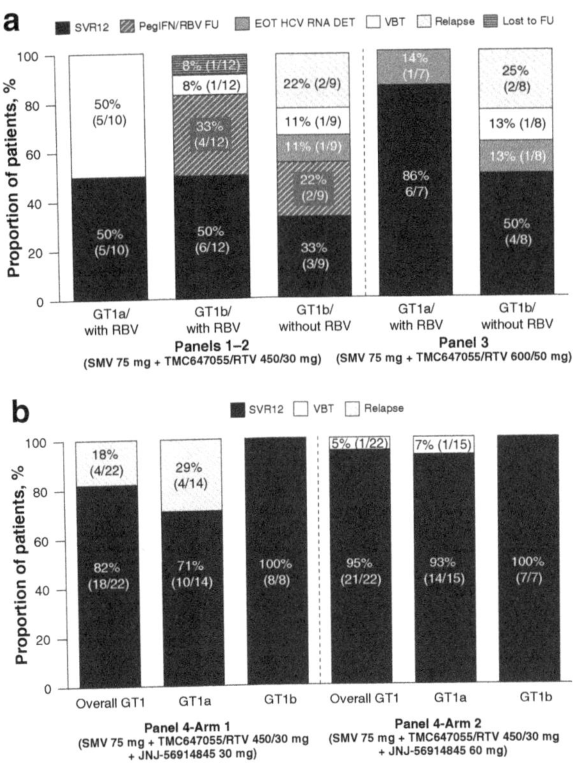

Fig. 3 Treatment outcome in (**a**) Panels 1–3, and (**b**) Panel 4. SVR12 data shown represent SVR12 achieved after treatment with only the combination of SMV + TMC647055/RTV ± RBV. In the Panel 2 GT1b/with RBV and GT1b/without RBV arms, four and two patients, respectively, had follow-up therapy with pegIFN/RBV and are, therefore, not included in the SVR12 category that focuses on SVR12 after 12 weeks of DAA treatment. Among them, five patients achieved SVR12 after completing follow-up therapy; one patient refused to receive follow-up treatment and was lost to follow-up. One additional patient in the Panel 2 GT1b/without RBV group had <25 IU/mL detectable HCV RNA at Week 4 and, therefore, met the criterion for the 12-week follow-up treatment with pegIFN/RBV; however, this patient refused to receive follow-up treatment. *DAA* direct-acting antiviral agent, *DET* detectable, *EOT* end of treatment, *FU* follow-up, *GT* genotype, *HCV* hepatitis C virus, *pegIFN* pegylated interferon α-2a, *RBV* ribavirin, *RTV* ritonavir, *SMV* simeprevir, *SVR12* sustained virologic response 12 weeks after end of treatment, *VBT* viral breakthrough

in Panel 4. Neither of the two GT1a-infected patients with baseline Q80K in Panel 1, and one of the two patients in Panel 4 achieved SVR12. In 5/42 (12%) patients with NS5A sequencing data available in Panel 4, baseline NS5A polymorphisms were detected at positions 28, 30, 31 and/or 93. Of those, only L31M ($n = 1$) and Y93C (in combination with M28V; $n = 1$), both detected in GT1a-infected patients, are associated with in vitro resistance to JNJ-56914845 [8]. Details on NS5B baseline polymorphisms are provided in Additional file 1.

Virologic failure (including the two patients who achieved SVR12 but had HCV RNA ≥25 IU/mL 24 weeks after end of treatment) was, in the majority of patients, associated with the emergence of simeprevir and TMC647055 resistance-associated variants (RAVs) in Panels 1–3 and simeprevir and JNJ-56914845 RAVs with or without TMC647055 RAVs in Panel 4 at time of failure. In line with the previously characterised simeprevir resistance profile, most GT1b-infected patients harboured an emerging mutation at NS3 position 168, while emerging mutations in GT1a-infected patients were mostly observed at NS3 position 155 (R155K alone or in combination with a Q80R; R155S) at time of failure. TMC647055 RAVs were only observed at NS5B position 495 (mainly P495L), consistent with the resistance profile of NNI-1 polymerase inhibitors. In all patients with virologic failure in Panel 4, emerging JNJ-56914845 RAVs at NS5A positions 30 and/or 31 were detected at time of failure. Treatment-emergent RAVs in NS3 and NS5B became undetectable in many of the patients after treatment was stopped, while emerging RAVs in NS5A could still be detected by population sequencing at the end of the study in the five patients who failed the 3-DAA treatment.

Pharmacokinetics

Co-administration of high-dose TMC647055/ritonavir (600/50 mg) increased simeprevir exposure compared with low-dose TMC647055/ritonavir (450/30 mg). Simeprevir C_{max} values were increased by 2.0-fold and AUC_{0-24h} values by 1.9- to 2.3-fold, respectively, following co-administration with TMC647055/ritonavir (600/50 mg vs 450/30 mg) with ribavirin (Panel 3-Arm 1 vs Panel 1) or without ribavirin (Panel 3-Arm 2 vs Panel 2-Arm 2) (Additional file 2: Figure S1a).

A more than dose-proportional increase in TMC647055 exposure occurred following co-administration of TMC647055/ritonavir 600 mg/50 mg once daily (Panel 3-Arm 2) compared with 450 mg/30 mg once daily (Panel 2-Arm 2) with simeprevir (C_{max}: 2.6-fold increase; AUC_{0-24h}: 2.4-fold increase) (Additional file 2: Figure S1b).

Co-administration of high-dose JNJ-56914845 60 mg once daily with simeprevir 75 mg once daily + TMC647055/ritonavir 450 mg/30 mg once daily increased simeprevir exposure (1.2-fold increase in both C_{max} and AUC_{0-24h} vs without JNJ-56914845) (Additional file 2: Figure S1a), but had minimal effect on TMC647055 and ritonavir exposure (Additional file 2: Figure S1b and c).

A dose-proportional increase in exposure to JNJ-56914845 60 mg versus 30 mg once daily was observed when co-administered with simeprevir 75 mg + TMC647055/ritonavir 450 mg/30 mg once daily (Panel 4-Arm 2 vs Panel 4-Arm 1: C_{max} 821 vs 389 ng/mL, AUC_{0-24h} 7747 vs 3358 ng · h/mL) (Additional file 2: Figure S1d; Additional file 3: Table S1).

No differences were observed in simeprevir, TMC647055 or ritonavir pharmacokinetics based on ribavirin use

(Additional file 4: Table S2, Additional file 5: Table S3 and Additional file 6: Table S4).

Safety

No patients discontinued any of the study drugs due to an AE, and there were no SAEs or deaths.

The incidence of AEs was similar between Panels 1 and 2, and Panel 3 (Table 2). In Panels 1 and 2, all reported AEs were Grade 1 or 2, and there were no clinically relevant differences among patients treated with ribavirin and those who did not receive ribavirin in terms of the incidence or severity of AEs. In Panel 3, all AEs were Grade 1 or 2, with the exception of one patient (GT1b/without ribavirin group) who experienced a Grade 3 AE (hypercholesterolaemia). This AE was not serious and was not considered related to simeprevir, TMC647055 or ritonavir by the investigator; the AE was ongoing at the time of the final analysis. A higher incidence of patients in Panel 3 treated with ribavirin experienced a Grade 1 or 2 AE compared with those who did not receive ribavirin. All AEs in Panel 4 were Grade 1 or 2, with the exception of one patient who experienced a Grade 3 increase in white blood cell count (not related to any study drug). There were no clinically relevant differences in the incidence of AEs between patients treated with JNJ-56914845 at either dose (Table 2).

The most frequently (in >20% of patients) reported AEs during the treatment phase were as follows; Panels 1 and 2: headache (14/31 [45%]), fatigue (9/31 [29%]) and influenza-like illness (7/31 [23%]); Panel 3: nausea (7/15 [47%]), headache (7/15 [47%]), diarrhoea (5/15 [33%]), fatigue (4/15 [27%]) and pruritus (4/15 [27%]); Panel 4: headache (15/44 [33%]), diarrhoea (14/44 [32%]) and fatigue (13/44 [30%]).

The majority of graded laboratory abnormalities were Grade 1 or 2 and were not clinically significant. Grade 3 or 4 laboratory abnormalities were observed in <10% of patients in all panels (further details are provided in Additional file 1). Hyperbilirubinaemia was reported as a laboratory-related AE in 1 (3%) patient in Panels 1 and 2 (considered possibly related to TMC647055 and simeprevir) and 1 (2%) patient in the 60-mg group in Panel 4 (considered possibly related to TMC647055, ritonavir and JNJ-56914845, and probably related to simeprevir). Both hyperbilirubinaemia AEs were Grade 1 or 2 in severity.

Discussion

This was a proof-of-concept study performed to explore the efficacy and safety of the 2-DAA combination of the HCV NS3/4A PI simeprevir and the HCV NS5B NNI TMC647055 administered with ritonavir ± ribavirin, and of the 3-DAA combination of simeprevir, TMC647055 and the HCV NS5A inhibitor JNJ-56914845 administered with ritonavir in HCV GT1-infected patients. The results suggest that the addition of JNJ-56914845 (60 mg) to the 2-DAA regimen of simeprevir and TMC647055 was highly beneficial in improving the efficacy of the combination treatment in patients with HCV GT1 infection.

Overall, the 2-DAA combination of low-dose TMC647055/ritonavir plus simeprevir, with or without ribavirin, did not demonstrate high efficacy in GT1-

Table 2 Summary of adverse events during the treatment phase (intent-to-treat population)

	Simeprevir 75 mg + TMC647055/ritonavir 450/30 mg			Simeprevir 75 mg + TMC647055/ritonavir 600/50 mg		Simeprevir 75 mg + TMC647055/ritonavir 450/30 mg + JNJ-56914845 30 mg	Simeprevir 75 mg + TMC647055/ritonavir 450/30 mg + JNJ-56914845 60 mg
	Panel 1	Panel 2		Panel 3		Panel 4	
	GT1a/with ribavirin (*n* = 10)	GT1b/with ribavirin (*n* = 12)	GT1b/without ribavirin (*n* = 9)	GT1a/with ribavirin (*n* = 7)	GT1b/without ribavirin (*n* = 8)	GT1a/b/other (*n* = 22)[a]	GT1a/b/other (*n* = 22)[b]
Any AE, n (%)	10 (100)	12 (100)	7 (78)	6 (86)	6 (75)	20 (91)	22 (100)
Worst Grade 1, n (%)	6 (60)	7 (58)	4 (44)	5 (71)	3 (38)	15 (68)	15 (68)
Worst Grade 2, n (%)	4 (40)	5 (42)	3 (33)	1 (14)	2 (25)	5 (23)	6 (27)
Worst Grade 3, n (%)	0 (0)	0 (0)	0 (0)	0 (0)	1 (13)[c]	0 (0)	1 (5)[d]
Worst Grade 4, n (%)	0 (0)	0 (0)	0 (0)	0 (0)	0 (0)	0 (0)	0 (0)
Leading to permanent stop of study drugs, n (%)	0 (0)	0 (0)	0 (0)	0 (0)	0 (0)	0 (0)	0 (0)
Serious AE, n (%)	0 (0)	0 (0)	0 (0)	0 (0)	0 (0)	0 (0)	0 (0)
Death, n (%)	0 (0)	0 (0)	0 (0)	0 (0)	0 (0)	0 (0)	0 (0)

AE adverse event, *GT* genotype

[a]GT1a/other, *n* = 14; GT1b, *n* = 8. GT1a/other includes one patient with HCV GT1c and one patient with GT1l, as determined by NS5B sequencing

[b]GT1a/other, *n* = 15; GT1b, *n* = 7

[c]Hypercholesterolaemia, not related to any study drug

[d]Increase in white blood cell count, not related to any study drug

infected patients (SVR12: 33%–50%). The SVR12 rate in HCV GT1a-infected patients treated with the 2-DAA combination and ribavirin was 86% (6/7) for the high dose of TMC647055/ritonavir, and 50% (5/10) for the low dose of TMC647055/ritonavir, indicating a dose-dependent increase in efficacy of TMC647055/ritonavir. The increased dose was not associated with an increase in AEs and there were no safety concerns regarding the use of ritonavir. Although the 2-DAA combination and the high dose of TMC647055/ritonavir demonstrated a higher SVR12 rate in GT1a-infected patients compared with the low dose of TMC647055/ritonavir, this was not observed in GT1b-infected patients who received the 2-DAA combination without ribavirin (SVR12 for the low- vs high-dose TMC647055/ritonavir: 33% [3/9] vs 50% [4/8], respectively). Although data are limited, these suggest the addition of ribavirin may be required to increase SVR12 in a 2-DAA regimen combining an NS3/4A PI and an NS5B NNI.

In Panel 1, neither of the two GT1a-infected patients with an NS3 Q80K polymorphism at baseline achieved SVR12. Moreover, viral breakthrough was frequently observed with the 2-DAA combination (ranging from 8–50%) compared with a frequency of 5% with the 3-DAA combination (1/22 patient who received the 3-DAA combination with JNJ-56914845 [60 mg]).

The 3-DAA combination resulted in an overall SVR12 rate of 95% with 60 mg JNJ-56914845. All GT1b-infected patients (7/7; 100%) treated with the 3-DAA combination achieved SVR12, and the majority of GT1a-infected patients (14/15; 93%) also achieved SVR12 following treatment with this regimen. The SVR12 rates observed with this combination therapy are consistent with those reported in Phase 3 studies that assessed the combination of the PI paritaprevir with the NNI dasabuvir and the NS5A inhibitor ombitasvir in treatment-naïve or treatment-experienced, non-cirrhotic, HCV GT1-infected patients [2, 10–12].

The simeprevir resistance profile observed in all panels in this study was similar to that observed in the simeprevir Phase 3 studies in the presence of pegIFN/ribavirin [13–15]. A genotypic and phenotypic analysis of baseline HCV isolates from all patients who participated in this study, as well as of isolates obtained at the time of failure and at the end of study from patients with virologic failure, are described in full in a separate paper (Leen Vijgen, Kim Thys, An Vandebosch, Pieter Van Remoortere, René Verloes, Sandra De Meyer. Virology analysis in HCV genotype 1-infected patients treated with the combination of simeprevir and TMC647055/ritonavir, with and without ribavirin, and JNJ-56914845, in preparation).

The interaction between the drugs assessed in this study had previously been evaluated in healthy volunteers [16]. In that study, co-administration of simeprevir increased exposure (AUC_{0-24h}) of JNJ-56914845 2.6-fold with no additional effect when TMC647055/ritonavir was added. Co-administration with JNJ-56914845 resulted in small increases in the plasma concentrations of simeprevir and TMC647055. These increases were not considered to be clinically relevant for either DAA [16]. In the current study, administration of simeprevir 75 mg once daily in combination with TMC647055/ritonavir in HCV-infected patients resulted in simeprevir exposures within the range observed in historical data for simeprevir when dosed at 150 mg once daily (data on file). In addition, high exposure to TMC647055 was achieved when administered in combination with ritonavir.

Both the 2-DAA and the 3-DAA regimens were well tolerated. There were no deaths, SAEs, Grade 4 AEs or AEs leading to temporary/permanent treatment discontinuation in any of the four panels. In addition, there were no Grade 3 or 4 laboratory-related AEs that were considered related to any of the study drugs. Differences in AE incidence among patients who received ribavirin and those who did not in Panels 1 and 2 (Table 2) were a result of ribavirin-related adverse drug reactions, as were the respective differences observed in the incidence of laboratory abnormalities in Panels 1–3 (see Additional file 1). A comparable safety profile was observed with TMC647055/ritonavir 450/30 mg and TMC647055/ritonavir 600/50 mg (Panels 1–3) and also between the JNJ-56914845 30-mg and 60-mg doses (Panel 4).

Conclusion

High SVR rates of 93% and 100% in GT1a- and GT1b-infected patients, respectively, were achieved in this study by combining simeprevir 75 mg with JNJ-56914845 60 mg and TMC647055/ritonavir 450/30 mg. Lower SVR rates were observed without the inclusion of JNJ-56914845. Based on the results of this study, the efficacy and safety of DAA-combination regimens targeting the same viral proteins as the drugs in this study (i.e., the HCV NS5B polymerase, the HCV NS5A protein and the HCV NS4/4A protease) are being investigated further.

Additional files

Additional file 1: Further information on the methods of the study, including dosing rationale and protocol deviations are included. In addition, further virologic resistance testing and safety results are included.

Additional file 2: Figure S1. Mean (SD) plasma concentration versus time profile for: (a) simeprevir; (b) TMC647055; and (c) ritonavir in Panels 1–4; and for (d) JNJ-56914845 in Panel 4. *RBV* ribavirin, *RTV* ritonavir, *SD* standard deviation, *SMV* simeprevir.

Additional file 3: Table S1. Week-4 JNJ-56914845 pharmacokinetic parameters after administration in Panel 4.

Additional file 4: Table S2. Week-4 simeprevir pharmacokinetic parameters after administration in (a) Panels 1–3 and (b) Panel 4.

Additional file 5: Table S3. Week-4 TMC647055 pharmacokinetic parameters after administration in (a) Panels 1–3 and (b) Panel 4.

Additional file 6: Table S4. Week-4 ritonavir pharmacokinetic parameters after administration in (a) Panels 1–3 and (b) Panel 4.

Abbreviations

AE: Adverse event; AUC_{0-24h}: Area under the plasma concentration–time curve over 24 h; BID: Twice daily; BQL: Below quantification limit; C_{max}: Maximum plasma concentration; C_{min}: Minimum plasma concentration; CYP: Cytochrome P450; DAA: Direct-acting-antiviral agent; DET: Detectable; EOT: End of treatment; EU: European Union; FU: Follow-up; GT: Genotype; HCV: Hepatitis C virus; HIV: Human immunodeficiency virus; IFN: Interferon; ITT: Intent-to-treat; LDL: Low-density lipoprotein; MCHC: Mean corpuscular haemoglobin concentration; NNI: Non-nucleoside inhibitor; OATP: Organic anion transporting polypeptide; pegIFN: Pegylated interferon α-2a; PI: Protease inhibitor; RAV: Resistance-associated variant; RBV: Ribavirin; RTV: Ritonavir; SAE: Serious adverse event; SD: Standard deviation; SMV: Simeprevir; SVR: Sustained virologic response; SVR12: Sustained virologic response 12 weeks after end of treatment; SVR24: Sustained virologic response 24 weeks after end of treatment; VBT: Viral breakthrough; WBC: White blood cell

Acknowledgements

The authors would like to thank the patients and investigators for their contributions to this study. Medical writing support was provided by Chrissie Kouremenou of Complete Medical Communications and funded by Janssen.

Funding

The study was funded by Janssen. Janssen were responsible for the study design and the collection and interpretation of data. Medical writing support was funded by Janssen.

Authors' contributions

SB, HW, CM, HO, FN, KA, YH, JMS, PB and SF were involved in the acquisition and interpretation of study data, and have been involved in the critical revision of the manuscript for important intellectual content. LV, TNK, EH, AV, BJ, PVR and RV were involved in the study concept and design, and the acquisition, analysis and interpretation of study data. They have also been involved in the critical revision of the manuscript for important intellectual content. DL provided statistical analysis of the study data, and has been involved in the critical revision of the manuscript for important intellectual content. All authors read and approved the final manuscript.

Competing interests

SB has received grants from Janssen, MSD and Roche, and has been on advisory boards for AbbVie, Bristol-Myers Squibb, Gilead Sciences, Janssen and MSD.
HW has received grants from Janssen.
CM has been an investigator for Roche, Schering-Plough, Gilead Sciences, Pfizer and Tibotec, has received research grants from Schering-Plough and Roche, has acted as an adviser/consultant for Janssen-Cilag and Schering-Plough, and as a speaker for Schering-Plough and Bristol-Myers Squibb.
HO has acted as a consultant for Janssen (National Advisory Board) for the past 3 years.
FN has received research grants from Roche, Astelles, Ferring, Novartis, Janssen-Cilag and AbbVie, and has consultancy agreements with CAF, Intercept, Gore, Bristol-Myers Squibb, AbbVie, Novartis, MSD, Janssen-Cilag, Promethera, Ono Pharma and Durect.
KA has received advisory and consultancy fees from Boehringer Ingelheim, Bristol-Myers Squibb, Gilead, Hexal and Merck, and has been a clinical investigator for Bionor, Boehringer Ingelheim, Bristol-Myers Squibb, Gilead, GlaxoSmithKline, Janssen, Merck and Pfizer.
YH has received grants from Janssen, Merck and Roche, and has been a clinical investigator and/or consultant for Vertex, Janssen, Bristol-Myers Squibb, Merck, Roche, Gilead, AbbVie and Boehringer Ingelheim.
JMS has received advisor and speaker fees from AbbVie, Bristol-Myers Squibb, Gilead, Janssen and Merck, and has been a clinical investigator for Boehringer Ingelheim, Gilead and Janssen.
PB has acted as a consultant for AbbVie, Bristol-Myers Squibb, Gilead, Janssen, Merz and MSD, and has given sponsored lectures for AbbVie, Bristol-Myers Squibb, Gilead, Falk, Janssen, Merck, Merz, MSD and Roche.
SF has nothing to disclose.
LV, TNK, EH, DL, AV, BJ, PVR and RV are employees of Janssen and may own stock in Johnson & Johnson.

Consent for publication

Not applicable.

Author details

[1]Department of Gastroenterology & Hepatology, ZNA Antwerp, Antwerpen, Belgium. [2]Department of Hepatology and Gastroenterology, Universitair Ziekenhuis Gent, Ghent, Belgium. [3]Liver Unit, CUB Hôpital Erasme, Université Libre de Bruxelles, Brussels, Belgium. [4]Department of Gastroenterology and Hepatology, AZ Sint-Jan AV Hospital, Bruges, Belgium. [5]Department of Liver and Biliopancreatic Disorders, University Hospitals KU Leuven, Leuven, Belgium. [6]EPIMED/Vivantes-Auguste-Viktoria-Klinikum, Berlin, Germany. [7]Hepato-gastroenterology, Cliniques Universitaires Saint-Luc, Université Catholique de Louvain, Brussels, Belgium. [8]Department of Medicine, University Medical Center Mainz, Mainz, Germany. [9]IFI, Liver Center Hamburg, Asklepiosklinik St. Georg, Hamburg, Germany. [10]Department of Gastroenterology and Hepatology, Universitair Ziekenhuis Antwerpen, Antwerp, Belgium. [11]Janssen Pharmaceutica NV, Beerse, Belgium. [12]Alios BioPharma Inc, South San Francisco, CA, USA. [13]Janssen Research & Development BVBA, Beerse, Belgium. [14]Janssen Pharmaceuticals LLC, Titusville, NJ, USA.

References

1. Florian J, Mishra P, Arya V, Harrington P, Connelly S, Reynolds KS, et al. Direct-acting antiviral drugs for the treatment of chronic hepatitis C virus infection: interferon free is now. Clin Pharmacol Ther. 2015;98:394–402.
2. Ferenci P, Bernstein D, Lalezari J, Cohen D, Luo Y, Cooper C, et al. ABT-450/r-ombitasvir and dasabuvir with or without ribavirin for HCV. N Engl J Med. 2014;370:1983–92.
3. Sanford M. Simeprevir: a review of its use in patients with chronic hepatitis C virus infection. Drugs. 2015;75:183–96.
4. Ouwerkerk-Mahadevan S, Snoeys J, Peeters M, Beumont-Mauviel M, Simion A. Drug-drug interactions with the NS3/4A protease inhibitor simeprevir. Clin Pharmacokinet. 2016;55:197–208.
5. Cummings MD, Lin TI, Hu L, Tahri A, McGowan D, Amssoms K, et al. Discovery and early development of TMC647055, a non-nucleoside inhibitor of the hepatitis C virus NS5B polymerase. J Med Chem. 2014;57:1880–92.
6. Bourgeois S, Reesink HW, Leempoels J, Vijgen L, Rouan MC, Marien K, et al. Combination therapy of TMC647055 with simeprevir (TMC435) in chronic hepatitis C patients [abstract]. J Hepatol. 2013;58:S483.
7. Gardner S, Cutrell A, Elko-Simms C, Adkison K, Hamatake R, Walker J, et al. A double-blind, randomized, placebo-controlled study to assess the safety, antiviral activity and pharmacokinetics of GSK2336805 when given as monotherapy and in combination with peginterferon alfa-2a and ribavirin in hepatitis C virus genotype 1-infected treatment-naive subjects. Liver Int. 2014;34:e89–95.
8. Walker J, Crosby R, Wang A, Woldu E, Vamathevan J, Voitenleitner C, et al. Preclinical characterization of GSK2336805, a novel inhibitor of hepatitis C virus replication that selects for resistance in NS5A. Antimicrob Agents Chemother. 2014;58:38–47.
9. Vanwelkenhuysen I, de Vries R, Timmerman P, Verhaeghe T. Determination of simeprevir: a novel, hepatitis C protease inhibitor in human plasma by high-performance liquid chromatography-tandem mass spectrometry. J Chromatogr B Analyt Technol Biomed Life Sci. 2014;958:43–7.

10. Andreone P, Colombo MG, Enejosa JV, Koksal I, Ferenci P, Maieron A, et al. ABT-450, ritonavir, ombitasvir, and dasabuvir achieves 97% and 100% sustained virologic response with or without ribavirin in treatment-experienced patients with HCV genotype 1b infection. Gastroenterology. 2014;147:359–65.
11. Feld JJ, Kowdley KV, Coakley E, Sigal S, Nelson DR, Crawford D, et al. Treatment of HCV with ABT-450/r-ombitasvir and dasabuvir with ribavirin. N Engl J Med. 2014;370:1594–603.
12. Zeuzem S, Jacobson IM, Baykal T, Marinho RT, Poordad F, Bourlière M, et al. Retreatment of HCV with ABT-450/r-ombitasvir and dasabuvir with ribavirin. N Engl J Med. 2014;370:1604–14.
13. Forns X, Lawitz E, Zeuzem S, Gane E, Bronowicki JP, Andreone P, et al. Simeprevir with peginterferon and ribavirin leads to high rates of SVR in patients with HCV genotype 1 who relapsed after previous therapy: a phase 3 trial. Gastroenterology. 2014;146:1669–79.
14. Jacobson IM, Dore GJ, Foster GR, Fried MW, Radu M, Rafalsky W, et al. Simeprevir with pegylated interferon alfa 2a plus ribavirin in treatment-naive patients with chronic hepatitis C virus genotype 1 infection (QUEST-1): a phase 3, randomised, double-blind, placebo-controlled trial. Lancet. 2014;384:403–13.
15. Manns M, Marcellin P, Poordad F, de Araujo ES, Buti M, Horsmans Y, et al. Simeprevir with pegylated interferon alfa 2a or 2b plus ribavirin in treatment-naive patients with chronic hepatitis C virus genotype 1 infection (QUEST-2): a randomised, double-blind, placebo-controlled phase 3 trial. Lancet. 2014;384:414–26.
16. Kakuda T, Spittaels K, Verloes R, Vanwelkenhuysen I, Truyers C, Van Remoortere P. Pharmacokinetics of simeprevir, JNJ-56914845 and ritonavir-boosted TMC647055 when co-administered in healthy volunteers. 2014. http://regist2.virology-education.com/abstractbook/2014_4.pdf. Accessed 23 Aug 2016.

4

Comparison of telbivudine and entecavir on the change of off-treatment eGFR after 3 years of treatment in non-cirrhotic chronic hepatitis B patients

Yang-Sheng Lin[1,2,3], Shou-Chuan Shih[1,3], Horng-Yuan Wang[1,2,3], Ching-Chung Lin[1,3], Chen-Wang Chang[1,2,3] and Ming-Jen Chen[1,2,3*]

Abstract

Background: The change of estimated glomerular filtration rate (eGFR) with off-treatment nucleos(t)ide analogues (NA) in chronic hepatitis B patients (CHB) is unclear. This study is aimed to evaluate the off-treatment eGFR after 3 years of therapy with telbivudine (LdT) or entecavir (ETV) and to assess predictive factors for eGFR improvement.

Methods: From January 2009 to December 2011, we identified NA-naïve patients who were at least 20 years of age diagnosed with compensated CHB. All patients received a 3-year NA treatment and 1 year off-treatment follow-up; the initial selection of patients for LdT or ETV treatment was at the physicians' discretion. An increase of more than 10% in eGFR from the baseline was identified as an improvement. The change of chronic kidney disease stages were recorded and compared with baseline at year 3 and year 4, respectively.

Results: This study included two groups consisting of 46 patients each (each with3 years of treatment with LdT or ETV). In LdT-treated patients, the mean eGFR increased from 94.3 ± 28.3 to 104.0 ± 31.2 mL/min/1.73 m^2 in year 3 ($p = 0.01$) and from 104.0 ± 31.2 to 104.0 ± 28.8 mL/min/1.73 m^2 in year 4 ($p = 0.99$). However, in ETV-treated patients, the mean eGFR decreased from 93.1 ± 26.1 to 85.5 ± 25.1 mL/min/1.73 m^2 in year 3 ($p = 0.0009$) and from 85.5 ± 25.1 to 87.7 ± 24.8 mL/min/1.73 m^2 in year 4 ($p = 0.2$). After a multivariate analysis, the predictors for the off-treatment eGFR improvement were the LdT treatment (odds ratio [OR], 3.97 (1.37–11.5), $p = 0.01$) and pre-treated eGFR (OR, 0.98 (0.95–1.00), $p = 0.04$).

Conclusions: At year 4, 48.8 and 21.3% patients had an improved eGFR from baseline in LdT and ETV patients, respectively. Telbivudine may have a protective renal effect that can last for one year after treatment in non-cirrhotic CHB patients without a virological breakthrough.

Keywords: Telbivudine, Entecavir, Chronic hepatitis B, Off-treatment, Renal function, eGFR

* Correspondence: mingjen.ch@msa.hinet.net
[1]Division of Gastroenterology, Department of Internal Medicine, MacKay Memorial Hospital, Taipei Campus, No. 92, Sec. 2, Chungshan North Road, 104 Taipei, Taiwan
[2]MacKay Junior College of Medicine, Nursing, and Management, Taipei, Taiwan

Background

Nucleos(t)ide analogs (NA) are widely used for the treatment of hepatitis B and have been shown to reverse fibrosis and cirrhosis, and reduce the risk of hepatic decompensation and hepatocellular carcinoma [1, 2]. Although NAs are effective in suppressing hepatitis B virus (HBV) replication, most patients require long-term treatment. Safety is one of the major considerations with a long-term and even life-long use of NAs and needs to gain more attention [3]. In particular, the effects of HBV infection or treatment agents on the renal dysfunction in CHB patients require further studies.

There are currently 5 oral antiviral agents for CHB: 2 nucleotides (adefovir and tenofovir) and 3 nucleosides (lamivudine, entecavir (ETV), and telbivudine (LdT)). All of these oral antiviral agents are primarily eliminated unchanged through the renal route, therefore, can have an effect on the mitochondrial or proximal tubular microstructures. The nephrotoxic potential seems to be more prevalent in nucleotides (adefovir and tenofovir) [3]. The exact mechanism is largely unknown and is likely to involve multiple pathophysiological pathways [3]. From a review article, during long-term therapy, minimal rates of eGFR decline have been reported, except for LdT [4]. Furthermore, retrospective analyses of LdT have demonstrated a potential renal improvement in a broad spectrum of CHB patients. In a large cohort of patients with CHB receiving LdT, the estimated GFR (eGFR) [using MDRD formula] increased by 14.9 mL/min or by 16.6% from baseline to year 4 [5].

This improvement in eGFR was more evident in the LdT-treated patients with stage 2 chronic kidney disease (i.e. eGFR 60–90 mL/min), wherein, 74% of the patients regained normal renal function (i.e. eGFR >90 mL/min) after 4 years of treatment [6]. This effect was maintained during long-term therapy and was also observed in patients after 2 years off treatment [6]. The mechanism of the beneficial effect of LdT therapy on renal function is still undetermined.

It is still unknown if the improvement in renal function is specific to LdT or what is the result of the maintenance after LdT off-treatment? As a hyperendemic area of CKD of 11.9% in general population [7], choice of NA with the potential renoprotection after off-treatment follow up is intriguing. In Taiwan, the Bureau of National Health Insurance reimburses NA treatment for up to 3 years in treatment-naïve CHB patients if there is no evidence of virological breakthrough during the treatment period. To the best of our knowledge, there is no published study comparing the effects of LdT and ETV on renal function after the treatment.

Methods

Patients

From January 2009 to December 2011, we identified NA-naïve patients who were at least 20 years of age and diagnosed with compensated CHB. All patients received a 3-year NA treatment and had a 1-year follow-up after off treatment; the initial selection of patients for LdT or ETV treatment was at the physicians' discretion. According to the current guidelines, antiviral treatment is recommended for HBeAg-negative patients with a HBV-DNA level over 2000 IU/mL and serum alanine transaminase (ALT) >2 x upper normal limit (ULN) for 3 months; all HBeAg-positive patients with HBV-DNA level over 20,000 IU/mL and serum ALT above >2 x ULN or any HBeAg-positive patients with ALT >5 x ULN).

We investigated the underlying diseases in the beginning of treatment including chronic kidney disease stages, hypertension, diabetes and prescribed potential renal toxicity agents such as nonsteroidal anti-inflammatory drugs (NSAIDs) or immunosuppressive agents. The patients were regularly followed up with abdominal sonography and serum HBV-DNA every 6 months during the treatment, and serum liver function tests and eGFR every 3 months for one year after the treatment according to the national guideline. If there were two more tests during the 3-month interval, we chose the test more closely to their respective check points (such as at year 3 or year 4).

The patients with coexisting HIV or HCV infection, prior NA therapy, liver cirrhosis or acute fulminant hepatitis, autoimmune disease, and malignancy were excluded from the study. The appropriate dosages (or dosing interval) of LdT and ETV were adjusted according to the patient's renal function. The study program was approved by the Institutional Review Board of MacKay Memorial Hospital (15MMH-ISO-014).

Assessments

Baseline data of patients were retrieved from the medical records that included age, sex, HBV DNA level (IU/mL), hepatitis B surface antigen/anti-HBs, hepatitis B e-antigen /anti-HBe, levels of ALT, albumin, total bilirubin and creatinine, and initial NA treatment. The renal function was estimated based on MDRD calculation for eGFR (mL/min/1.73 m^2): 186 x creatinine $(mg/dL)^{-1.154}$ x $age^{-0.203}$ x 0.742 (if female). An eGFR more than 90 mL/min/1.73 m^2 was classified as chronic kidney disease 1 (CKD stage 1). An eGFR of 60–89 mL/min/1.73 m^2 was classified as CKD stage 2. An eGFR of 30–59 mL/min/1.73 m^2 was classified as CKD stage 3. An eGFR of 15–29 mL/min/1.73 m^2 was classified as chronic kidney disease CKD stage 4.

As compared to the baseline, patients with an increasing eGFR >10% was seen as an improvement. The number of patient changing CKD stages compared with baseline at year 3 and year 4 were recorded in each groups. Factors such as age, sex, NA, HBV DNA, HBeAg status, and baseline eGFR were evaluated to predict improvement in eGFR at year 3 and year 4, respectively.

Statistical analysis

Continuous variables were expressed as mean ± standard deviation (SD) and compared using the Student's *t*-test. Categorical data were compared using the Fisher's exact test or $\chi 2$ test, as appropriate. Continuous variables that were not normally distributed were evaluated using Mann-Whitney's *U*-test. We used SPSS version 12.0 (SPSS Inc., Chicago, IL, USA) for all statistical analyses. All statistical tests were two-tailed, and $P < 0.05$ was considered statistically significant. We included all the covariates for the logistic regression analysis and a multivariate analysis was also performed to assess the predictive factors.

Results

The demographics and characteristics of 92 HBV patients assigned to treat with LdT or ETV

A total of 180 CHB patients were enrolled in this retrospective study, of which 89 patients were treated with LdT and 91 patients were treated with ETV according to the Taiwanese Health Insurance Guidelines. The initial selection of NA for treatment was at the physicians' discretion. Nineteen patients in the LdT group had a virological breakthrough during the 3-year treatment period, 15 patients decided to continue the treatment with self-paid medicine, and 9 patients had a viral breakthrough within 1 year after treatment following 3 years of therapy. Two patients in the ETV group changed to another NA due to headache and intent to become pregnant, 38 patients decided to continue the treatment with self-paid medicine, and 5 patients experienced viral breakthrough within 1 year after the treatment.

In total, 2 groups of 46 patients with HBV treated with LdT or ETV, respectively, were analyzed in this study (Fig. 1). The dosages and dosing interval were adjusted according to the patient's renal function. Only one patient in the ETV group modified the dosing interval every two days according to his creatinine clearance (25 mL/min), which was less than 50 mL/min.

The mean age of patients who completed 3 years of treatment with LdT and ETV were 46.3 and 51.3 years, respectively. The baseline demographic data were balanced at baseline for age, sex, comorbidity of chronic kidney disease stages, hypertension, and diabetes and prescribed with potential renal toxicity agents (Table 1). There were 63% (29 of 46) and 60.1% (28 of 46) HBeAg-positive patients in the LdT-treated group and ETV-treated groups, respectively ($p = 0.57$). Nonsteroidal anti-inflammatory drugs (NSAIDs) were used in 2.2% of the ETV group and 8.8% in the LdT group; immunosuppressive agents were used in 2.2% of the ETV group and 2.2% in the LdT group.

The change of eGFR at the end of 3 years of treatment with LdT and ETV compared with baseline

At the end of year 3, mean eGFR increased from 94.3 ± 28.3 to 104.0 ± 31.2 (mL/min/1.73 m^2) ($p = 0.01$) in LdT-treated patients, whereas it decreased from 93.1 ± 26.1 to 85.5 ± 25.1 (mL/min/1.73 m2) ($p = 0.0009$) in ETV-treated patients (Fig. 2). In addition, 23 of 46 (50.0%) patients had 10% more eGFR improvement compared to baseline in LdT patients. Similarly, 6 of 46 patients (13.1%) showed an improvement in the ETV group.

Eleven patients improved their CKD stages (8 patients from stage 2 to stage 1 and 3 patients from stage 3 to stage 2) and 2 patients worsened their CKD stages (one from stage 2 to stage 3 and one from stage 1 to stage 2) in the LdT group, one patient improved his CKD stage from stage 2 to stage 1 and 8 patients worsened their CKD stages (7 patients from stage 1 to stage 2 and one patient from stage 2 to stage 3) in the ETV group at year 3, compared to the baseline, respectively ($p = 0.004$) (Table 2).

After a multivariate analysis of patients' age, sex, pretreatment eGFR, HBeAg status, HBV DNA levels, NA, and nephrotoxic agents, the predictors for an eGFR improvement at the end of 3-year were the LdT treatment (odds ratio [OR], 7.97 [2.46–25.7], $p = 0.001$) (Table 3).

The change of eGFR 1 year after the off-treatment period compared with baselines

The present analyses focused on key therapeutic endpoints at 1 year after the off-treatment period. During the fourth year without viral breakthrough, the eGFR increased from 94.3 ± 28.3 to 104.0 ± 28.8 mL/min/1.73 m^2 in LdT patients and decreased from 85.5 ± 25.1 mL/min/1.73 m2 to 87.7 ± 24.8 mL/min/1.73 m^2 in ETV patients (Fig. 2). Overall, 21 of 46 (48.8%) patients in the LdT group and 10 of 46 (21.3%) in the ETV group showed an improved renal function 1 year after the treatment compared with baseline. Eleven patients improved their CKD stages (8 patients from stage 2 to stage 1 and 3 patients from stage 3 to stage 2) and 2 patients worsened their CKD stages (1 from stage 2 to stage 3 and 1 from stage 1 to stage 2) in the LdT group, 4 patients improved their CKD stages (1 patient from stage 3 to stage 2 and 3 patients from stage 2 to stage 1) and 9 patients worsened their CKD stages from stage 1 to stage 2 in the ETV group at year 4, compared to the baseline, respectively ($p = 0.07$) (Table 2). There was no significant change in

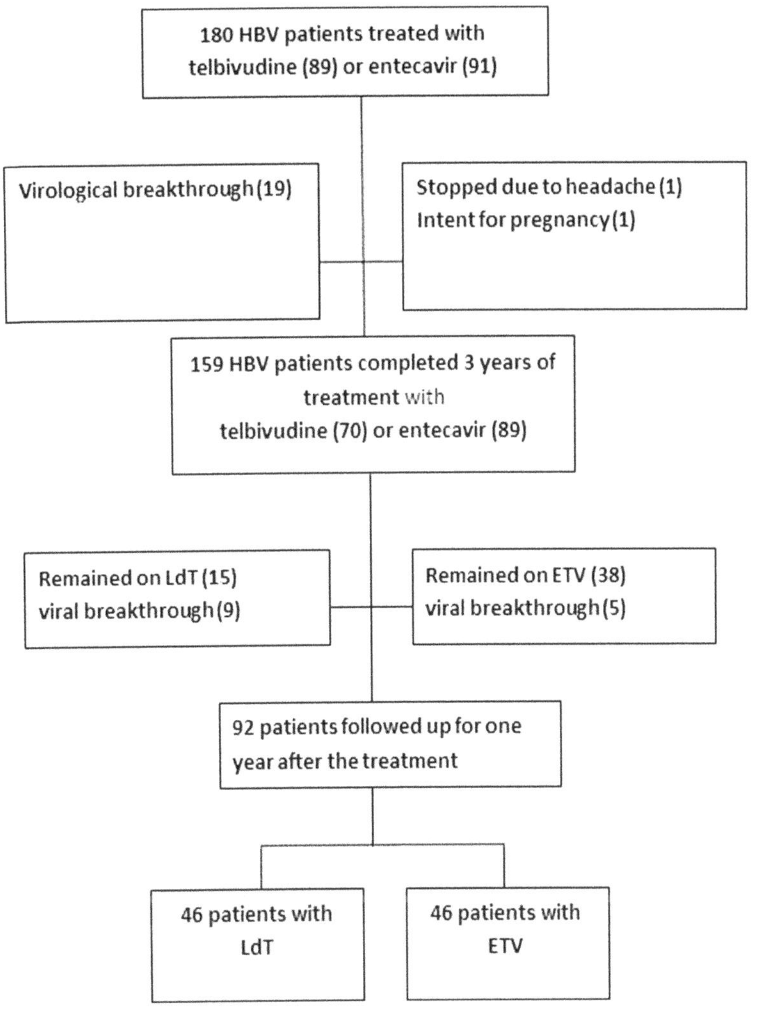

Fig. 1 Flow chart of the treatment

eGFR from the 3rd to the 4th year of treatment in the LdT group (104.0 – 104.0 mL/min/1.73 m^2, $p = 0.99$) and ETV group (85.5 ± 25.1 – 87.7 mL/min/1.73 m^2, $p = 0.2$). After a multivariate analysis, the predictors for off-treatment eGFR improvement were the LdT treatment (OR, 3.97 (1.37–11.5), $p = 0.01$) and pre-treated eGFR (OR, 0.98 [0.95–1.00], $p = 0.04$) (Table 4).

Discussion

Nucleos(t)ides are generally safe and well-tolerated, but side effects have been reported including nephrotoxicity, neuropathy, myopathy, lactic acidosis, and a decrease in bone mineral density. Of these, nephrotoxicity associated with nucleotide treatment has received the most attention. The GLOBE trial, which was composed of about 65% Asian patients treated with LdT, demonstrated the safety profile of renal function [5]. The renal function measured by eGFR increased from baseline and remained the same during continuous treatment for up to 6 years and also in the off-treatment period [6]. However, the promising results could not be extrapolated to a wider spectrum of patients in clinical and real-life practice. Post-marketing real-life observational studies are needed to demonstrate the effectiveness of these agents in different regions. The mechanism responsible for the change of renal function during long-term NA treatment is still under investigation and the effect of maintenance after the off-treatment follow-up is unknown. To the best of our knowledge, there is no published study comparing the effects of LdT and ETV on off-treatment renal function.

This study aimed to compare LdT versus ETV off-treatment effects on the changes in eGFR. Entecavir is very potent and maintains a high genetic barrier to HBV resistance, and thus, is widely prescribed. As inferred from the literature, ETV was highly effective in suppressing the HBV DNA replication at undetectable levels and had a very low resistance rate (1.2%) in NA-naive

Table 1 The demographics and change of CKD stages of 92 HBV patients assigned to be treated with LdT or ETV

	LdT (*n* = 46)	ETV (*n* = 46)	*P*-value
Age (mean ± SD)	46.3 ± 13.4	51.3 ± 11.5	0.06
Sex (M) (%)	35 (76.1)	35 (76.1)	1
CKD stages (%)			0.31
CKD 1	23 (50.0)	20 (43.5)	
CKD 2	19 (41.3)	24 (52.2)	
CKD 3	4 (8.7)	1 (2.2)	
CKD 4	0 (0)	1 (2.2)	
Diabetes (%)	11 (23.9)	8 (17.4)	0.44
Hypertension (%)	15 (32.6)	8 (17.4)	0.09
Nephrotoxic agents (%)	13 (28.3)	10 (21.7)	0.47
Cyclophosphamide (%)	1 (2.2%)	1 (2.2%)	
NSAID (%)	4 (8.8%)	1 (2.2%)	
HBV DNA (log IU/mL) (IQR)	6.6 (1.9)	6.2 (2.5)	0.93
HBe Ag (+) (%)	29 (63.0)	28 (60.1)	0.57
eGFR (± SD) (mL/min/1.73 m^2)			
Baseline	94.3 ± 28.3	93.1 ± 26.1	0.87
Year 3	104.0 ± 31.2	85.5 ± 25.1	0.005
Year 4	104.0 ± 28.8	87.7 ± 24.8	0.04

The age and eGFR were analyzed with Student's *t*-test. The sex, diabetes, hypertension and nephrotoxic agents, HBeAg status and CKD stages were analyzed with $\chi 2$ test and the others were analyzed with Mann-Whitney's *U*-test

HBeAg-negative patients for up to 5 years [7]. Telbivudine has renal protection potential but is less potent compared to ETV. The rationale of comparing LdT to ETV is that we want to know whether the potential renal protective effect is dependent on its antiviral effect. A question remains as to why tenofovir is not chosen for treatment. This is because some patients with potential renal risk or renal dysfunction at baseline were excluded from tenofovir clinically due to its renal toxicity [3].

All international guidelines indicate that the primary goal of CHB treatment is to permanently suppress the HBV replication to anti-HBe seroconversion, HBsAg loss, or anti-HBs seroconversion with undetectable HBV DNA [1, 2, 8]. However, in Taiwan, the health insurance reimburses NA treatment for up to 3 years in patients with naïve CHB if there is no virological breakthrough during the treatment period regardless of meeting the treatment stopping criteria because of medical resource constraints. This restricted therapy policy allows us to select a relatively homogenous CHB patients (viremia $<0^6$ for HBeAg negative or $<10^8$ for HBeAg positive) treating group according to the national guideline with a defined (3-year) treatment period to evaluate the change in eGFR after off-treatment.

After 1 year off-treatment, their eGFR remained stable, as seen during the end of 3-year therapy. In LdT-treated patients, the mean eGFR increased from 94.3 to 104.0 mL/min/1.73 m2 in year 4. However, in ETV-treated patients, the mean eGFR decreased from 93.1 to 87.7 mL/min/1.73 m^2 in year 4. In the fourth year, 48.8 and 21.3% patients had an improved eGFR from the baseline in LdT-treated and ETV-treated patients,

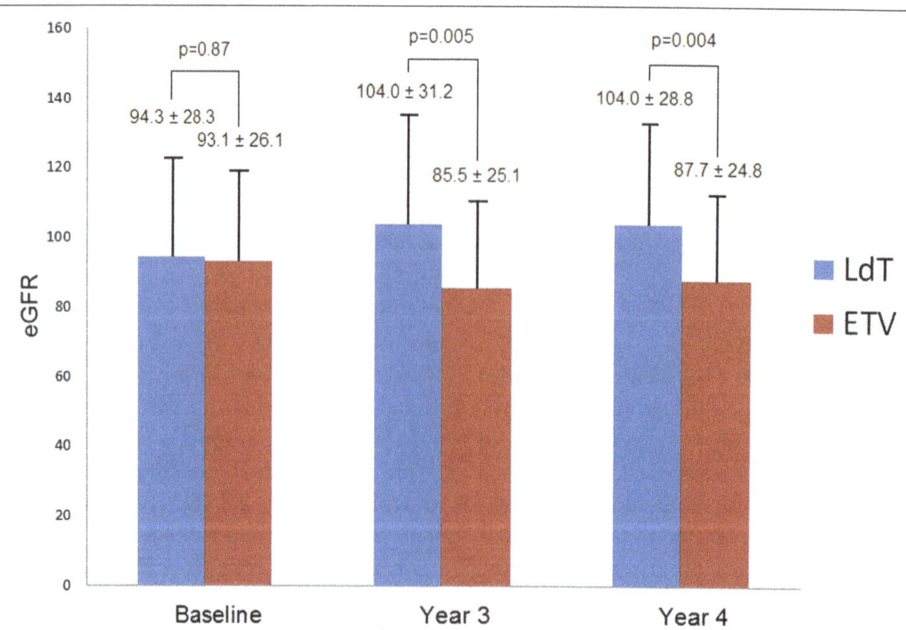

Fig. 2 Change of eGFR at the end of 3-years of treatment and 1 year after the treatment in LdT and ETV groups compared to the baseline

Table 2 The change of CKD stages compared with baseline at year 3 and year 4 with LdT or ETV

	LdT (*n* = 46)	ETV (*n* = 46)	*P*-value
Year 3 compared with baseline			
CKD stages (%)			0.004
CKD improved	11 (24.0)	1 (2.2)	
CKD no changed	32 (69.6)	37 (80.4)	
CKD worsen	3 (6.5)	8 (17.4)	
Year 4 compared with baseline			
CKD stages (%)			0.07
CKD improved	11 (23.9)	5 (10.9)	
CKD no changed	32 (69.6)	32 (69.6)	
CKD worsen	3 (6.5)	9 (19.6)	

The CKD status was analyzed with $\chi 2$ test

respectively. The benefit of LdT on the off-treatment eGFR improvement is unique from that of ETV because the effect is not related to viral suppression. It also indicates that the increase in eGFR was influenced by LdT itself rather than the control of HBV infection. Chan et al. suggested that the direct mechanism responsible for the improvement of renal function could be the increased blood flow by LdT that improves the tubular dysfunction [9]. A possible effect of LdT could be on the kidney structures or inflammatory/fibrotic pathways. The mechanisms of NA excretion of the kidney should also be explored by studying the expression of transport pumps (e.g., hOAT1, hOAT3, MRP4) in cells of the proximal tubules [10, 11]. A previous study reported that the LdT treatment can affect the angiotensin-converting enzyme that can control the renin-angiotensin aldosterone regulatory system. However, further investigations are required to study this phenomenon under the pharmaco-pathophysiology [12]

In some real-life cohort studies, long-term LdT therapy resulted in an improved eGFR, while ETV therapy did not significantly influence eGFR [13–16]. However, in our study, ETV group showed a slight decline of eGFR in year 3 and during the maintenance effect 1 year after treatment. This may be attributed to the small sample size or selection biases.

Multivariate analysis of baseline factors in the GLOBE study that predicted a shift in eGFR from baseline of 60–90 to 90 mL/min/1.73 m^2 in year 2 were the LdT treatment (OR, 2.51), younger age (OR, 0.94), and non-Caucasian race (OR, 0.34). In our study, we found similar results. A shift in eGFR from baseline of CKD stage 2 (60–90 mL/min/1.73 m^2) to CKD stage 1 (>90 mL/min/1.73 m^2) in year 3 was 8 of 19 (42%) patients in LdT group and 1 of 24 (4.1%) in ETV group. Multivariate analysis of baseline viral or host factors in our study that predicted a maintenance of eGFR improvement in year 4 were LdT treatment (OR, 3.97 (1.37–11.5) $p = 0.01$) and insufficient pre-treated eGFR (OR, 0.98 (0.95–1.00), $p = 0.04$), which is similar to previous studies [17, 18]. The lack of association between the change in eGFR and on-treatment virologic or serologic response would support a direct beneficial effect on the kidneys rather than an indirect effect from the HBV suppression [17].

The improvement of glomerular filtration is particularly important in patients with a slightly abnormal eGFR at baseline and could have important clinical implications. In our study, 11 patients improved their CKD stages and 2 patients worsened their CKD stages in the LdT group; one patient improved his CKD stage and 8 patients worsened their CKD stages in the ETV group at year 3 compared to baseline, respectively. ($p = 0.004$). Nevertheless, several concerns have been raised regarding the potential use of LdT as the first-line NA in CHB. Although its use has been associated with an improvement of renal function, it remains a low genetic barrier NA to overcome drug resistance in CHB patients and neuromuscular adverse effects [18].

There are many limitations in our study. First, there was a small sample size, retrospective design, and selection bias in choosing the initial medication. Second, it is still unclear the optimum level of eGFR change considered as clinically significant. Recent evidence suggests that a 30% decline of eGFR over 2 years is strongly and consistently associated with the risk of end-stage renal

Table 3 The predictors for eGFR improvement at the end of 3-years of treatment with LdT and ETV compared with baseline

	Univariate logistic regression			Multivariate logistic regression		
	OR	95% CI	*p*-value	OR	95% CI	*p*-value
Age	0.99	0.96–1.03	0.75	0.98	0.94–1.03	0.48
Sex	0.77	0.26–2.22	0.62	1.09	0.28–4.21	0.90
LdT	6.67	2.37–18.8	0.0001	7.97	2.47–25.7	0.001
HBV DNA	1	1	0.83	1	1	0.26
HBeAg	0.50	0.20–1.27	0.13	0.33	0.09–1.24	0.10
Baseline eGFR	0.98	0.96–1.00	0.067	0.98	0.96–1.00	0.08
Nephrotoxic agents	1.70	0.36–8.15	0.51	1.15	0.17–7.61	0.89

Table 4 The predictors for eGFR improvement 1 year after offtreatment with LdT and ETV compared with baseline

	Univariate logistic regression			Multivariate logistic regression		
	OR	95%CI	*P*-value	OR	95%CI	*P*-value
Age	1.03	0.99–1.07	0.10	1.03	0.98–1.08	0.20
Sex	0.50	0.16–1.51	0.22	0.86	0.23–3.19	0.82
LdT	3.02	1.22–7.51	0.02	3.97	1.37–11.5	0.01
HBV DNA	1	1	0.50	1	1	0.70
HBeAg	0.43	0.17–1.10	0.08	0.64	0.19–2.15	0.47
Baseline eGFR	0.98	0.96–1.00	0.03	0.98	0.95–1.00	0.04
Nephrotoxic agents	1.53	0.32–7.29	0.60	1.04	0.17–11.0	0.97

disease and mortality [19]. However, we do not know how much improvement is clinically relevant. Most clinical studies use eGFR >10% as a standard, although this needs to be further confirmed. Finally, we have only described the differences in the eGFR between the 2 treated groups to hypotheses a direct influence on eGFR without a relevant pathophysiologic theory. Clinical trials with a large sample size, randomized controlled design, dose dependence analysis, and long-term follow-up period are needed to confirm our findings.

Conclusions

The mechanism behind the potential renal protective effect of LdT is still unclear, although it appears to be independent of its antiviral effect on HBV. Our findings show that LdT may have a protective renal effect that can last for one year after the treatment in selected non-cirrhotic CHB patients without a virological breakthrough.

Abbreviations

ALT: Alanine transaminase; CHB: Chronic hepatitis B patients; CKD: Chronic kidney disease; eGFR: Estimated glomerular filtration rate; ETV: Entecavir; HBV: Hepatitis B virus; LdT: Telbivudine; NA: Nucleos(t)ide analogs; NSAIDs: Nonsteroidal anti-inflammatory drugs

Acknowledgements

The authors want to thank Miss Yu-Yun Ting for preparing the documents and providing technical assistance.

Funding

No funding.

Authors' contributions

LYS and CMJ designed the study and wrote this article. WHY, CCW and LCC participated in data analysis, and discussion. LYS and CCH conducted the literature review. SCS supported this work and performed critical reading of the manuscript. All authors read and approved the final manuscript.

Competing interests

The authors declare that they have no competing interests.

Consent for publication

Not applicable.

Author details

[1]Division of Gastroenterology, Department of Internal Medicine, MacKay Memorial Hospital, Taipei Campus, No. 92, Sec. 2, Chungshan North Road, 104 Taipei, Taiwan. [2]MacKay Junior College of Medicine, Nursing, and Management, Taipei, Taiwan. [3]MacKay Medical College, New Taipei City, Taiwan.

References

1. Liaw YF, Kao JH, Piratvisuth T, Chan HL, Chien RN, Liu CJ, et al. Asian-Pacific consensus statement on the management of chronic hepatitis B: a 2012 update. Hepatol Int. 2012;6:531–61.
2. European Association For The Study Of The L. EASL clinical practice guidelines: Management of chronic hepatitis B virus infection. J Hepatol. 2012;57:167–85.
3. Fung J, Seto WK, Lai CL, Yuen MF. Extrahepatic effects of nucleoside and nucleotide analogues in chronic hepatitis B treatment. J Gastroenterol Hepatol. 2014;29:428–34.
4. Pipili C, Cholongitas E, Papatheodoridis G. Review article: nucleos(t)ide analogues in patients with chronic hepatitis B virus infection and chronic kidney disease. Aliment Pharmacol Ther. 2014;39:35–46.
5. Wang Y, Thongsawat S, Gane EJ, Liaw YF, Jia J, Hou J, et al. Efficacy and safety of continuous 4-year telbivudine treatment in patients with chronic hepatitis B. J Viral Hepat. 2013;20:e37–46.
6. Hsu CW, Chen YC, Liaw YF. Prolonged efficacy and safety of 3 years of continuous telbivudine treatment in pooled data from Globe and 015 studies in chronic hepatitis B patients. J Hepatol. 2009;50:S331–7.
7. Wen CP, Cheng TYD, Tsai MK, Chang YC, Chan HT, Tsai SP, et al. All-cause mortality attributable to chronic kidney disease: a prospective cohort study based on 462 293 adults in Taiwan. Lancet. 2008;371:2173–82.
8. Tujios SR, Lee WM. Update in the management of chronic hepatitis B. Curr Opin Gastroenterol. 2013;29:250–6.
9. Chan HL, Chen YC, Gane EJ, Sarin SK, Suh DJ, Piratvisuth T, et al. Randomized clinical trial: efficacy and safety of telbivudine and lamivudine in treatment-naive patients with HBV-related decompensated cirrhosis. J Viral Hepat. 2012;19:732–43.
10. Izzedine H, Launay-Vacher V, Deray G. Antiviral drug-induced nephrotoxicity. Am J Kidney Dis. 2005;45:804–17.
11. Izzedine H, Hulot JS, Villard E, Goyenvalle C, Dominguez S, Ghosn J, et al. Association between ABCC2 gene haplotypes and tenofovir-induced proximal tubulopathy. J Infect Dis. 2006;194:1481–91.
12. Liang KH, Chen YC, Hsu CW, Chang ML, Yeh CT. Decrease of serum Angiotensin converting enzyme levels upon telbivudine treatment for chronic hepatitis B virus infection and negative correlations between the enzyme levels and estimated glumerular filtration rates. Hepat Mon. 2014;14:e15074.
13. Qi X, Wang JY, Mao RC, Zhang JM. Impact of nucleos(t)ide analogues on the estimated glomerular filtration rate in patients with chronic hepatitis B: a prospective cohort study in China. J Viral Hepat. 2015;22:46–54.

14. Koklu S, Gulsen MT, Tuna Y, Koklu H, Yuksel O, Demir M, et al. Differences in nephrotoxicity risk and renal effects among anti-viral therapies against hepatitis B. Aliment Pharmacol Ther. 2015;41:310–9.
15. Tsai MC, Chen CH, Hung CH. Case control study comparing renal function with telbivudine vs entecavir treatment in chronic hepatitis B patients in real-world clinical practice. Hepatol Int. 2013;7:S210–1.
16. Tsai MC, Chen CH, Tseng PL, Hung CH, Chiu KW, Wang JH, et al. Comparison of renal safety and efficacy of telbivudine, entecavir and tenofovir treatment in chronic hepatitis B patients: real world experience. Clin Microbiol Infect. 2016;95:e1–7.
17. Gane EJ, Deray G, Liaw YF, Lim SG, Lai CL, Rasenack J, et al. Telbivudine improves renal function in patients with chronic hepatitis B. Gastroenterology. 2014;146:138–146 e5.
18. Lee S, Park JY, Song K, Kim do Y, Kim BK, Kim SU, et al. Comparison of the effects of telbivudine and entecavir treatment on estimated glomerular filtration rate in patients with chronic hepatitis B. Gut Liver. 2015;9:776–83.
19. Rebholz CM, Grams ME, Matsushita K, Selvin E, Coresh J. Change in novel filtration markers and risk of ESRD. Am J Kidney Dis. 2015;66:47–54.

5

A preliminary investigation on single nucleotide polymorphism rs2287622 of bile salt export pump gene in patients with chronic hepatitis C virus infection in Hunan, China

Jian-Hua Lei*, Xu Yang, Xin-Qiang Xiao, Zi Chen and Feng Peng

Abstract

Background: European researchers have underscored associations between single nucleotide polymorphism (SNP) rs2287622 of the hepatobiliary bile salt export pump (BSEP) gene and the risk of hepatitis C virus (HCV) infection. The distributions of SNP rs2287622 are racially specific. This study was aimed to preliminarily investigate the distribution of BSEP gene SNP rs2287622 in the Han patients with chronic HCV-infection (CHC) in Hunan, China.

Methods: BSEP gene SNP rs2287622 of 165 CHC patients, 99 patients with chronic hepatitis B virus infection (CHB) and 99 healthy individuals were analyzed by polymerase chain reaction-restriction fragment length polymorphism analysis and nucleotide sequencing.

Results: The overall frequencies of the C allele of BESP gene SNP rs2287622 in the CHC patients, CHB patients and healthy individuals were 74.2, 72.7 and 74.2%, respectively ($P > 0.05$). The overall odds ratios (ORs) aiming at predicting CHC risk by comparing the ratios of the frequency distribution of alleles or genotypes in the CHC group with those in the non-CHC group had no statistical significance ($P > 0.05$). However, the CHC ORs of CC vs TT, TC vs TT and CC + CT vs TT among the individuals aged over 40 years were 2.680, 3.122 and 2.824 respectively ($P < 0.05$), and the higher risk did not relate to gender, HCV genotypes and presence of HCV-related liver cirrhosis.

Conclusions: Among the Han individuals aged over 40 years in Hunan, China, genotype CC or CT of BSEP gene SNP rs2287622 may correlate with higher risk of CHC in comparison with genotype TT. Further study with a larger cohort is essential.

Keywords: Single nucleotide polymorphism, Bile salt export pump, Hepatitis C virus, Chronic infection, China

Background

Hepatitis C is a global pandemic disease. About 185 million people are or have previously been infected with hepatitis C virus (HCV), most of whom develop chronic hepatitis. Besides, new infections are emerging [1]. Hepatitis C is more prevalent in East Asia, especially in China, with an estimated prevalence rate of 3.2% in the general population [2, 3]. Most HCV-infected persons are unaware that they are at risk for hepatitis C-related life-threatening diseases such as liver cirrhosis and hepatocellular carcinoma, whose incidences are predicted to rise in the coming decade [1, 2].

Although it remains unclear, host genetic diversity is believed to contribute to the susceptibility to HCV infection or HCV clearance in vivo. In recent years, researches on different related genetic variants have been published [4–11]. Since 2009, single nucleotide polymorphisms (SNPs) of the interleukin-28B gene have been identified as accurate predictors for therapy response and spontaneous clearance of HCV infection [4, 5]. Significant associations

* Correspondence: leijianhua73@163.com
Department of Infectious Diseases, the Second Xiangya Hospital, Central South University, No.139 Middle Renmin Road, Changsha, Hunan 410011, People's Republic of China

of estrogen receptor α or Toll-like receptor 7 genetic polymorphisms with HCV infection susceptibility or viral clearance among Han Chinese population have been reported [6, 7].

Since 2011, several European researches have underscored associations between a certain SNP, V444A (HGVS name: NM_003742.2: c.1331 T > C; ref SNP: rs2287622) in exon 13 of the hepatobiliary bile salt export pump (BSEP) gene, and the risk of HCV infection, progression of liver fibrosis and even the virological response during anti-HCV therapy [8–11]. But their findings need to be validated by investigation on extended population, especially on population of different races. So far, studies on the SNPs of BSEP gene in the chronic HCV-infected population have been rarely reported in China. The aim of the present study was to make a preliminary investigation on the distribution of SNP rs2287622 of BSEP gene in Han patients with chronic HCV-infection in Hunan, China.

Methods

Patients and control cohort

Random sampling was carried out on patients with confirmed diagnosis of chronic HCV infection in Liver Disease Research Center, the Second Xiangya Hospital, Central South University during 2012 and 2013. The sample size was estimated by the formula $N = Z^2 \times P \times (1-P)/E^2$. The annual amount of the HCV-infected patients visiting the center is about 1000. The frequency of allele C in exon 13 c.1331 of BESP gene in Chinese and Japanese is about 0.70 [12–14]. When the confidence level was set at 95% ($Z_{0.05} = 1.96$) and the sampling error at 10% (E = 0.10), the sample size worked out was 75 for each year. Additional 10% of the sample size was recruited, and finally 82 and 83 cases were respectively sampled from the patients in 2012 and 2013. All the 165 patients were of the Han nationality.

The diagnostic criteria for the chronic HCV infection (CHC) were based on the combination of clinical history, physical examination, imaging and laboratory data and/or histology. All of the patients finally enrolled in the study were positive for serum anti-HCV antibodies and had detectable serum HCV-RNA for at least 6 months. One hundred and seven of them had abnormal liver function indicated by elevated aspartate aminotransferase (AST) and alanine aminotransferase (ALT) before anti-HCV treatment. One hundred and thirty-three cases had ever received systematic anti-HCV therapy by combination of recombinant interferon-alpha (INF-α) and ribavirin (RBV). Twenty-six of them adopted common INF-α/RBV therapeutic scheme and 107 adopted polyethyleneglycolated INF-α (Peg-INF-α)/RBV therapeutic scheme. Twenty-six of the 165 CHC patients were diagnosed as HCV-related liver cirrhosis and 10 of them had been treated with adjusted low dose Peg-INF-α/RBV therapy.

A total of 99 healthy individuals of the Han nationality without evidences of hepatitis B virus (HBV) or HCV infections available at the Physical Examination Center of the hospital on two randomly chosen days (November 21th, 2012 and January 15th, 2013) served as the health control. Their blood specimens, clinical features and demographic data were collected.

On January 15th, 2013, 99 chronic hepatitis B (CHB) cases of Han nationality, including 30 CHB related liver cirrhosis cases, were randomly selected from the opening CHB case database in our center, severing as the CHB control. The database had collected the demographic data, clinical features and genomic DNA specimens of more than 1500 CHB patients visiting our center since 2010, all of whom had been HBV surface antigen (HBsAg) positive for over six months and had detectable serum HBV DNA when their genomic DNA samples were collected. Inclusion of hepatitis B patients into the controls was based on two facts. Firstly, HBV and HCV are both hepatotropic viruses and share similar transmission routes and clinical manifestations. Secondly, having CHB patients as controls is popular in professional researches on CHC, so is in the similar European research [10].

One hundred and sixty-five CHB and 99 CHB cases finally enrolled in the study were all confirmed to have no evidence of co-infection with hepatitis A virus, hepatitis E virus, Epstein-Barr virus, cytomegalovirus or human immunodeficiency virus, no detectable anti-delta antibodies, or no evidence of other chronic liver disease (autoimmune chronic liver disease, alcoholic liver disease, drug-induced liver injury, hemochromatosis, Wilson's disease, or α1-antitrypsin deficiency). None of the 165 CHC or 99 CHB cases was co-infected with HCV and HBV.

The collection of all the demographic data, clinical features and biological specimens including genomic DNA from the peripheral blood of the research objects fulfilled the requirements of medical ethics. The ethical review committees of the Second Xiangya Hospital of Central South University approved this study. Guidelines of the Declaration of Helsinki set by the committees were strictly followed. Written informed consent was obtained from all participants.

Clinical features of the patients and control cohort

Serum ALT, AST and total bilirubin of the patients were measured by a 7600 Series automatic analyzer (Hitachi High-Tech Co., Japan) according to the manufacturer's instructions. Serum anti-HCV was assessed by an enzyme linked immunosorbent assay (ELISA) diagnostic kit (Zhuhai Livzon Diagnostics Inc., China), and HBsAg was tested by another ELISA diagnostic kit (Shanghai Kehua Bio-engineering Co., Ltd., China) according to the manufacturer's instructions. Quantitation of plasma HCV RNA was assessed in 7500 real-time PCR system (Applied Biosystems Inc., USA) by using HCV RNA quantitative fluorescence diagnostic kit (Sansure biotech Inc. Ltd, China), and the lower limit of the detection was 25 IU/mL. Quantitation of serum HBV DNA was assessed in StepOnePlus real-time PCR system (Applied Biosystems Inc., USA) by using HBV DNA quantitative fluorescence diagnostic kit (Sansure biotech Inc. Ltd, China), and the lower limit of the detection was 10 IU/mL.

Liver cirrhosis was diagnosed by liver biopsy, or FibroScan liver stiffness more than 13 kilopascal (kPa) together with Child-Turcotte-Pugh score more than 7, or FibroScan liver stiffness more than 13 kPa together with any two of the following criteria: the presence of ascites, hepatic encephalopathy, upper gastrointestinal bleeding, endoscopic detection of gastroesophageal varices, radiologic imaging of nodular liver or splenomegaly and peripheral blood platelet count below 100×10^9/L in the absence of other explanations. Liver stiffness was measured by the FibroScan® 502 transient elastography device (Echosens, Paris, France), and the liver stiffness values were expressed in units of kPa, ranging from 2.5 to 75 kPa. Percutaneous liver histological examination was performed from the right lobe under real-time ultrasound guidance, and the inflammation grades and fibrosis stages of the biopsy samples were interpreted by two experienced hepatopathologists who were blinded to the clinical data.

Based on the assessment of hepatic encephalopathy grade, ascites, prothrombin activity, serum albumin and bilirubin levels, liver cirrhosis severity was assessed in the cirrhotic cases using a modified Child-Pugh's classification system [15, 16]: 5–6 points, grade A; 7–9 points, grade B; 10–15 points, grade C.

Collection of genomic DNA from peripheral blood

About 5 mL peripheral blood was collected from each patient into elhylene diamine tetraacetic acid (EDTA)-containing vacationer tubes. Plasma was stored at –70 °C until HCV RNA loading analysis. Peripheral blood monouclear cells (PBMCs) were isolated from EDTA-treated blood by lymphocyte separation medium (Tianjin Haoyang Biological manufacture Co., Ltd., China) by centrifugation over density gradient. PBMCs were then washed three times with phosphate-buffered saline (pH =7.4), counted and stored at –70 °C for later detection.

Genomic DNA was isolated from a pellet of approximately $3–5 \times 10^6$ PBMCs using EZHighTM-TG DNA Extraction Kit (Texas BioGene, Inc. USA) according to the manufacturer's instructions. The concentrations of DNA samples were measured using the T6 spectrophotometer (Beijing Purkinje General Instrument Co., Ltd., China), then the DNA samples were diluted to 10 ng/μl.

Confirmation of SNP rs2287622 genotypes by polymerase chain reaction-restriction fragment length polymorphism analysis (PCR-RFLP)

The sequences of the oligonucleotide primers using for PCR amplification of exon 13 of BSEP gene were 5′-CACACAGACACCGAGTATCAACACA-3′ (sense) and 5′-CAGGACAGTCTCAATGTATGCTACACCT-3′ (antisense).

PCR was performed in a total volume of 30 μl containing 60 ng genomic DNA, 0.3 pmol of each primer, 15 μl 2 × Taq MasterMix (0.05 U/μl Taq DNA polymerase, reaction buffer, 4 mM $MgCl_2$, and 0.4 mM of each dNTP; Beijing ComWin Biotech Co., Ltd., China), 0.75 units Pfu DNA Polymerase (recombinant; Beijing ComWin Biotech Co., Ltd., China) and sterile deionized nuclease-free water. A PTC-100TM Programmable thermal controller (MJ Research, Inc., USA) was used for PCR with the following cycling conditions: initial denaturation at 94 °C for 3 min, followed by 35 cycles consisting of denaturation at 94 °C for 30 s, annealing at 60 °C for 30 s, extension at 72 °C for 30 s, and a final extension step at 72 °C for 5 min followed by cooling to 25° for 5 min. The PCR amplicon fragment was 333 base pairs in length.

10 μL PCR products were digested by HaeIII restriction endonuclease and buffer R (Fermentas Inc., USA) at 37 °C for 12 h, then the restriction digestion products for each were separated on 1.5% agarose gel stained with ethidium bromide for visualization on a ultraviolet transilluminatior. HaeIII digestion of allele CC yielded fragments of 127 and 206 base pairs, whereas PCR amplicons containing the allele TT polymorphism maintained 333 base pairs and amplicons containing the allele TC polymorphism yielded fragments of 127, 206 and 333 base pairs. All of the tests were performed in duplicate.

Nucleotide sequencing

In order to confirm the accuracy of the detection results of SNP rs2287622 genotypes by PCR-FRLP, PCR was performed in triplicate on the genomic DNA samples of the 165 chronic HCV infection patients, 33 samples randomly chosen from the 99 chronic HBV infection patients and 33 from the 99 healthy individuals. The PCR products were purified with Wizard® SV Gel and PCR Clean-Up System (Promega Biotech Co., Ltd, USA) according to the manufacturer's instructions. Direct sequencing of the purified products was performed by Shanghai Sangon Biotech Co., Ltd., China, with 3730xl DNA Analyzer and ABI BigDye® Terminator v3.1 Cycle

Sequencing kit (Applied Biosystems Inc., USA). The sequences obtained were compared with the BSEP reference sequence derived from publicly available databases provided by NCBI (http://www.ncbi.nlm.nih.gov/) to confirm the SNP rs2287622 genotypes.

Statistical analysis

All statistical analyses were performed with IBM® SPSS® Statistics version 20.0. The BSEP SNP rs2287622 genotypes and clinical features were compared between patients and control cohort. Chi-squared test, Analysis of Variance and Student *t*-test were used for comparisons between groups and Hardy-Weinberg equilibrium tests of the genotyping results. Allelic discrimination assay and association case–control analysis based on gender-, age-, HCV genotype- or liver cirrhosis-stratified analyses were performed to investigate the role of the BSEP SNP rs2287622 genotyping in the susceptibility to HCV infection, and odds ratios (ORs) were given with 95% confidence intervals (CIs). For all these tests, P value less than 0.05 was considered statistically significant.

Results

Demographic characteristics and clinical parameters of the study subjects

Overall, 165 patients with chronic HCV infection, 99 patients with chronic HBV infection and 99 healthy individuals were included in this study. A summary of demographic data and clinical parameters of the study subjects was given in Table 1. All of the participants were aged 18 years or above. Among the three groups, gender was equally distributed and average age and BMI was not significantly different. Serum ALT and AST levels were comparable between HCV-infected and HBV-infected patients.

Among the 26 cirrhotic CHC cases, 10 were assessed as Child-Pugh (C-P) grade A and were treated with low dose Peg-INF-α/RBV therapy. Nine cases with C-P grade B and seven cases with C-P grade C received symptomatic and supportive treatment other than Peg-IFN-α/RBV combination therapy. Among the 30 cirrhotic CHB cases, 12 were assessed as C-P grade A, 10 as grade B and 8 as grade C. The severity of liver cirrhosis was statistically comparable between cirrhotic CHC and cirrhotic CHB cases.

Confirmation of SNP rs2287622 genotypes of BSEP gene by PCR-RFLP and nucleotide sequencing

The exon 13 and 5′ flanking region of BSEP gene of all samples were successfully amplified by PCR. RFLP analysis and nucleotide sequencing of the PCR products confirmed the SNP rs2287622 genotypes TT, CC and TC, as the codon of the 444th amino acid had three polymorphisms as GTC, GCC and heterozygote (see Fig. 1). Identification findings of the SNP rs2287622 genotypes by PCR-RFLP were completely consistent with the results by the triplicate PCR and nucleotide sequencing.

Frequency distribution of BSEP rs2287622 alleles and genotypes

Frequency distribution of BSEP rs2287622 genotypes

The frequency distribution of BSEP SNP rs2287622 in the research objects with different ages accorded with Hardy-Weinbery genetic equilibrium law ($P > 0.05$), suggesting that the cohorts were representative of the targeted population (Table 2).

Frequency distribution of BSEP SNP rs2287622 alleles and genotypes on age stratification basis

The frequency distribution of BSEP SNP rs2287622 alleles and genotypes in the research subjects was described on age stratification basis (Table 2). The overall frequencies of the C allele of BESP gene SNP rs2287622 in the CHC patients, CHB patients and healthy individuals were 74.2, 72.7 and 74.2%, respectively, indicating

Table 1 Demographic characteristics and clinical parameters of the study subjects

Parmeter	CHC	CHB	Healthy	*P* value
n	165	99	99	–
Gender male (n, %)	88 (53.3)	50 (50.5)	50 (50.5)	NS
Age, years (mean ± SD, range)	43.3 ± 11.9 (18–70)	43.5 ± 12.3 (22–67)	40.3 ± 12.2 (18–68)	NS
BMI (mean ± SD, range)	23.2 ± 3.9 (16.5–34.6)	22.6 ± 3.5 (18.4–33.9)	23.8 ± 3.4 (17.1–32.3)	NS
ALT, IU/L (median ± SD, IQR)	82.0 ± 62.0 (70.2)	94.1 ± 65.1 (83.6)	normal	NS[b]
AST, IU/L (median ± SD, IQR)	65.6 ± 40.4 (50.1)	77.4 ± 42.0 (68.0)	normal	NS[b]
HCV RNA level, log IU/mL (median ± SD, IQR)	6.08 ± 1.35 (1.51)	—	—	—
HBV DNA level, log IU/mL (median, IQR)	—	5.97 ± 1.21 (1.43)	—	—

BMI body mass index, *SD* standard deviation, *IQR* interquartile range, *NS* non-significant, $P > 0.05$

[a]The clinical data of the patients treated with anti-HCV or anti-HBV therapy were collected at the start point of the treatment, while data of the other patients were collected on the day when the genomic DNA were collected

[b]Comparisons of serum aminotransferase levels were carried out only between patients with chronic HCV infection and those with chronic HBV infection

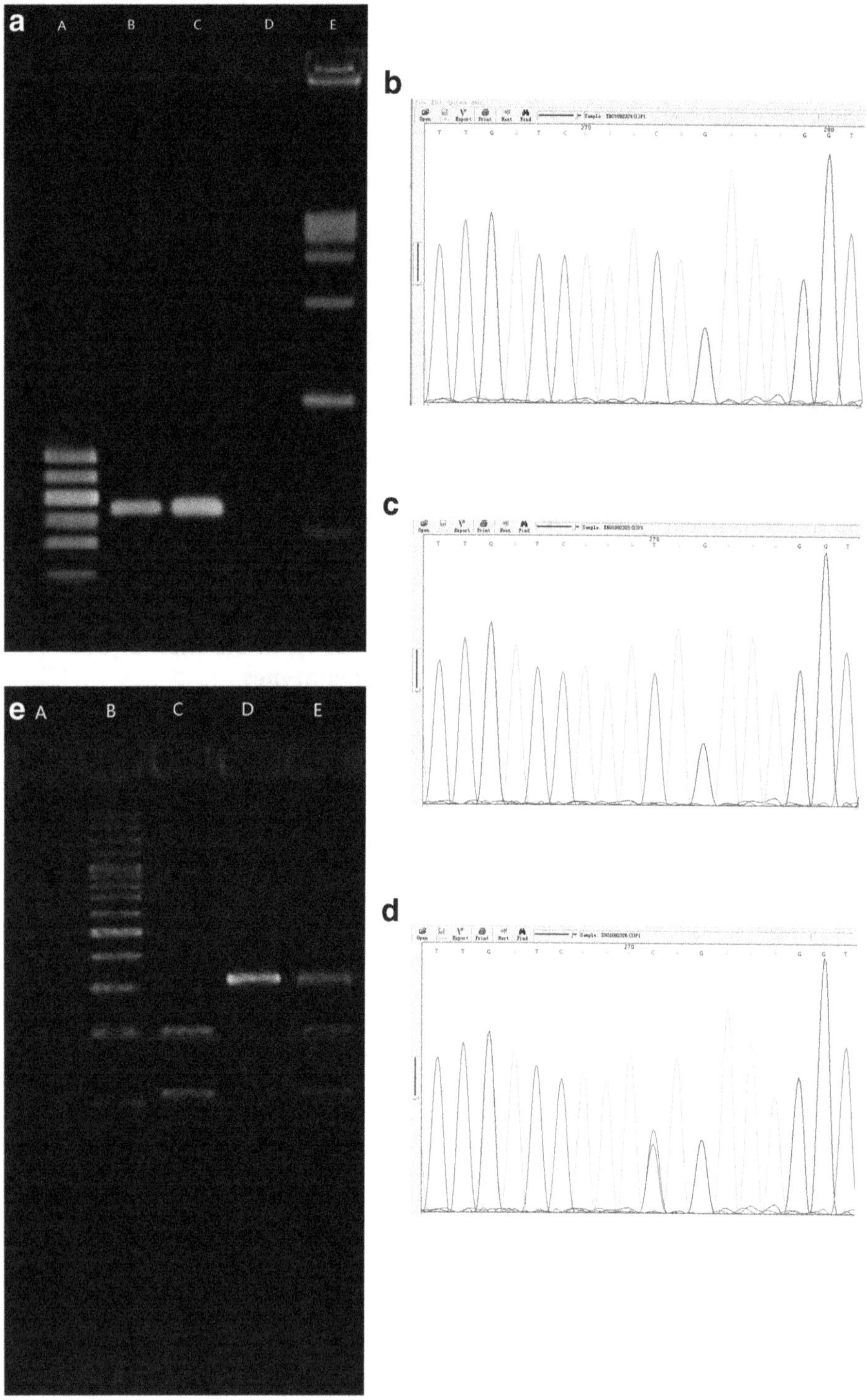

Fig. 1 PCR amplification products of exon 13 of BSEP gene and confirmation of the SNP rs2287622 genotypes by nucleotide sequencing and RFLP. 1.1 amplification product of exon 13 of BSEP gene. **a**.DNA Marker I (Shanghai yuanye biotechnology Co., Ltd., China); **b**, **c**:cases; **d**:blank; **e**:DNA MarkerVI (Shanghai yuanye bio-technology Co., Ltd., China). 1.2 CC 1.3 TT 1.4 TC: Confirmation of rs2287622 genotypes by nucleotide sequencing. 1.5 Confirmation of rs2287622 genotypes by RFLP. **a**.blank; **b**.100bp DNA Ladder Marker (Beijing BLKW biotechnology Co., Ltd., China); **c**. rs2287622 genotype CC; **d**. rs2287622 genotype TT; **e**.rs2287622 genotype TC

Table 2 Frequency distribution of BSEP SNP rs2287622 genotypes in the research subjects of different age groups

Genotypes	18-years old			30-years old			40-years old			50-years old			60-years old		
	Non-CHC		CHC	Non-CHC		CHC	Non-CHC		CHC	Non-CHC		CHC	Non-CHC		CHC
	Health	CHB		Health	CHB		Health	CHB		Health	CHB		Health	CHB	
CC	16	10	12	19	14	18	11	14	37	9	13	20	5	6	7
TT	2	1	1	2	2	6	5	5	4	2	3	3	1	1	0
TC	6	5	10	9	9	11	6	7	17	4	6	11	2	3	8

Table 3 Frequency distribution of BSEP SNP rs2287622 alleles and genotypes in the research subjects on age stratification basis (n, %)

Alleles or genotypes		Overall			18- years old			40- years old		
		Non-CHC		CHC ($n = 165$)	Non-CHC		CHC ($n = 58$)	Non-CHC		CHC ($n = 107$)
		Health ($n = 99$)	CHB ($n = 99$)		Health ($n = 54$)	CHB ($n = 41$)		Health ($n = 45$)	CHB ($n = 58$)	
Alleles	C	147 (74.2)	144 (72.7)	245 (74.2)	85 (78.7)	62 (75.6)	81 (69.8)	62 (68.9)	82 (70.7)	164 (76.6)
	T	51 (25.8)	54 (27.3)	85 (25.8)	23 (21.3)	20 (24.4)	35 (30.2)	28 (31.1)	34 (29.3)	50 (23.4)
Genotypes	CC	60 (60.6)	57 (57.6)	94 (57.0)	35 (64.8)	24 (58.5)	30 (51.7)	25 (55.6)	33 (56.9)	64 (59.8)
	TT	12 (12.1)	12 (12.1)	14 (8.5)	4 (7.4)	3 (7.3)	7 (12.1)	8 (17.8)	9 (15.5)	7 (6.5)
	TC	27 (27.3)	30 (30.3)	57 (34.5)	15 (27.8)	14 (34.1)	21 (36.2)	12 (26.7)	16 (27.6)	36 (33.6)
Alleles analysis	Overall									
	Chi-square	0.172			2.391			2.517		
	P value	0.918			0.302			0.284		
	CHC vs Non-CHC									
	Chi-square	0.053			2.156			2.433		
	P value	0.817			0.142			0.119		
	Risk of CHC OR (95%CI) (C vs T)	1.040 (0.746–1.450)			0.677 (0.402–1.141)			1.412 (0.914–2.181)		
Genotypes analysis	Overall									
	Chi-square	2.379			2.340[a]			5.516		
	P value	0.666			0.674			0.238		
	CHC vs Non-CHC									
	Chi-square	2.157			1.892			5.388		
	P value	0.340			0.388			0.068		
	Risk of CHC									
	CC vs TT									
	Chi-square	0.779			1.395			4.355		
	P value	0.377			0.238			0.037		
	OR (95%CI)	1.377 (0.675–2.809)			0.508 (0.163–1.584)			2.680 (1.037–6.924)		
	CC + TC vs TT									
	Chi-square	1.270			0.957			5.146		
	P value	0.260			0.328			0.023		
	OR (95%CI)	1.488 (0.743–2.979)			0.580 (0.192–1.746)			2.824 (1.118–7.130)		
	TT + TC vs CC									
	Chi-square	0.166			1.595			0.264		
	P value	0.683			0.207			0.607		
	OR (95%CI)	1.091 (0.718–1.658)			1.530 (0.790–2.963)			0.866 (0.500–1.499)		
	TC vs TT									
	Chi-square	1.982			0.284			5.124		
	P value	0.159			0.594			0.024		
	OR (95%CI)	1.714 (0.806–3.645)			0.724 (0.221–2.377)			3.122 (1.138–8.567)		

CHC patients with chronic HCV infection, *CHB* patients with chronic HBV infection, *Healthy* Healthy individuals, *OR* odds ratio, *CI* confidence interval
[a]Continuity Corrected Chi-square

Table 4 Frequency distribution of BSEP SNP rs2287622 alleles and genotypes on gender stratification basis

Alleles or genotypes		Overall							40- years old						
		Non-CHC				CHC		*P* value	Non-CHC				CHC		*P* value
		CHB		Healthy					CHB		Healthy				
		Male	Female	Male	Female	Male	Female		Male	Female	Male	Female	Male	Female	
Alleles	C	69	75	78	69	132	113	NS	41	41	20	42	78	86	NS
	T	31	23	24	27	44	41		19	15	16	12	22	28	
Genotypes	CC	26	31	33	27	51	43	NS	16	17	12	13	31	33	NS
	TT	7	5	6	6	7	7		5	4	5	3	3	4	
	CT	17	13	12	15	30	27		9	7	6	6	16	20	
P value			NS		NS		NS			NS		NS		NS	

CHC patients with chronic HCV infection, *CHB* patients with chronic HBV infection, *Healthy* Healthy individuals, *NS* non-significant
All $P > 0.05$

no statistical difference ($P > 0.05$). The odds ratios (ORs) aiming at predicting CHC risk by comparing the ratios of the frequency distribution of allele C to T, of genotype CC, TC or CC + CT to TT, and of genotype TT, TC or TT + TC to CC in the CHC group with those in the non-CHC group had no statistical significance ($P > 0.05$) (Table 3). However, further data analysis found that when the research subjects were stratified into 18- and 40- years old age groups, the ORs of genotype CC to TT, TC to TT and CC + CT to TT in the 40- years old age group all had statistical significance (CC vs TT, OR = 2.680, 95%CI:1.037–6.924, $P = 0.037$;TC vs TT, OR = 3.122, 95%CI: 1.138–8.567, $P = 0.024$; CC+ CT vs TT, OR = 2.824, 95%CI:1.118–7.130, $P = 0.023$), indicating that homozygous and heterozygous presence of C allele was associated with CHC infection. Nevertheless, for the subjects aged 18- years, it was not the case.

Frequency distribution of BSEP SNP rs2287622 alleles and genotypes on gender stratification basis

Further analysis was conducted to explore the CHC risk of C allele in 40- years old subgroup. First, the gender differences of the frequency distributions of BSEP SNP rs2287622 alleles and genotypes were examined. The analysis showed that there were no statistical differences in the frequencies of the alleles and genotypes of BESP SNP rs2287622 between males and females, either for the overall population or for the 40- years old subgroup (all $P > 0.05$) (Table 4).

Frequency distribution of BSEP SNP rs2287622 alleles and genotypes on HCV genotype basis

As described in Table 5, the HCV genotypes distributed differently between CHC patients aged 18- years and those aged 40- years, and the proportion of type 1 HCV infection was statistically higher in CHC patients aged 40- years (Chi-square =14.035, $P = 0.001$). So the role of HCV genotypes in the higher presence of SNP rs2287622 allele C and genotypes CC and TC in CHC cases aged 40 years and above was explored. Further analysis was made to explore whether the higher presence of SNP rs2287622 allele C and genotypes CC and TC in CHC cases aged 40- years were associated with HCV type 1 infection. Therefore, the distribution of the frequencies of the genotypes of BESP gene SNP rs2287622 was compared among HCV type 1 infected patients, non HCV type 1 infected cases and those with unknown genotype. No significant difference was found, either for the overall, or for the 18- or 40- years age groups (all $P > 0.05$) (Table 5).

Table 5 Frequency distribution of BSEP SNP rs2287622 genotypes on HCV genotype stratification basis (n, %)

HCV genotypes	Overall				18- years old				40- years old			
	n	CC	TT	CT	n	CC	TT	CT	n	CC	TT	CT
Type 1	59	32 (54.2)	6 (10.2)	21 (35.6)	14	6 (42.9)	1 (7.1)	7 (50.0)	45	26 (57.8)	5 (11.1)	14 (31.1)
Non type 1	20	13 (65.0)	2 (10.0)	5 (25.0)	14	9 (64.3)	2 (14.3)	3 (21.4)	6	4 (66.7)	0 (0.0)	2 (33.3)
Unknown	86	49 (57.0	6 (7.0)	31 (36.0)	30	15 (50.0)	4 (13.3)	11 (36.7)	56	34 (60.7)	2 (3.6)	20 (35.7)
Total	165	94 (57.0)	14 (8.5)	57 (34.5)	58	30 (51.7)	7 (12.1)	21 (36.2)	107	64 (59.8)	7 (6.5)	36 (33.6)
Chi-square	1.388[a]					2.617[a]				2.827[a]		
P value	0.846					0.624				0.572		

[a]Continuity Corrected Chi-square

Table 6 Frequency distribution of BSEP SNP rs2287622 alleles and genotypes on cirrhosis stratification basis in CHC and CHB patients (n, %)

Groups	Cirrhosis	Alleles		Genotypes			
		C	T	CC	TT	TC	Total
CHC	no	204	74	77 (55.4)	12 (8.6)	50 (36.0)	139 (100)
	yes	41	11	17 (65.4)	2 (7.7)	7 (26.9)	26 (100)
	Total	245	85	94 (57.0)	14 (8.5)	57 (34.5)	165 (100)
CHB	no	99	39	39 (56.5)	9 (13.0)	21 (30.4)	69 (100)
	yes	45	15	18 (60.0)	3 (10.0)	9 (30.0)	30 (100)
	Total	144	54	57 (57.6)	12 (12.1)	30 (30.3)	99 (100)

All $P > 0.05$

Frequency distribution of BSEP SNP rs2287622 alleles and genotypes on cirrhosis stratification basis in CHC and CHB patients

Among all the 165 CHC cases, 26 had clinical diagnosis of liver cirrhosis, among which 22 were older than 40 years. So the association of the alleles and genotypes of BESP SNP rs2287622 with liver cirrhosis was explored to find whether the predilection potential of C in CHC cases was due to its close relationship with liver cirrhosis. No significant differences in the frequencies of the alleles and genotypes of BESP gene SNP rs2287622 were found between CHC and CHB patients with and without liver cirrhosis (all $P > 0.05$, Table 6).

Discussion

BSEP is a hepatobiliary bile salt transporter on human hepatocellular canalicular membrane, one of the members of ATP-binding protein super family. Bile salts are transported to hepatocytes by Na^+-taurocholate cotransporting polypeptide (NTCP) and sodium-independent organic anion transporting polypeptide (OATP), while they are transported from hepatocytes into bile canaliculus mainly by BSEP. BSEP plays an important role in the metabolism of hepatocellular bile acid [17, 18].

BSEP gene is located in the long arm of human chromosome 2, 2q24-31. It transcribes an mRNA of 5.5 kb. The expression of BSEP gene is mainly regulated by the farnesoid X receptor (FXR). Expression and activation of FXR in the cell is the key to the transcriptional activation of BSEP gene [18]. There are FXR binding elements in the promoter of BSEP gene. Many bile acid components, such as chenodeoxycholic acid (CDCA), lithocholic acid (LCA), deoxycholic acid (DCA) and cholic acid (CA), represent the native activators of FXR, among which CDCA can induce the strongest activation. The metabolic balance of bile acid in the hepatocytes is maintained by positive regulation on BSEP expression through activating FXR by bile acid.

In vitro experiments, studies have demonstrated that DCA and CDCA at physiological concentration increased the levels of HCV RNA and proteins up to five to ten folds, while the antagonist of the bile acid receptor or siRNA targeted at the gene of the bile acid receptor would reduce the bile acid-mediated increase of HCV RNA [19–21]. It has been reported that multiple bile acid components could increase HCV replication by activating FXR or EGFR/ERK pathway [21–23]. Meanwhile, they up-regulated apolipoprotein CII and activated a rate-limiting enzyme associated with the activation of the lipoprotein lipase. In these ways, they changed the course of HCV entering the host cells and the secretion of the virus particles from the host cells [21–23].

The clinical data indicated that elevated serum bile salt levels were significantly associated with increased risk of cirrhosis in patients with chronic HCV infection, and decreased sustained virological response (SVR) rate in patients treated with pegylated interferon-α and ribavirin. The mechanism may involve the block of the signal pathway of interferon, which is independent of FXR. Hydrophobic bile acids will inhibit Jak1- and Tyk2-phosphorylation, resulting in a decreased mRNA and protein expression of IFN-stimulated genes such as myxovirus resistance protein A (MxA) or dsRNA-activated protein kinase (PKR) thereby explaining interferon-α resistance [24].

It has been reported that the polymorphism of BSEP gene might affect the expression and distribution of BSEP and transportation of bile acid, and eventually change the acid bile pool [17, 18, 25]. Studies on patients with intrahepatic cholestasis or idiopathic cholestasis during pregnancy indicated that polymorphism c.1331 T > C (p.V444A) (SNP rs2287622) in exon 13 of BSEP gene would lead to inhibition of the transportation of bile acid out of the hepato cytes [17, 25, 26].

In view of these, the effects of BSEP on the occurrence, progression and antiviral treatment response in chronic hepatitis C were studied. Europeans researches suggested that the polymorphism of BSEP V444A might be associated with the HCV infection development, liver fibrosis progression and long-term treatment response [8–11]. The few studies needed to be further supported by researches on extended population.

So far, no researches on the association between BSEP polymorphism and HCV infection in Chinese population were reported. Our preliminary study indicated that the frequency of allele C in BESP exon 13 c.1331 in Han patients with chronic HCV infection, chronic HBV infection and healthy individuals were 74.2, 72.7 and 74.2%, respectively, and the distributions of the alleles in the three groups were in accordance with Hardy-Weinberg equilibrium. The frequencies of allele C in the three groups were not statistically different. Our study suggested that the distributions of the polymorphism of BSEP SNP rs2287622 in the Han nationality in Hunan, China had different characteristics from those of Europeans. However, it had similar findings with the studies in the people without HCV infection in Chinese Taiwan and the mainland, and in a Japanese population, with frequencies of allele C in BESP exon 13 c.1331 of 75.6, 74.5 and 73.7%, respectively [12–14]. Similar genetic background in Chinese and Japanese supported the credibility of our findings.

Our research illustrated that the polymorphism of BSEP SNP rs2287622 was statistically correlated with chronic HCV infection in Han population aged 40 years and above. Interestingly, the correlation was not found in HCV patients aged 18–<40 years. Many gene polymorphisms or mutations, and their corresponding protein functions, and even the presence of clinical features, are age specific. The reasons for the age-related difference in frequency distribution of the alleles and genotypes of BSEP SNP rs2287622 were not included in this study. But further stratification analysis found that there were no statistical differences in the frequencies of the alleles and genotypes of BESP gene SNP rs2287622 between males and females, among CHC patients with different HCV genotypes, or between CHC patients with and without liver cirrhosis. It is speculated that BSEP might change the components of the bile acid pool in serum and liver cells to modify the chronicity process of HCV infection. Further study with a larger cohort of research subjects is essential.

Conclusions

Among the Han individuals aged over 40 years in Hunan, China, genotype CC or CT of BSEP gene SNP rs2287622 may correlate with higher risk of CHC in comparison with genotype TT. Further study with a larger cohort is essential.

Abbreviations

ALT: Alanine aminotransferase; AST: Aspartate aminotransferase; ATP: Adenosine triphosphate; BSEP: Bile salt export pump; CA: Cholic acid; CDCA: Chenodeoxycholic acid; CHB: Chronic HBV-infection; CHC: Chronic HCV-infection; CI: Confidence interval; DCA: Deoxycholic acid; DNA: Deoxyribonucleic acid; EDTA: Elhylene diamine tetraacetic acid; FXR: The farnesoid X receptor; HBsAg: HBV surface antigen; HBV: Hepatitis B virus; HCV: Hepatitis C virus; INF-α: Interferon-alpha; IQR: Interquartile range; LCA: Lithocholic acid; NS: Non-significant; OR: Odds ratio; PBMC: Peripheral blood monouclear cell; PCR: Polymerase chain reaction; RBV: Ribavirin; RFLP: Restriction fragment length polymorphism analysis; RNA: Ribonucleic acid; RT-PCR: Reverse transcription-PCR; SD: Standard deviation; SNP: Single nucleotide polymorphism; SVR: Sustained virological response; UTR: Untranslated region

Acknowledgements

HCV genotyping was carried out at Shenyou Bio-Technology Co., Ltd., Shanghai, China, and Sansure biotech Inc. Ltd., Hunan, China.

Funding

Design of the study and collection, analysis, and interpretation of data and publication of the manuscript were funded by the Second Xiangya Hospital, Central South University.

Authors' contributions

JHL designed the research. JHL and XY managed and followed up the patients. JHL, ZC and FP collected the data and established the database. XQX genotyped BSEP SNP rs2287622. JHL, ZC and FP analyzed the data statistically. JHL drafted the manuscript. ZC participated in paper modification and revised the manuscript for English writing. All authors read and approved the final manuscript.

Competing interests

The authors declare that they have no competing interests.

Consent for publication

Not applicable

References

1. Mohd Hanafiah K, Groeger J, Flaxman AD, Wiersma ST. Global epidemiology of hepatitis C virus infection: new estimates of age-specific antibody to HCV seroprevalence. Hepatology. 2013;57(4):1333–42.
2. Thomas DL. Global control of hepatitis C: where challenge meets opportunity. Nat Med. 2013;19(7):850–8.
3. Cui Y, Jia J. Update on epidemiology of hepatitis B and C in China. J Gastroenterol Hepatol. 2013;28 Suppl 1:7–10.
4. Ge D, Fellay J, Thompson AJ, Simon JS, Shianna KV, Urban TJ, Heinzen EL, Qiu P, Bertelsen AH, Muir AJ, Sulkowski M, McHutchison JG, Goldstein DB. Genetic variation in IL28B predicts hepatitis C treatment-induced viral clearance. Nature. 2009;461(7262):399–401.
5. Rauch A, Kutalik Z, Descombes P, Cai T, Di Iulio J, Mueller T, Bochud M, Battegay M, Bernasconi E, Borovicka J, Colombo S, Cerny A, Dufour JF, Furrer H, Günthard HF, Heim M, Hirschel B, Malinverni R, Moradpour D, Müllhaupt B, Witteck A, Beckmann JS, Berg T, Bergmann S, Negro F, Telenti A, Bochud PY, Swiss Hepatitis C Cohort Study; Swiss HIV Cohort Study. Genetic variation in IL28B is associated with chronic hepatitis C and treatment failure: a genome-wide association study. Gastroenterology. 2010;138(4):1338–45.
6. Tang S, Yue M, Wang J, Su J, Yu R, Zhou D, Xu K, Cai L, Zhang Y, Wang J. Association of genetic variants in estrogen receptor α with HCV infection susceptibility and viral clearance in a high-risk Chinese population. Eur J Clin Microbiol Infect Dis. 2014;33(6):999–1010.
7. Yue M, Gao CF, Wang JJ, Wang CJ, Feng L, Wang J, Yu RB, Peng ZH, Xue XX, Cai L, Fan NJ, Zhang Y, Deng XZ. Toll-like receptor 7 variations are associated with the susceptibility to HCV infection among Chinese females. Infect Genet Evol. 2014;27:264–70.
8. Iwata R, Stieger B, Mertens JC, Müller T, Baur K, Frei P, Braun J, Vergopoulos A, Martin IV, Schmitt J, Goetze O, Bibert S, Bochud PY, Müllhaupt B, Berg T, Geier A, Swiss Hepatitis C Cohort Study Group. The role of bile acid retention and a common polymorphism in the ABCB11 gene as host factors affecting antiviral treatment response in chronic hepatitis C. J Viral Hepat. 2011;18(11): 768–78.
9. Kubitz R, Brinkmeyer C, Sagir A, Herebian D, Häussinger D. Genetic variants of the bile salt export pump: inducers and modifiers of liver diseases. Dig Dis. 2011;29(1):89–92.
10. Müllenbach R, Weber SN, Krawczyk M, Zimmer V, Sarrazin C, Lammert F, Grünhage F. A frequent variant in the human bile salt export pump gene ABCB11 is associated with hepatitis C virus infection, but not liver stiffness in a German population. BMC Gastroenterol. 2012;12:63–8.
11. Iwata R, Baur K, Stieger B, Mertens JC, Daly AK, Frei P, Braun J, Vergopoulos A, Stickel F, Sabrane K, Martin IV, Schmitt J, Goetze O, Day CP, Müllhaupt B, Geier A, Swiss Hepatitis C Cohort Study Group. A common polymorphism in the ABCB11 gene is associated with advanced fibrosis in hepatitis C but not in non-alcoholic fatty liver disease. Clin Sci (Lond). 2011;120(7):287–96.

12. Chen HL, Liu YJ, Su YN, Wang NY, Wu SH, Ni YH, Hsu HY, Wu TC, Chang MH. Diagnosis of BSEP/ABCB11 mutations in Asian patients with cholestasis using denaturing high performance liquid chromatography. J Pediatr. 2008;153(6):825–32.
13. Kim SR, Saito Y, Itoda M, Maekawa K, Kawamoto M, Kamatani N, Ozawa S, Sawada J. Genetic variations of the ABC transporter gene ABCB11 encoding the human bile salt export pump (BSEP) in a Japanese population. Drug Metab Pharmacokinet. 2009;24(3):277–781.
14. Hu G, He P, Liu Z, Chen Q, Zheng B, Zhang Q. Diagnosis of ABCB11 gene mutations in children with intrahepatic cholestasis using high resolution melting analysis and direct sequencing. Mol Med Rep. 2014;10(3):1264–74.
15. Tarantino G, Citro V, Conca P, Riccio A, Tarantino M, Capone D, Cirillo M, Lobello R, Iaccarino V. What are the implications of the spontaneous spleno-renal shunts in liver cirrhosis? BMC Gastroenterol. 2009;9:89.
16. Tarantino G, Citro V, Esposito P, Giaquinto S, de Leone A, Milan G, Tripodi FS, Cirillo M, Lobello R. Blood ammonia levels in liver cirrhosis: a clue for the presence of portosystemic collateral veins. BMC Gastroenterol. 2009;9:21.
17. Kubitz R, Dröge C, Stindt J, Weissenberger K, Häussinger D. The bile salt export pump (BSEP) in health and disease. Clin Res Hepatol Gastroenterol. 2012;36(6):536–53.
18. Halilbasic E, Claudel T, Trauner M. Bile acid transporters and regulatory nuclear receptors in the liver and beyond. J Hepatol. 2013;58(1):155–68.
19. Chang KO, George DW. Bile acids promote the expression of hepatitis C virus in replicon-harboring cells. J Virol. 2007;81(18):9633–40.
20. Chhatwal P, Bankwitz D, Gentzsch J, Frentzen A, Schult P, Lohmann V, Pietschmann T. Bile acids specifically increase hepatitis C virus RNA-replication. PLoS One. 2012;7(4):e36029.
21. Scholtes C, Diaz O, Icard V, Kaul A, Bartenschlager R, Lotteau V, André P. Enhancement of genotype 1 hepatitis C virus replication by bile acids through FXR. J Hepatol. 2008;48(2):192–9.
22. André P, Ramière C, Scholtes C, Curtil C, Lotteau V. Role of nuclear receptors in hepatitis B and C infections. Clin Res Hepatol Gastroenterol. 2011;35(3):169–75.
23. Patton JB, George D, Chang KO. Bile acids promote HCV replication through the EGFR/ERK pathway in replicon-harboring cells. Intervirology. 2011;54(6):339–48.
24. Graf D, Haselow K, Münks I, Bode JG, Häussinger D. Inhibition of interferon-α-induced signaling by hyperosmolarity and hydrophobic bile acids. Biol Chem. 2010;91(10):1175–87.
25. Byrne JA, Strautnieks SS, Ihrke G, Pagani F, Knisely AS, Linton KJ, Mieli-Vergani G, Thompson RJ. Missense mutations and single nucleotide polymorphisms in ABCB11 impair bile salt export pump processing and function or disrupt pre-messenger RNA splicing. Hepatology. 2009;49(2):553–67.
26. Krawczyk M, Grünhage F, Langhirt M, Bohle RM, Lammert F. Prolonged cholestasis triggered by hepatitis A virus infection and variants of the hepatocanalicular phospholipid and bile salt transporters. Ann Hepatol. 2012;11(5):710–4.

6

Comparison of the long-term efficacy between entecavir and tenofovir in treatment-naïve chronic hepatitis B patients

Ji Won Park[1,2], Kyeong Min Kwak[3,4], Sung Eun Kim[1], Myoung Kuk Jang[5], Ki Tae Suk[6], Dong Joon Kim[6], Sang Hoon Park[7], Myung Seok Lee[7], Hyoung Su Kim[5*] and Choong Kee Park[1]

Abstract

Background: There have been limited studies directly comparing the long-term efficacy between entecavir (ETV) and tenofovir disoproxil fumarate (TDF). This study was aimed to compare the long-term efficacy between them in treatment-naïve chronic hepatitis B (CHB).

Methods: Out of 345 CHB patients who received first line therapy with ETV ($n = 200$) or TDF ($n = 145$) in a cohort, 210 patients were analyzed using propensity score matching, at a ratio of 1:1.

Results: Two groups showed no difference in baseline characteristics. During the follow-up of 12 months, HBV DNA levels were similarly suppressed in both groups (ETV vs. TDF; −5.01 vs. -5.242 $\log_{10}$IU/mL, $P = 0.559$). At month 12, both groups showed no difference in terms of the serologic, biochemical and virologic (VR) response. In multivariate analysis, the initial virologic response at 3 months (IVR-3) was independent factor for VR at 1 year. During the long-term follow-up, HBV DNA levels were more strongly suppressed by TDF than ETV in hepatitis B e antigen (HBeAg) positive patients ($P = 0.035$), especially with high viral load ($P = 0.012$), although there was no significant difference in overall VR between two groups. The type of antivirals was not an independent factor for long-term VR.

Conclusions: Although either ETV or TDF, overall, may show a comparable long-term antiviral efficacy in treatment-naïve CHB, TDF might be better regimen than ETV in the subgroup of HBeAg-positive CHB, especially with a higher HBV DNA levels.

Keywords: Entecavir, Tenofovir, Hepatitis B virus

Background

Approximately 350 million people are estimated to be chronically infected with hepatitis B virus (HBV), which may result in serious complications, such as hepatic failure, advanced cirrhosis, and/or hepatocellular carcinoma (HCC) in 15–40% of patients [1–3]. In addition to clinical host factors, such as age, family history, and alcohol abuse, many HBV-related factors themselves, which include HBV mutations of precore/core promoter regions, HBV genotype C, and high serum HBV DNA levels (viral factors), contribute to the critical progression of chronic liver diseases [4–6]. Although factors such as mutations or genotypes are not changed by antivirals, serum HBV DNA levels, e.g., HBV replication, can be sustainably suppressed by anti-HBV therapies to prevent and/or retard cirrhosis and subsequently HCC. To date, oral antiviral drugs such as lamivudine, adefovir, entecavir, telbivudine and tenofovir have been widely used in clinical settings [4, 7, 8].

According to several international guidelines, entecavir (ETV) or tenofovir disoproxil fumarate (TDF) are recommended as first line therapy in the treatment of naïve CHB because of their higher antiviral potency and higher genetic

* Correspondence: hskim@hallym.or.kr
[5]Department of Internal Medicine, Kangdong Sacred Heart Hospital of Hallym University Medical Center, 18, Cheonho-daero 173-gil, Gangdong-gu, Seoul 05355, Republic of Korea

barriers than other antiviral agents [9–13]. In reality, ETV and TDF showed high virologic responses of up to 93% and 100%, respectively, and a rare genotypic resistance of only 1.2% and 0%, respectively, during the 5- year follow-up in a cohort study [14, 15].

Although there have been a few reports comparing the short-term efficacy directly between TDF and ETV in treatment-naïve CHB, there is still little available clinical information about the long-term efficacy. Therefore, we performed this study to compare the long-term efficacy between TDF and ETV in treatment-naïve CHB patients.

Methods

Patients and study design

A total of 345 treatment-naïve CHB patients who received a single regimen of either TDF ($n = 145$) or ETV ($n = 200$) for at least 12 months were consecutively enrolled from 4 tertiary university hospitals in Korea between January 2011 and December 2014. Because TDF or ETV use was not randomly assigned, potential confounding and selection biases were accounted for by developing a propensity score. Among a total of 345 patients, 210 patients were selected using propensity score match, at a ratio of 1:1. Patients with the following characteristics were excluded: 1) other viral infections such as HCV, HDV and HIV, 2) other concomitant liver diseases such as alcoholic liver disease and autoimmune liver disease, or 3) HCC. Patients were monitored by clinical examination and biochemical and virologic assessments at least every 3 to 4 months during the antiviral therapy.

The study protocol was approved by the Hallym University Medical Center Institutional Review Boards (IRB No. 13-1-49).

Serum assay and methodology

Biochemistry was performed using standard laboratory procedures. Hepatitis B surface antigen (HBsAg), antibody to HBsAg (anti-HBs), HBeAg, and antibody to HBeAg (anti-HBe) were measured using microparticle enzyme immunoassay (Abbott Laboratories, North Chicago, IL, USA). Serum HBV DNA levels were measured using a COBAS TaqMan PCR assay (Roche, Branchburg, NJ, USA; lower limit of detection 20 IU/mL).

Definitions

Primary non-response was defined as a failure to reduce serum HBV DNA levels by >1 $\log_{10}$ IU/mL after 3 months of therapy [16]. A high HBV DNA level was defined as a serum HBV DNA level greater than 6 $\log_{10}$ IU/mL. Initial virologic response at 3 months (IVR-3) and virologic response (VR) were defined as an HBV DNA level <3.3 $\log_{10}$ IU/mL after 3 months of therapy [17, 18] and an undetectable HBV DNA level (<20 IU/mL) during the therapy, respectively. A biochemical response was defined as a normalization of the serum alanine aminotransferase (ALT) levels. Virologic breakthrough (VBT) was defined as an increase over 1 $\log_{10}$ IU/mL of serum HBV DNA levels from the nadir during the therapy or serum HBV DNA levels >200 IU/mL in patients who experienced VR.

Statistical analyses

HBV DNA levels were logarithmically transformed for analysis. The Mann–Whitney U-test for continuous variables and chi-squared test for categorical variables were used in the analyses as appropriate. A repeated measures analysis was used to compare HBV DNA reduction according to the drug used. Cumulative VR and VBT rates were calculated using the Kaplan-Meier method, and the difference was determined by a log-rank test. The multivariate logistic regression model and Cox proportional hazards model were used to identify the independent risk factors significantly associated with short-term and long-term VR, respectively. Candidate variables with a P value of < 0.1 on univariate analysis were entered into the regression analysis. A P-value of less than 0.05 was considered significant. Statistical analyses were performed using SPSS, version 16 (SPSS, Inc, Chicago, IL).

To reduce and control any confounding factors before receiving the treatment, we used the propensity scores to match TDF users to ETV users. A macro (available at: http://www2.sas.com/proceedings/sugi26/p214-26.pdf) was used to develop the propensity scores.

Results

Baseline patient characteristics

Among 345 patients, the propensity-matched 105 patients in each group were included (1:1). The baseline characteristics of the study population are summarized in Table 1.

One hundred thirty one (62.4%) patients were men and the mean age was 46.2 ± 12.0 years. Eighty four patients (40%) had had cirrhosis and 121 patients (57.6%) were positive for HBeAg. The mean HBV DNA levels and ALT levels were 6.61 ± 1.30 $\log_{10}$ IU/mL and 205.9 ± 351.5 IU/L, respectively. There was no difference in the baseline characteristics between the TDF and ETV groups. On average, patients were treated for 25.3 (12–39) months.

Therapeutic responses

Figure 1 shows the changes in the mean HBV DNA levels during the first 12 months. Overall, serum HBV DNA levels continuously declined, and the overall mean changes at months 3, 6 and 12 were −4.26 $\log_{10}$ IU/mL, −4.89 $\log_{10}$ IU/mL and −5.12 $\log_{10}$ IU/mL, respectively (Fig. 1a). The mean reduction in serum HBV DNA levels from baseline to month 12 was similar in the ETV and TDF groups (−5.01 vs.−5.22 $\log_{10}$ IU/mL, $P = 0.559$) using a repeated measure analysis (Fig. 1b). During the first year

Table 1 Baseline characteristics of the patients

Variables	ETV ($n = 105$)	TDF ($n = 105$)	*P*
Age (years)	47.0 ± 12.0	45.5 ± 11.9	0.396
Sex (male, %)	64 (61.0)	67 (63.8)	0.776
HBeAg-positive (%)	58 (55.2)	63 (50.0)	0.577
Disease status; CHB/LC (%)	62/43 (59.0/41.0)	64/41 (61.0/39.0)	0.888
MELD (<7/7-13/>13, %)	73/26/6 (69.5/24.8/5.7)	71/33/1 (67.6/31.4/1.0)	0.800
Serum ALT (IU/L)	179.5 ± 253.0	232.3 ± 427.7	0.278
Serum total bilirubin (mg/dL)	1.20 ± 1.74	1.06 ± 1.29	0.507
Serum albumin (g/dL)	4.11 ± 0.56	4.10 ± 0.53	0.905
INR	1.12 ± 0.19	1.11 ± 0.17	0.927
Serum HBV DNA level (log_{10} IU/mL)	6.56 ± 1.33	6.66 ± 1.26	0.564
Duration of follow-up (months)	27.0 ± 7.2	23.6 ± 5.2	

Continuous variables were expressed as mean ± standard deviation
ALT alanine aminotransferase, *CHB* chronic hepatitis B, *ETV* entecavir, *HBeAg* hepatitis B e antigen, *HBV* hepatitis B virus, *INR* international normalized ratio, *LC* liver cirrhosis, *MELD* model for end stage liver disease, *TDF* tenofovir

of therapy, VR (HBV DNA levels < 20 IU/mL) and primary non-response were observed in 161 (76.7%) and 0 patients (0%), respectively. One hundred fifty of 184 patients who had shown elevated serum ALT levels at baseline achieved a normalization of serum ALT levels (81.5%). During the first year of therapy, HBeAg loss/seroconversion occurred in 18 of 121 (14.9%) HBeAg-positive patients.

There were no significant differences in the virologic, serologic and biochemical responses at year 1 between two groups (Table 2). The mean reduction in serum HBV DNA levels from baseline to month 12 was similar between the ETV and TDF groups (−5.54 vs.−5.78 log_{10} IU/mL, $P = 0.159$), even in the HBeAg-positive patients (Fig. 2a). Although HBV DNA levels were more strongly suppressed by TDF than by ETV (−5.92 vs. −5.78 log_{10} IU/mL, $P = 0.022$) in the HBeAg-positive subgroup with higher HBV DNA levels (Fig. 2b), the type of antiviral used was not an independent factor for VR. During the mean long-term therapy period of 25.3 months, the virologic and serologic responses were additionally achieved in 22 and 10 patients, respectively. Persistent viremia was observed in 26 patients, consisting of 17 patients (16.2%, 17/105) in the ETV group and 9 patients (8.6%, 9/105) in the TDF group.

The cumulative VR rates at 3, 6, 12, 24 and 36 months were 20%, 54%, 79%, 86% and 91%, respectively, during the follow-up period (Fig. 3a). The cumulative VR rates in the ETV group at 3, 6, 12, 24 and 36 months were 21%, 55%, 75%, 84% and 87%, respectively, whereas, in the TDF group, the rates at 3, 6, 12, 24 and 36 months were 19%, 52%, 83%, 91% and 94%, respectively. These differences were not significant (Fig. 3b, $P = 0.222$). The cumulative VR rates in the HBeAg-negative subgroup also showed no significant difference between the ETV and TDF groups (89%, 96% and 100% vs. 76%, 98% and 100% at 6, 12 and 24 months, respectively, $P = 0.819$). However, in the HBeAg-positive subgroup, the cumulative VR rates in the ETV group at 6, 12, 24 and 36 months were 28%, 57%, 70% and 77%, respectively, whereas the rates in the TDF group at 6, 12, 24 and 36 months were 37%, 73%, 84% and 91%, respectively, with significant difference between two groups ($P = 0.035$, Fig. 3c). This finding was conspicuous in another subgroup of HBeAg-positive CHB with higher HBV DNA levels (20%, 53%, 68% and 68% at 6, 12, 24 and 36 months in ETV group vs. 32%, 71%, 83% and 90% at 6, 12, 24 and 36 months in TDF group, respectively, $P = 0.012$, Fig. 3d).

Predictive factors for virologic response

A multivariate logistic regression model was used to identify the independent risk factors significantly associated

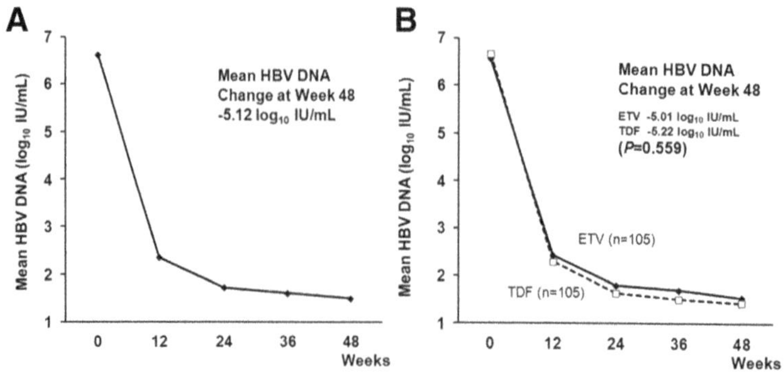

Fig. 1 Change of HBV DNA during follow-up period. **a** The changes in the mean hepatitis B virus (HBV) DNA levels from baseline through week 48. The overall mean changes at weeks 12, 24 and 48 were −4.26 log_{10} IU/mL, −4.89 log_{10} IU/mL and −5.12 log_{10} IU/mL, respectively. **b** The mean reduction in serum HBV DNA levels from baseline to week 48 was similar in tenofovir and entecavir group (−5.22 vs. −5.01 log_{10} IU/mL, $P = 0.559$) by repeated measure analysis

Table 2 Virologic, serologic and biochemical response at week 48

	Baseline	Week 24	Week 48	Total	*P*
Mean HBV DNA ($\log_{10}$ IU/mL)	6.61	1.72	1.49	5.12↓	0.559
ETV (*n* = 105)	6.56	1.80	1.55	5.01↓	
TDF (*n* = 105)	6.66	1.64	1.44	5.22↓	
HBV DNA negativity by PCR				161(76.7%)	0.192
ETV (*n* = 105)		58 (55.2%)	76 (72.4%)		
TDF (*n* = 105)		56 (53.3%)	85 (81.0%)		
HBeAg loss/seroconversion				18 (14.9%)	0.452
ETV (*n* = 58)			7 (12.1%)		
TDF (*n* = 63)			11 (17.5%)		
Biochemical response				150 (81.5%)	0.647
ETV (*n* = 92)			77 (83.7%)		
TDF (*n* = 92)			73 (79.3%)		

Data are expressed mean or number
ETV entecavir, *HBeAg* hepatitis B e antigen, *HBV* hepatitis B virus, *TDF* tenofovir

with VR during the first year. In a univariate analysis, disease status (CHB vs. cirrhosis), HBeAg status, serum HBV DNA levels and IVR-3 were candidate variables for the multivariate analysis. Of the clinical features, cirrhosis, HBeAg negativity, low serum HBV DNA levels and IVR-3 were considered favorable factors for VR, while other factors, including the type of antiviral used (ETV vs. TDF), were not significantly associated with VR (Table 3). In the multivariate analysis, only IVR-3 remained independent predictors for one year VR (Table 4).

A cox proportional hazards model was used to identify the independent factors for long-term VR. In the multivariate analysis, HBeAg status, serum HBV DNA levels and IVR-3 were identified as predictive factors for long-term VR (Table 5).

Predictive factors on the long-term efficacy

Sixty seven patients (31.9%) had low baseline serum HBV DNA levels (<6 $\log_{10}$ IU/mL), 173 patients (82.4%) showed IVR-3 and 89 patients (42.4%) were negative for HBeAg. The patients with low serum HBV DNA levels, IVR-3 or HBeAg negativity had a significantly higher probability of achieving a VR. In patients with low baseline serum HBV DNA levels, the cumulative VR rates were 84%, 94%, 97% and 100% at 6, 12, 24 and 36 months, which were in contrast with the rates, 40%, 72%, 80% and 83% in patients with high baseline serum HBV DNA levels ($P < 0.001$, Fig. 4a). The cumulative VR rates were 64%, 89%, 94% and 100% in patients with IVR-3 and 5%, 32%, 46% and 51% in patients without IVR-3 at 6, 12, 24 and 36 months, respectively (P <0.001, Fig. 4b). A similar pattern was observed according to HBeAg status ($P < 0.001$).

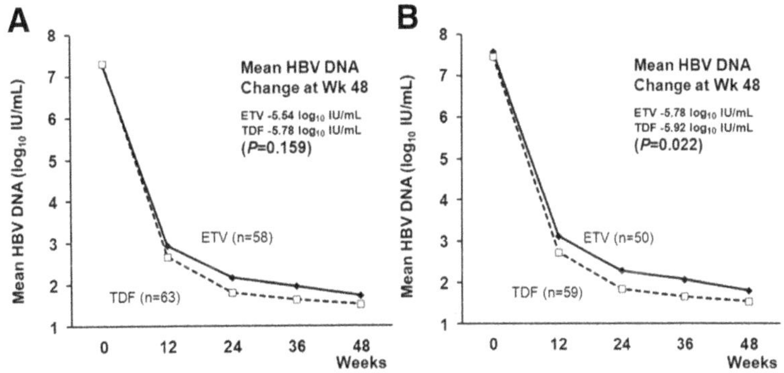

Fig. 2 Change of HBV DNA in HBeAg-positive patients. **a** The mean reduction in serum hepatitis B virus (HBV) DNA levels from baseline to month 12 was similar in tenofovir and entecavir group (−5.88 vs. −5.54 $\log_{10}$ IU/mL, $P = 0.159$) in the hepatitis e antigen (HBeAg) positive patients. **b** Serum HBV DNA levels were more strongly suppressed by tenofovir than entecavir (−5.92 vs. −5.78 $\log_{10}$ IU/mL, $P = 0.022$) in the HBeAg-positive patients with a higher HBV DNA levels

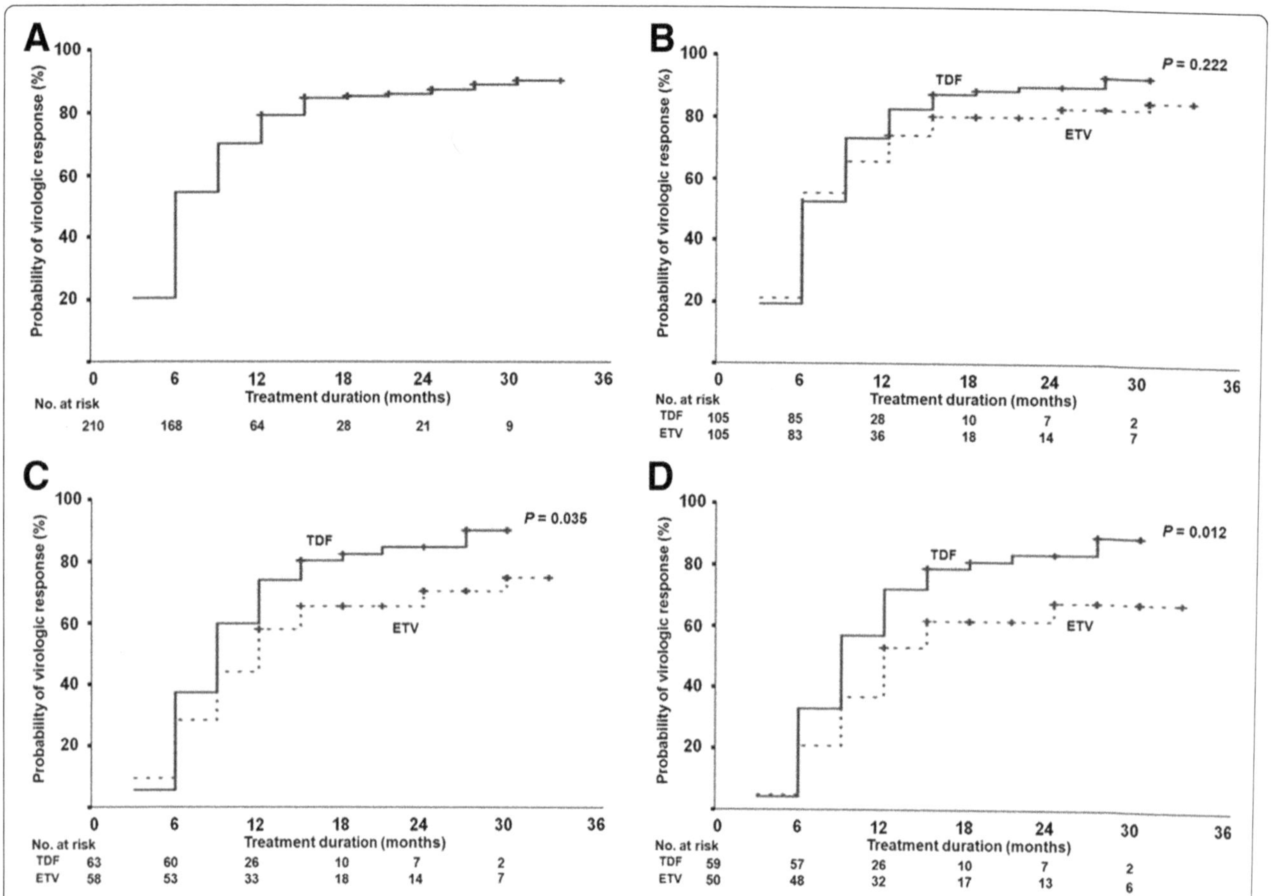

Fig. 3 Cumulative virologic response (VR) rate. **a** Cumulative VR rates at 3, 6, 12, 24 and 36 months were 20%, 54%, 79%, 86% and 91%, respectively. **b** Cumulative VR rates were not significant different between the two groups ($P = 0.222$). **c** Cumulative VR rates of tenofovir group were higher than those of entecavir group, in the hepatitis B e antigen (HBeAg) positive patients. **d** The difference of cumulative VR rates was more evident in HBeAg-positive patients with a higher hepatitis B virus DNA levels (>6 log_{10} IU/mL)

Virologic breakthrough during long-term therapy

VBT was experienced in 13 patients, with cumulative rates of 1%, 4% and 11% at 12, 24 and 36 months, respectively. There was no significant difference in the cumulative rates between the ETV and TDF groups (2%, 5% and 12% vs. 1%, 4% and 7% at 12, 24 and 36 months, respectively, $P = 0.333$). VBT developed in 9 cases in the ETV group and in 4 cases in the TDF group. The majority (11/13, 85%) of VBT was related to medication adherence. As expected, mutations associated with drug resistance were detected in 2 patients in the ETV group (L180M+ M204V + S202G).

Adverse effects

No serious adverse effects such as lactic acidosis or increase in serum creatinine levels were reported in any of the patients in either treatment group. No adverse effects leading to discontinuation of therapy occurred during the whole treatment period. During the follow-up period, 6 patients (5.7%) in TDF group and 7 (6.7%) in ETV group were diagnosed with HCC. The incidence of HCC according to the type of treatment was not different. All of them except two patients were already cirrhotic patients before antiviral treatment, the patients diagnosed with HCC were significantly older than without HCC at the beginning of antiviral treatment (54.2 ± 8.5 vs. 45.7 ± 12.0, $P = 0.014$).

Discussion

The risk of cirrhosis and/or HCC in CHB increases proportionally as serum HBV DNA levels increase [5, 6]. This finding suggests that sustained suppression of HBV replication with anti-HBV therapy may successfully prevent the progression of chronic liver diseases. Thus, the suppression of HBV replication should be considered the most important therapeutic goal for CHB patients in clinical settings. Currently, ETV and TDF are the most commonly used HBV drugs due to their excellent potency and higher genetic barrier. However, there is limited information on the comparative efficacy of these drugs, and only one drug-to-drug comparison study has been conducted thus far [19]. Although there have been,

Table 3 Comparison of clinical features between the groups according to one year virologic response

Variables	Patients with VR (*n* = 161)	Patients without VR (*n* = 49)	*P*
Age (years)	46.8 ± 11.0	44.4 ± 14.7	0.285
Sex (male, %)	99 (61.5)	32 (65.3)	0.737
HBeAg-positive (%)	77 (47.8)	44 (89.8)	<0.001
Disease status; CHB/LC (%)	85/76 (52.8/47.2)	41/8 (83.7/16.3)	<0.001
MELD (<7/7-13/>13, %)	109/47/5 (67.7/29.2/3.1)	35/12/2 (71.4/24.5/4.1)	0.768
Serum ALT (IU/L)	198.0 ± 305.7	231.8 ± 475.0	0.557
Serum total bilirubin (mg/dL)	1.12 ± 1.46	1.19 ± 1.77	0.774
Serum albumin(g/dL)	4.10 ± 0.53	4.11 ± 0.60	0.952
INR	1.12 ± 0.17	1.09 ± 0.21	0.319
IVR-3 (−/+)	12/149(7.5/92.5)	25/24 (51.0/49.0)	<0.001
Serum HBV DNA level (log_{10} IU/mL)	6.30 ± 1.23	7.61 ± 0.97	<0.001
Treatment regimens			0.192
ETV (*n* = 105, %)	76 (72.4)	29 (27.6)	
TDF (*n* = 105, %)	85 (81.0)	20 (19.0)	

Data are expressed as mean ± standard deviation or number
ALT alanine aminotransferase, *CHB* chronic hepatitis B, *ETV* entecavir, *HBeAg* hepatitis B e antigen, *HBV* hepatitis B virus, *INR* international normalized ratio, *IVR-3* initial virologic response at 3 months, *LC* liver cirrhosis, *MELD* model for end stage liver disease, *TDF* tenofovir, *VR* virologic response

so far, a few studies evaluating the efficacy of ETV and TDF in treatment-naïve CHB, they included only a limited number of patients or only showed a short-term efficacy [20–25]. Futhermore, most previous studies were retrospective and not randomized, some of them showed different baseline characteristics-such as age, gender or liver disease severity. The present study was also not a randomized controlled trial, but the limitation was complemented by using propensity score. The present study enrolled an adequate number of the treatment-naıve CHB patients and followed these patients for a sufficient time period (up to 39 months) to directly compare the efficacy between ETV and TDF. Of note, in this study, the majority of patients had a VR over 90% after 36 months of therapy. Among HBeAg-positive patients, the cumulative VR rates at month 12 in our study (75% in ETV and 83% in TDF) are comparable with previous global multicenter trials of 67% and 76%, respectively. These results were also comparable in HBeAg-negative patients (97% vs. 90% in ETV; 98% vs. 93% in TDF, respectively) [9, 10, 12].

Table 4 Multivariate analyses of clinical factors affecting one year virologic response

Factors	RR	95% CI	*P*
Disease status (CHB/LC)	0.559	0.205–1.521	0.255
IVR-3 (+/−)	6.214	2.500–15.443	<0.001
HBeAg (−/+)	3.184	0.977–10.377	0.055
Serum HBV DNA level (log_{10} IU/mL)	0.605	0.357–1.023	0.061

RR, relative risk, *95% CI* 95% confidence interval, *CHB* chronic hepatitis B, *HBeAg* hepatitis B e antigen, *HBV* hepatitis B virus, *IVR-3* initial virologic response at 3 months, *LC* liver cirrhosis

In this study, ETV and TDF showed similar overall antiviral efficacy both for one year and during the long-term follow-up. These results were similar to previous studies [21–23, 25]. However, our subgroup analysis indicated that TDF was significantly better than ETV for suppressing HBV DNA in HBeAg-positive patients, especially with higher HBV DNA levels. There were a few studies which TDF showed more potent antiviral efficacy than ETV in HBeAg-positive patients [24, 26]. When comparing our study with these previous studies, the present study included only treatment-naïve patients and who had been adherent to medication therapy for at least one year. Patient adherence may contribute to achieve comparable overall VR at month 12 and during long-term period in both groups.

Another interesting finding in the present study is the prognostic role of IVR-3, which is a good predictive factor for both short-term and long-term VR. Higher baseline ALT, lower HBV DNA levels and HBeAg-negative status are already well known to be associated with VR. In addition to these factors, our finding suggested that IVR-3 was also able to predict VR very well. In fact, cumulative VR rates in patients achieving IVR-3 was significantly higher than in patients without IVR-3 (100% vs. 51% at 36 months, RR 3.403, 95% CI 1.977–5.849, $P < 0.001$). Surprisingly, the predictive value of IVR-3 was much higher than those of previously known factors, such as HBeAg status and HBV DNA levels. Pragmatically, IVR-3 combined with HBeAg and HBV DNA levels may help to predict

Table 5 Factors associated with long-term virologic response

Factors	Univariate analysis			Multivariate analysis		
	RR	95% CI	*P*	RR	95% CI	*P*
Age (years)	1.007	0.995–1.018	0.262			
Sex (female/male)	1.009	0.747–1.363	0.952			
HBeAg-positive (−/+)	3.031	2.209–4.158	<0.001	1.834	1.246–2.698	0.002
Disease status (LC/CHB)	1.577	1.172–2.121	0.003	1.028	0.748–1.411	0.867
MELD (<7/≥7)	0.923	0.676–1.260	0.613			
INR	1.020	0.469–2.218	0.961			
Serum ALT (IU/L)	1.000	1.000–1.000	0.890			
Serum total bilirubin (mg/dL)	1.005	0.918–1.101	0.908			
Serum albumin (g/dL)	1.077	0.824–1.406	0.588			
IVR-3 (+/−)	4.851	2.902–8.109	<0.001	3.403	1.977–5.859	<0.001
Serum HBV DNA level (log_{10} IU/mL)	0.638	0.569–0.715	<0.001	0.817	0.696–0.958	0.013
Therapy regimens (TDF/ETV)	1.162	0.868–1.555	0.313			

RR relative risk, *95% CI* 95% confidence interval, *ALT* alanine aminotransferase, *CHB* chronic hepatitis B, *ETV* entecavir, *HBeAg* hepatitis B e antigen, *HBV* hepatitis B virus, *INR* international normalized ratio, *IVR-3* initial virologic response at 3 months, *LC* liver cirrhosis, *MELD* model for end stage liver disease, *TDF* tenofovir

long-term VR and determine whether to maintain primary therapy or switch to other regimens.

Multi-center, long-term studies using ETV and/or TDF have shown excellent safety and tolerance with little antiviral resistance (1.2% in ETV and 0% in TDF up to 5 years). In our study, there was no serious clinical adverse reaction in the two treatment groups. However, even though the patient had achieved VR, HCC was developed in 5.7% of patients receiving TDF and 6.7% of ETV. Considering the risk of developing HCC is appears to be greatest among individuals with the highest serum HBV DNA levels, the introduction of nucleos(t)ide analogues has contributed to reduce the risk of HCC. The reason why the incidence of HCC was higher than previous studies was that the present study included a large number of cirrhotic patients. Cirrhosis has been well known risk factor for HCC. Actually, all patients diagnosed with HCC in this study were cirrhotic patients, except two patients. Our finding confirmed that old and cirrhotic patients should be carefully undergone surveillance for HCC regardless of achieving VR.

It should be considered that poor medication adherence is a major cause of suboptimal response and/or VBT that tends to be increasingly prevalent in proportion to the duration of therapy [27–31]. In the current study, overall cumulative VBT rates were 1%, 4% and 11% at 12, 24 and 36 months, respectively, which was primarily related to medication adherence. Only two patients showed resistance in the ETV group.

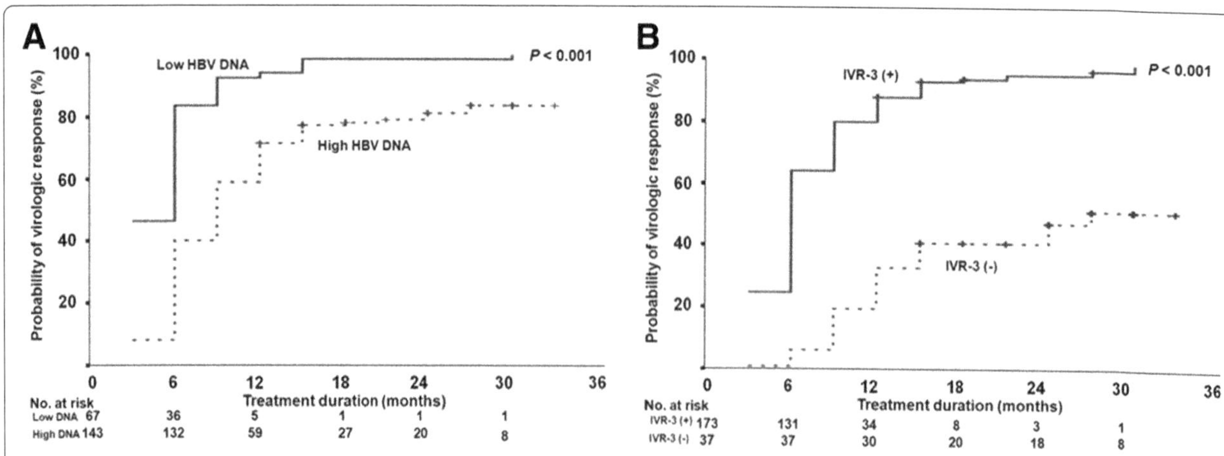

Fig. 4 Cumulative virologic response (VR) rate according to HBV DNA levels and IVR-3. **a** Cumulative VR rates in the patients with high baseline serum HBV DNA levels at 6, 12, 24 and 36 months were 40%, 72%, 80% and 83%, respectively. They were 84%, 94%, 97% and 100%, respectively, in the patients with low baseline serum HBV DNA levels. **b** Cumulative VR rates in the patients without IVR-3 at 6, 12, 24 and 36 months were 5%, 32%, 46% and 51%, respectively. And in the patients with IVR-3, they were 64%, 89, 94 and 100%, respectively

Our study has some limitations. First, the study was retrospective and non-randomized. However, we adjusted this shortcoming by using propensity score to minimize the influence of the baseline characteristics. This process made our outcomes to be more reliable. Second, in the process of matching the patients, the sample size was decreased and the follow-up period was shortened. Nevertheless, each group included over 100 patients and the follow-up period was up to 39 months. This is comparable with the most recently published, randomized controlled trial to compare treatment efficacy of ETV and TDF in treatment-naïve CHB patients [32]. Third, the study may not be generalizable to other ethnic groups because we included only Asian patients (Koreans) who were infected by mainly HBV genotype C.

To date, randomized controlled or well matched comparative studies regarding the efficacy of TDF or ETV in treatment-naïve CHB patients were very rare. Therefore, it is necessary to conduct direct comparisons of a prospective nature with larger numbers of patients and longer period of treatment.

Conclusions

TDF and ETV showed comparable efficacy and safety during 3 years in treatment-naïve CHB patients. We found that IVR-3 was predictive factor on long-term efficacy in addition to HBV DNA levels and HBeAg status. The present study suggested that TDF might be the more potent option in a subgroup of HBeAg-positive CHB, especially with higher HBV DNA levels. VBT occurred with similar rates in both groups, and was primarily the result of medication nonadherence. Old and cirrhotic patients should be carefully undergone surveillance for HCC regardless of achieving VR.

Abbreviation

ALT: Alanine aminotransferase; anti-HBe: Antibody to hepatitis B e antigen; anti-HBs: Antibody to hepatitis B surface antigen; CHB: Chronic hepatitis B; ETV: Entecavir; HBeAg: Hepatitis B e antigen; HBsAg: Hepatitis B surface antigen; HBV: Hepatitis B virus; HCC: Hepatocellular carcinoma; IVR-3: Initial virologic response at 3 months; TDF: Tenofovir; VBT: Virologic breakthrough; VR: Virologic response

Acknowledgments

Not Applicable.

Funding

The authors who have taken part in this study declare that they do not have anything to disclose regarding funding. No grants or financial support were received for this study.

Authors' contributions

HSK, DJK and CKP designed the study. JWP, SEK, MSL, SHP and KTS carried out the extraction of data. KMK, MKJ and HSK carried out the statistical analysis of studies. JWP wrote the paper. All authors read and approved the final manuscript.

Competing interests

The authors declare that they have no competing interests.

Consent for publication

Not Applicable.

Author details

[1]Department of Internal Medicine, Hallym University Sacred Heart Hospital of Hallym University Medical Center, 22, Gwanpyeong-ro 170 beon-gil, Dongan-gu, Anyang-si, Gyeonggi-do 14068, Republic of Korea. [2]Department of Biomedical Gerontology, Graduate School of Hallym University, 1 Hallymdaehak-gil, Chuncheon-si, Gangwon-do 24252, Republic of Korea. [3]Department of Occupational and Environmental Medicine, Hallym University Sacred Heart Hospital of Hallym University Medical Center, 22, Gwanpyeong-ro 170 beon-gil, Dongan-gu, Anyang-si, Gyeonggi-do 14068, Republic of Korea. [4]Department of Environmental Health, Seoul National University School of Public Health, 1, Gwanak-ro, Gwanak-gu, Seoul 08826, Republic of Korea. [5]Department of Internal Medicine, Kangdong Sacred Heart Hospital of Hallym University Medical Center, 18, Cheonho-daero 173-gil, Gangdong-gu, Seoul 05355, Republic of Korea. [6]Department of Internal Medicine, Chuncheon Sacred Heart Hospital of Hallym University Medical Center, 77, Sakju-ro, Chuncheon-si, Gangwon-do 24253, Republic of Korea. [7]Department of Internal Medicine, Kangnam Sacred Heart Hospital of Hallym University Medical Center, 1, Singil-ro, Yeongdeungpo-gu, Seoul 07441, Republic of Korea.

References

1. Safileas M, Lygidakis NJ, Manti C. Hepatitis B today. Hepatogastroenterology. 2007;54:545–8.
2. Lavanchy D. Hepatitis B, virus epidemiology, disease burden, treatment, and current and emerging prevention and control measures. J Viral Hepat. 2004;11:97–107.
3. Bosch FX, Ribes J, Cleries R, Diaz M. Epidemiology of hepatocellular carcinoma. Clin Liver Dis. 2005;9:191–211.
4. Lok AS, McMahon BJ. Chronic hepatitis B: update 2009. Hepatology. 2009;50:661–2.
5. Chen CJ, Yang HI, Su J, Jen CL, You SL, Lu SN, et al. Risk of hepatocellular carcinoma across a biological gradient of serum hepatitis B virus DNA level. JAMA. 2006;295:65–73.
6. Iloeje UH, Yang HI, Su J, Jen CL, You SL, Chen CJ. Predicting cirrhosis risk based on the level of circulating hepatitis B viral load. Gastroenterology. 2006;130:678–86.
7. Liaw YF. Hepatitis B, virus replication and liver disease progression: the impact of antiviral therapy. Antivir Ther. 2006;11:669–79.
8. Chang TT, Liaw YF, Wu SS, Schiff E, Han KH, Lai CL, et al. Long-term entecavir therapy results in the reversal of fibrosis/cirrhosis and continued histological improvement in patients with chronic hepatitis B. Hepatology. 2010;52:886–93.
9. Chang TT, Gish RG, de Man R, Gadano A, Sollano J, Chao YC, et al. A comparison of entecavir and lamivudine for HBeAg-positive chronic hepatitis B. N Engl J Med. 2006;354:1001–10.
10. Lai CL, Shouval D, Lok AS, Chang TT, Cheinguer H, Goodman Z, et al. Entecavir versus lamivudine for patients with HBeAg-negative chronic hepatitis B. N Engl J Med. 2006;354:1011–20.
11. Leung N, Peng CY, Hann HW, Sollano J, Lao-Tan J, Hsu CW, et al. Early hepatitis B virus DNA reduction in hepatitis B e antigen-positive patients with chronic hepatitis B: A randomized international study of entecavir versus adefovir. Hepatology. 2009;49:72–9.
12. Marcellin P, Heathcote EJ, Buti M, Gane E, de Man RA, Krastev Z, et al. Tenofovir disoproxil fumarate versus adefovir dipivoxil for chronic hepatitis B. N Engl J Med. 2008;359:2442–55.
13. European Association for the Study of the Liver. EASL clinical practice guidelines: management of chronic hepatitis B virus infection. J Hepatol. 2012;57:167–85.
14. Tenney DJ, Rose RE, Baldick CJ, Pokornowski KA, Eggers BJ, Fang J, et al. Long-term monitoring shows hepatitis B virus resistance to entecavir in nucleoside-naïve patients is rare through 5 years of therapy. Hepatology. 2009;49:1503–14.

15. Kitrinos KM, Corsa A, Liu Y, Flasherty J, Snow-Lampart A, Marcellin P, et al. No detectable resistance to tenofovir disoproxil fumarate after 6 years of therapy in patients with chronic hepatitis B. Hepatology. 2014;59:434–42.
16. Zoulim F, Locarnini S. Hepatitis B virus resistance to nucleos(t)ide analogues. Gastroenterology. 2009;137:1593–608.
17. Park JW, Kim HS, Seo DD, Jang JS, Shin WG, Kim KH, et al. Long-term efficacy of entecavir in adefovir-refractory chronic hepatitis B patients with prior lamivudine resistance. J Viral Hepat. 2011;18:e475–81.
18. Lee JM, Kim HJ, Park JY, Lee CK, Kim DY, Kim JK, et al. Rescue monotherapy in lamivudine-resistant hepatitis B e antigen-positive chronic hepatitis B: adefovir versus entecavir. Antivir Ther. 2009;14:705–12.
19. Murat K, Fatma S, Yesim A, Nail O, Ahmet TE, Deniz S. Head-to-head comparison of two years efficacy of entecavir and tenofovir in patients with treatment-naïve chronic hepatitis B-The real life data. Hepatogastroenterology. 2015;62:982–6.
20. Ha NB, Trinh HN, Rosenblatt L, Nghiem D, Nguyen MH. Treatment outcomes with first-line therapies with entecavir and tenofovir in treatment-naive chronic hepatitis B patients in a routine clinical practice. J Clin Gastroenterol. 2016;50:169–74.
21. Idilman R, Gunsar F, Koruk M, Keskin O, Meral CE, Gulsen M, et al. Long-term entecavir or tenofovir disoproxil fumarate therapy in treatment-naïve chronic hepatitis B patients in the real-world setting. J Viral Hepat. 2015;22:504–10.
22. Batirel A, Guclu E, Arslan F, Kocak F, Karabay O, Ozer S, et al. Comparable efficacy of tenofovir versus entecavir and predictors of response in treatment-naïve patients with chronic hepatitis B: a multicenter real-life study. Int J Infect Dis. 2014;28:153–9.
23. Ozaras R, Mete B, Ceylan B, Ozgunes N, Gunduz A, Karaosmanoglu H, et al. First-line monotherapies of tenofovir and entecavir have comparable efficacies in hepatitis B treatment. Eur J Gastroenterol Hepatol. 2014;26:774–80.
24. Gao L, Trinh HN, Li J, Nguyen MH. Tenofovir is superior to entecavir for achieving complete viral suppression in HBeAg-positive chronic hepatitis B patients with high HBV DNA. Aliment Pharmacol Ther. 2014;39:629–37.
25. Doğan ÜB, Kara B, Gümürdülü Y, Soylu A, Akin MS. Comparison of the efficacy of tenofovir and entecavir for the treatment of nucleos(t)ide-naive patients with chronic hepatitis B. Turk J Gastroenterol. 2012;23:247–52.
26. López Centeno B, Collado Borrell R, Pérez Encinas M, Gutiérrez García ML, Sanmartin FP. Comparison of the effectiveness and renal safety of tenofovir versus entecavir in patients with chronic hepatitis B. Farm Hosp. 2016;40:279–86.
27. Hongthanakorn C, Chotiyaputta W, Oberhelman K, Fontana RJ, Marrero JA, Licari T, et al. Virological breakthrough and resistance in patients with chronic hepatitis B receiving nucleos(t)ide analogues in clinical practice. Hepatology. 2011;53:1854–63.
28. Sogni P, Carrieri MP, Fontaine H, Mallet V, Vallet-Pichard A, Trabut JB, et al. The role of adherence in virological suppression in patients receiving anti-HBV analogues. Antivir Ther. 2012;17:395–400.
29. Chotiyaputta W, Hongthanakorn C, Oberhelman K, Fontana RJ, Licari T, Lok AS. Adherence to nucleos(t)ide analogues for chronic hepatitis B in clinical practice and correlation with virological breakthroughs. J Viral Hepat. 2012;19:205–12.
30. Kamezaki H, Kanda T, Arai M, Wu S, Nakamoto S, Chiba T, et al. Adherence to medication is a more important contributor to viral breakthrough in chronic hepatitis B patients treated with entecavir than in those with Lamivudine. Int J Med Sci. 2013;10:567–74.
31. Chien RN, Peng CY, Kao JH, Hu TH, Lin CC, Hu CT, et al. Higher adherence with 3-year entecavir treatment than lamivudine or telbivudine in treatment-naive Taiwanese patients with chronic hepatitis B. J Gastroenterol Hepatol. 2014;29:185–92.
32. Sriprayoon T, Mahidol C, Ungtrakul T, Chun-On P, Soonklang K, Pongpun W, et al. Efficay and safety of entecavir versus tenofovir treatment in chronic hepatitis B patients: A randomized controlled trial. Hepatol Res. 2016. doi: 10.1111/hepr.12743.

7

Telbivudine treatment started in early and middle pregnancy completely blocks HBV vertical transmission

Weihui Sun[1*], Shangfei Zhao[2], Lei Ma[1], Anhua Hao[1], Bo Zhao[1], Lin Zhou[1], Fengzhu Li[1] and Mingquan Song[2]

Abstract

Background: To evaluate the efficacy and safety of treating HBV-positive mothers with telbivudine in early and middle pregnancy to prevent mother-to-infant HBV transmission.

Methods: The subject population comprised pregnant women with chronic hepatitis B (CHB; $n = 188$) from January 2013 to June 2015, with HBV DNA $\geq 1.0 \times 10^7$copies/mL and increased alanine aminotransferase levels. Groups A ($n = 62$) and B ($n = 61$) were treated with telbivudine starting at 12 weeks or 20–28 weeks after gestation, respectively. Telbivudine was discontinued at postpartum 12 weeks. Group C ($n = 65$) received no antiviral. All infants were vaccinated with hepatitis B immunoglobulin (200 IU) and HBV vaccine (20 with hepatitis B The maternal HBV DNA levels of the groups were compared. Mother-to-infant transmission of HBV was indicated by the presence of HBsAg in infants 7 months after birth.

Results: Before treatment, the HBV DNA levels of the 3 groups were similar. Before delivery and 12 weeks after delivery, the HBV DNA levels of groups A and B were similar, but both were significantly lower than that of group C ($P < 0.01$, all). No infants in groups A and B were HBsAg-positive, but the infection rate of group C was 18.4% ($P < 0.01$). The HBV infection rate of infants was positively associated with the HBV DNA levels of the pregnant mothers.

Conclusion: Administration of telbivudine to HBV-infected mothers, started during early and middle pregnancy, completely blocked mother-to-infant HBV transmission.

Keywords: Telbivudine, Hepatitis B virus, Mother-to-infant transmission, Fetus safety, Drug efficacy

Background

Chronic hepatitis B virus (HBV) infection is a serious health problem in many parts of the world. Persistent HBV infection can cause chronic liver injury that may advance to cirrhosis and hepatocellular carcinoma [1].

In regions where HBV infection is endemic, the main transmission route is mother to infant, and may be intrauterine, perinatal, or lactational [2]. Although passive and active immunoprophylaxis is widely implemented at birth (i.e., hepatitis B immunoglobulin and HBC vaccine), HBV transmission still occurs in 5% to 10% of immunized infants [3]. A risk factor for immunization failure is high maternal HBV load [4]. Therefore, antiviral therapy to reduce maternal HBV DNA levels during pregnancy has been employed to block mother-to-infant transmission.

Telbivudine is a synthetic thymidine nucleoside analogue that is approved as a pregnancy category B medicine for treating chronic hepatitis B [4, 5]. Many studies have reported that telbivudine administrated during the second and third trimester of pregnancy is highly safe for effectively interrupting mother-to-infant HBV transmission [6, 7]. However, the efficacy and safety of telbivudine treatment in early pregnancy has not been adequately investigated.

To identify effective approaches for preventing mother-to-infant transmission of HBV, the present study evaluated the efficacy and safety of telbivudine, begun in

* Correspondence: qdscyrmyy@sina.com
[1]Department of Hepatology, Chengyang People's Hospital of Qingdao, Qingdao 266109, Shandong Province, China

early and middle pregnancy, for treating HBV-positive pregnant women.

Methods

Patients

The Institutional Review Board of Qingdao Municipal Hospital had approved the study. Pregnant women (n = 188) at Chengyang People's Hospital of Qingdao, China from January 2013 to June 2015 who met the following inclusion criteria were enrolled on a voluntary basis: 20 to 35 years old; 12 weeks or 20–28 weeks gestation; HBsAg- and HBeAg-positive, and HBV DNA $\geq 1.0 \times 10^7$ copies/mL; elevated alanine aminotransferase (ALT), 40 to 400 U/L.

Criteria for exclusion were: received previous treatment with interferon or nucleos(t)ide analogs, coinfection with hepatitis A, C, D, or E virus, human immunodeficiency virus, rubella virus, cytomegalovirus, or simple herpes virus, syphilis, or *Toxoplasma gondii*; other antiviral drug medication, immunosuppressive or cytotoxic drugs, or corticosteroids during pregnancy; fetal deformity indicated by ultrasound examination; genetic disease; gestational diabetes or severe respiratory, urinary, or neurological co-morbidity or severe gastrointestinal diseases which may affect drug absorption.

Grouping and management

The women were allocated to 3 groups, A ($n = 62$), B ($n = 61$), and C ($n = 65$). In groups A and B, the women were at 12 weeks and 20 to 28 weeks of gestation, respectively; and all were given oral telbivudine 600 mg daily beginning immediately after the enrollment until week 12 postpartum. Group C received no antiviral therapy. All the women received glycyrrhizin to protect the liver. Maternal blood samples were collected before treatment, prior to delivery, and at postpartum 12 weeks to detect HBV DNA and ALT levels.

All infants born to the enrolled women were vaccinated with 200 IU of hepatitis B immunoglobulin within 6 h and at 30 days after birth, and 20 μg of hepatitis B vaccine within 12 h after birth, and at postpartum 4 and 24 weeks. The following infant data was collected at birth: height, weight, chest, and head circumference, 1-min Apgar score, and birth defects (the presence of any deformities). In addition, adverse pregnancy events (e.g., eclampsia, premature rupture of membranes, and premature delivery), postpartum hemorrhage, and cesarean section were recorded. Serum HBV DNA and HBsAg in infants were tested at week 28 postpartum.

Statistical analyses

The data were analyzed using software SPSS 17.0. The chi-squared test was applied to compare categorical variables among groups. Continuous variables are presented as mean ± standard deviation. Differences among groups were compared with ANOVA test. $P < 0.05$ was considered statistically significant. The statistical analyses were performed by Li-Ping Su, Department Of Education, Chengyang People's Hospital of Qingdao.

Results

Pregnancy characteristics

Groups A, B, and C were statistically similar with regard to age, infection duration, gravidity, delivery time, and gestational age at delivery (Table 1).

Serum HBV DNA levels before and after treatment

Before treatment with telbivudine, the serum HBV DNA levels of the 3 groups were statistically similar (Table 2). Before delivery, the serum HBV DNA levels of groups A and B were significantly lower than that of group C ($P < 0.01$, both). At week 12 postpartum, the differences in HBV DNA levels between groups A and C, and between groups B and C, were significantly different ($P < 0.01$; $P < 0.01$). There were no significant differences in HBV DNA levels between groups A and B before delivery or at 12 weeks postpartum ($P = 0.934$ and $P = 0.923$, respectively).

ALT levels

Before treatment with telbivudine, there were no significant differences in ALT levels among groups A, B, and C ($P > 0.05$; Table 2). The differences between A and C, and between B and C were statistically significant before delivery ($P < 0.01$; $P < 0.01$), as well at week 12 postpartum ($P < 0.01$; $P < 0.01$). There were no significant differences in ALT levels between groups A and B before delivery or at postpartum 12 weeks ($P = 0.104$ and $P = 0.488$, respectively).

Table 1 Pregnancy characteristics and safety rates of the 3 groups

	Group A	Group B	Group C	P
Subjects, n	62	61	65	-
Age, y	28.9 ± 11.8	29.7 ± 9.8	27.5 ± 12.9	0.559
Infection duration, y	15.3 ± 10.9	16.1 ± 9.9	15.7 ± 11.5	0.919
Gravidity, n	1.8 ± 1.2	1.8 ± 1.1	1.8 ± 1.3	0.369
Delivery, n	1.1 ± 0.2	1.1 ± 0.1	1.1 ± 0.4	0.369
Gestational age, wk	39.0 ± 1.0	39.3 ± 1.2	39.2 ± 1.1	0.308
Adverse pregnancy, %	12.9(8/62)	11.4(7/61)	13.8(9/65)	0.923
Postparum hemorrhage, %	17.7(11/62)	14.7(9/61)	18.4(12/65)	0.844
Cesarean section, %	19.3(12/62)	16.4(10/61)	20.0(13/65)	0.859

Table 2 Average HBV DNA and ALT levels before and after treatment

	Group A	Group B	Group C	P
Sujects, n	62	61	65	
HBV DNA viral load, log_{10} copies/ml				
Before treatment	7.79 ± 0.22	7.75 ± 0.19	7.74 ± 0.22	0.373
Before delivery	0.51 ± 1.44	0.49 ± 1.26	7.64 ± 0.24	<0.001
Postpartum 12 weeks	0.38 ± 1.12	0.35 ± 1.28	7.85 ± 0.27	<0.001
ALT levels, IU/mL				
Before treatment	125.3 ± 57.6	132.3 ± 52.9	128.5 ± 48.7	0.766
Before delivery	63.8 ± 15.6	59.5 ± 13.4	112.7 ± 24.1	<0.001
Postpartum 12 weeks	48.9 ± 18.2	51.3 ± 20.1	84.1 ± 32.5	<0.001

Infant HBV infection rate at week 28 postpartum

The HBsAg positivity rates of infants in groups A, B, C at postpartum 28 weeks was 0%, 0%, and 18.4%, respectively (Table 3). The differences in HBV infection rate between groups A and C and between groups B and C were statistically significant ($P < 0.01$ and $P < 0.01$, respectively). The HBV DNA level of infants with HBsAg(+) was 6.04 ± 0.15 log copies/mL.

Safety profile of telbivudine administrated during pregnancy

There were no significant differences in neonatal gestational age, body weight, height, head circumference, or Apgar score among the infants born to mothers in the 3 groups (Table 3). Among the 3 groups, there were no significant differences in the incidence of adverse pregnancy events (including eclampsia, premature rupture of membranes, premature birth), or in the rates of postpartum hemorrhage or cesarean section (Table 1). Among the patients enrolled, there were no virologic resistance found assessed by evaluating genotypic changes using HBV polymerase/reverse transcriptase assay, with absence of genotypic resistance in the telbivudine treatment.

Table 3 General conditions and HBV infection of infants in the 3 groups

	Group A	Group B	Group C	P
Sujects, n	62	61	65	
Gestational age, wk	39.1 ± 1.1	39.2 ± 1.2	39.0 ± 1.1	0.613
Weight, g	3465.78 ± 408.5	3475.4 ± 398.4	3468.6 ± 401.3	0.991
Length, cm	50.4 ± 1.1	50.5 ± 1.3	50.6 ± 1.4	0.677
Head circumference, cm	33.5 ± 1.2	33.7 ± 1.1	33.3 ± 1.3	0.179
Apgar score	9.95 ± 0.2	9.97 ± 0.17	9.98 ± 0.18	0.648
HBV infection, n(%)	0	0	12(18.4)	<0.001

Discussion

In this study, we treated HBeAg-positive pregnant women with telbivudine beginning at 12 weeks or 20–28 weeks gestation until 28 weeks postpartum. All infants born to telbivudine-treated mothers were HBV-infection free, while the HBV infection rate of infants born to untreated mothers was 18.4%. Early treatment of HBV-positive pregnant women with telbivudine was effective and safe.

Chronic HBV infection in the Chinese general population is ~7.2% [8], and a significant portion of HBV-infected individuals are fertile women. The main route of HBV transmission is from mother to infant, and can occur during pregnancy or lactation. Combined passive and active immunization is unable to block completely this vertical HBV transmission. The reported mother-to-infant transmission rate can be as high as 15% [4], and was 18.4% in untreated pregnant women in the present study. This is consistent with the latest paper published in *N Engl J Med* by Pan et al. [9], the mother-to-infant transmission rate of the control group is 18%. The high mother-to-infant transmission rate was positively associated with serum HBV DNA levels in pregnant women prior to delivery [10]. This highlights the challenge of completely protecting infants from HBV infection.

Intrauterine transmission is an important cause for immunization failure, but the mechanisms for intrauterine infection are unclear. Viral, placental, and genetic factors, as well peripheral mononuclear cells are likely involved in intrauterine transmission. In early pregnancy, HBV can directly infect the fetus because the placental barrier has not formed. Even after formation of the placenta, abnormal pregnancy events such as maternal systemic toxemia can damage the placental barrier, leading to intrauterine HBV infection in early pregnancy [11].

As reported by Zou et al. [10], the HBV mother-to-infant transmission rate was positively associated with serum HBV DNA levels in pregnant women prior to delivery. If the HBV DNA load was effectively reduced during pregnancy, the intrauterine infection rate decreased [10]. In addition, pregnant women with active HBV replication may experience a flare-up of liver injury that can endanger the lives of both mother and fetus [12]. These circumstances support the antiviral treatment of HBV-positive women. We reasoned that earlier treatment may be more effective for blocking intrauterine HBV infection.

Telbivudine is an approved L-nucleoside drug for treating chronic HBV infection. Structurally, it is similar to lamivudine. Several studies have reported that telbivudine can effectively block mother-to-infant transmission in late pregnancy, with good tolerance and safety [6, 7, 13]. However, the efficacy and safety of telbivudine in treating HBV-positive women during early pregnancy has not been established. To our knowledge, our present study is the first report concerning early treatment of pregnant women with telbivudine. Consistent with our previous study [14], administration of telbivudine during early and middle pregnancy can reduce the rate of mother-to-infant transmission. Telbivudine treatment was also associated with normalized ALT, once HBV replication was at a low level, and an improved liver function fully supports successful pregnancy and delivery.

We found that the HBV DNA load of pregnant women prior to delivery and the HBsAg-positive rate of infants at 28 weeks postpartum were positively associated. In our study, the rate of vertical transmission in groups A and B was 0%, suggesting that telbivudine treatment was 100% effective in blocking HBV infection. There was no difference in the efficacy of telbivudine between groups A and B. This indicates that telbivudine treatment begun during middle pregnancy can be as effective as that started during early pregnancy. Because of the relatively small sample size in this study, our findings need to be verified in large cohorts.

Telbivudine is a pregnancy category B medication, and in preclinical studies showed no significant carcinogenic or teratogenic effects, nor organ, mitochondrial, or embryo-fetal toxicity. Furthermore, telbivudine inhibits viral DNA replication without affecting cellular DNA synthesis [15–17]. Some studies recommend initiating oral nucleoside analog therapy during the second or third trimester of pregnancy [18, 19]. Development of the vital organs of a fetus is essentially completed within the first 15 to 16 weeks of gestation [6]. Many studies have reported a safe profile for telbivudine used in the second and third trimester of pregnancy [6, 7]. Liu et al. [20] found that telbivudine used throughout pregnancy did not increase congenital malformations, indicated that its use was safe during early pregnancy. In the present study, we found no congenital deformity, severe adverse events, or complications in infants born to mothers who received telbivudine during early and middle pregnancy. Our findings further support the safe profile of telbivudine for pregnant women and their fetuses and infants.

The experience of drug related viral resistance is an important incident in anti-HBV treatment. Study have recognized that resistance may result in primary non-response or virologic breakthrough on therapy [21]. In addition, Nucleos(tide) analogs-related HBV resistance is associated with prior treatment with Nucleos(tide) analogs or treatment-naïve patients with high viral load [22]. A genotypic resistance test was performed in our included patients and data indicated that no patients enrolled developed with viral resistance. this may be because the limited period of antiviral treatment. All the patients stop antiviral treatment at 12 weeks after delivery. Study had reported that there were about 5% patients developing telbivudine related viral resistance during first year of treatment [23]. Therefore, whether or not to continue telbivudine treatment after delivery requires careful consideration.. Tenofovir is another pregnancy category B medication with high barrier of resistance [23]. Change from telbivudine with tenofovir after delivery if patients need prolong antiviral treatment may be a good clinical decision. However, there are still lack of evidence of safety data of tenofovir during lactation. Lamivudine is a well-tolerated anti-HBV Nucleoside analogues. It is effective in HBV suppression, ALT normalization and histologic improvement. However, viral breakthrough and drug resistance may occur after a long time LAM therapy with rtM204I/V ± rtL180M [24, 25]. HBV with substitutions rtM204I/V ± rtL180M has cross-resistance to telbivudine [21]. Patients with prior lamivudine exposure may not suitable use telbivudine treatment to blocks HBV vertical transmission. Although in our study, all patients included were treatment-naïve patients without potential lamivudine exposure and no patients found that experienced with telbivudine resistance during pregnancy. It still need to be concern the effective intervention to blocks HBV vertical transmission among CHB patients with potential prior lamivudine exposure or development of telbivudine resistance mutations during pregnancy. Tenofovir, the pregnancy category B nucleotide analogue that effective for both HBV and HIV, has shown to have superior HBV DNA suppression. Tenofovir is highly effective in the treatment of patients with rtM204I/V ± rtL180M HBV substitutions [21]. For blocks HBV vertical transmission among CHB patients with potential prior lamivudine exposure or development of telbivudine resistance mutations during pregnancy, initial tenofovir treatment or switch to tenofovir after telbivudine resistance may be a proper medical intervention. However, more clinical evidences are needed.

This study has a few limitations. Firstly, the sample size was relatively small, with only 188 subjects. Secondly, it was a single-center study, which requires verification in multi-center based investigations. Thirdly, we only studied the short-term safety of telbivudine for infants and a long-term follow-up is needed.

Conclusions

Telbivudine administrated during early and middle pregnancy can completely block HBV mother-to-infant transmission. Early telbivudine treatment is safe for both pregnant mothers and their infants up to at least 28 weeks postpartum.

Abbreviations

ALT: Alanine aminotransferase; CHB: Chronic hepatitis B; HBV: Hepatitis B virus

Acknowledgements
We thank Li-Ping Su, Department Of Education, Chengyang People's Hospital of Qingdao, for the contribution to statistical analyses. We are grateful to the doctors and nurses working in Chengyang People's Hospital of Qingdao, China for the help in conducting of this study.

Funding
None.

Authors' contributions
SWH, SMQ, and ZSF designed the research; ZL, ML, HAH, ZB, and LFZ performed the research; SWH and SMQ analyzed the data; ML and ZL checked accuracy of the data; and SWH, SMQ, and ZSF wrote the paper. All authors read and approved the final manuscript.

Competing interests
The authors declare that they have no competing interests.

Consent for publication
Not applicable.

Author details
[1]Department of Hepatology, Chengyang People's Hospital of Qingdao, Qingdao 266109, Shandong Province, China. [2]Department of Gastroenterology, The Affiliated Hospital of Qingdao University, Qingdao 266011, Shandong Province, China.

References

1. Ma L, Alla NR, Li X, Mynbaev OA, Shi Z. Mother-to-child transmission of HBV: review of current clinical management and prevention strategies. Rev Med Virol. 2014;24:396–406.
2. Pan CQ, Duan ZP, Bhamidimarri KR, Zou HB, Liang XF, Li J, et al. An algorithm for risk assessment and intervention of mother to child transmission of hepatitis B virus. Clin Gastroenterol Hepatol. 2012;10:452–9.
3. Guo Z, Shi XH, Feng YL, Wang B, Feng LP, Wang SP, et al. Risk factors of HBV intrauterine transmission among HBsAg-positive pregnant women. J Viral Hepat. 2013;20:317–21.
4. Yin Y, Wu L, Zhang J, Zhou J, Zhang P, Hou H. Identification of risk factors associated with immunoprophylaxis failure to prevent the vertical transmission of hepatitis B virus. J Infect. 2013;66:447–52.
5. Hoofnagle JH, Doo E, Liang TJ, Fleischer R, Lok AS. Management of hepatitis B: summary of a clinical research workshop. Hepatology. 2007;45:1056–75.
6. Han GR, Cao MK, Zhao W, Jiang HX, Wang CM, Bai SF, et al. A prospective and open-label study for the efficacy and safety of telbivudine in pregnancy for the prevention of perinatal transmission of hepatitis B virus infection. J Hepatol. 2011;55:1215–21.
7. Pan CQ, Han GR, Jiang HX, Zhao W, Cao MK, Wang CM, et al. Telbivudine prevents vertical transmission from HBeAg-positive women with chronic hepatitis B. Clin Gastroenterol Hepatol. 2012;10:520–6.
8. Liang X, Bi S, Yang W, Wang L, Cui G, Cui F, et al. Epidemiological serosurvey of hepatitis B in China–declining HBV prevalence due to hepatitis B vaccination. Vaccine. 2009;27:6550–7.
9. Pan CQ, Duan Z, Dai E, Zhang S, Han G, Wang Y, et al. Tenofovir to prevent Hepatitis B transmission in mothers with high viral load. N Engl J Med. 2016;374:2324–34.
10. Zou H, Chen Y, Duan Z, Zhang H, Pan C. Virologic factors associated with failure to passive-active immunoprophylaxis in infants born to HBsAg-positive mothers. J Viral Hepat. 2012;19:e18–25.
11. Bai GQ, Li SH, Yue YF, Shi L. The study on role of peripheral blood mononuclear cell in HBV intrauterine infection. Arch Gynecol Obstet. 2011;283:317–21.
12. Sinha S, Kumar M. Pregnancy and chronic hepatitis B virus infection. Hepatol Res. 2010;40:31–48.
13. Deng Y, Wu W, Zhang D, Hu P, Kang J, Yang Y, et al. The safety of telbivudine in preventing mother-to-infant transmission of hepatitis B virus in pregnant women after discontinuation. Zhonghua Gan Zang Bing Za Zhi. 2015;23:586–9.
14. Sun W, Ma L, Hao A, Liu W, Song M, Li M, et al. Predictive value of telbivudine in preventing mother-to-infant transmission of hepatitis B virus in pregnant women with high viremia. Zhonghua Gan Zang Bing Za Zhi. 2015;23:180–3.
15. Liaw YF, Gane E, Leung N, Zeuzem S, Wang Y, Lai CL, et al. 2-Year GLOBE trial results: telbivudine Is superior to lamivudine in patients with chronic hepatitis B. Gastroenterology. 2009;136:486–95.
16. Dienstag J, Easley C, Kirkpatrick P. Telbivudine. Nat Rev Drug Discov. 2007;6:267–8.
17. Ruiz-Sancho A, Sheldon J, Soriano V. Telbivudine: a new option for the treatment of chronic hepatitis B. Expert Opin Biol Ther. 2007;7:751–61.
18. Keeffe EB, Dieterich DT, Han SH, Jacobson IM, Martin P, Schiff ER, et al. A treatment algorithm for the management of chronic hepatitis B virus infection in the United States: 2008 update. Clin Gastroenterol Hepatol. 2008;6:1315–41. quiz 1286.
19. Liaw YF, Leung N, Kao JH, Piratvisuth T, Gane E, Han KH, et al. Asian-Pacific consensus statement on the management of chronic hepatitis B: a 2008 update. Hepatol Int. 2008;2:263–83.
20. Liu M, Cai H, Yi W. Safety of telbivudine treatment for chronic hepatitis B for the entire pregnancy. J Viral Hepat. 2013;20 Suppl 1:65–70.
21. Zoulim F, Locarnini S. Management of treatment failure in chronic hepatitis B. J Hepatol. 2012;56 Suppl 1:S112–22.
22. Cai S, Yu T, Jiang Y, Zhang Y, Lv F, Peng J. Comparison of entecavir monotherapy and de novo lamivudine and adefovir combination therapy in HBeAg-positive chronic hepatitis B with high viral load: 48-week result. Clin Exp Med. 2016;16:429–36.
23. Liaw YF, Kao JH, Piratvisuth T, Chan HL, Chien RN, Liu CJ, et al. Asian-Pacific consensus statement on the management of chronic hepatitis B: a 2012 update. Hepatol Int. 2012;6:531–61.
24. Zeng J, Cai S, Liu J, Xue X, Wu X, Zheng C. Dynamic changes in liver stiffness measured by transient elastography predict clinical outcomes among patients with chronic Hepatitis B. J Ultrasound Med. 2017;36:261–8.
25. Cai SH, Lv FF, Zhang YH, Jiang YG, Peng J. Dynamic comparison between Daan real-time PCR and Cobas TaqMan for quantification of HBV DNA levels in patients with CHB. BMC Infect Dis. 2014;14:85.

8

Accuracy of M2BPGi, compared with Fibro Scan®, in analysis of liver fibrosis in patients with hepatitis C

Hongqin Xu[1,3†], Wenli Kong[1†], Lei Liu[1], Xiumei Chi[1,3], Xiaomei Wang[1,3], Ruihong Wu[1,3], Xiuzhu Gao[1,3], Huan Wang[1], Limei Qu[4], Yue Qi[1], Yu Pan[1*†] and Junqi Niu[1,2,3*†]

Abstract

Background: Mac-2 Binding Protein Glycosylation isomer (M2BPGi) is a novel serological glyco-biomarker for staging liver fibrosis. Here, we aimed to evaluate the efficiency of serum M2BPGi in identifying liver fibrosis stages in Chinese patients with chronic hepatitis C infection.

Methods: Serum M2BPGi levels were evaluated in 680 patients with chronic hepatitis C and 164 healthy controls who underwent the Fibro Scan® test of liver fibrosis. The diagnostic accuracy of serum M2BPGi values was compared to that of other fibrosis markers, including Fibro Scan®, the aspartate transaminase to platelet ratio index (APRI), the fibrosis index based on four factors (FIB4), and the gamma-glutamyltranspeptidase to platelet ratio (GPR).

Results: Among the chronic hepatitis C patients, the median serum M2BPGi level increased with increasing fibrosis score as follows: 0.88 (≤F2), 1.70 (F2/F3), and 5.68 (cirrhosis). M2BPGi concentrations could also distinguish between healthy controls (0.38 ± 0.24) and hepatitis C patients (1.57 ± 2.28). After adjusting for potential confounders, M2BPGi was the most significant factor associated with the liver stiffness measurement (effect size = 0.275, $P < 0.001$). The optimum cutoff values of serum M2BPGi for patients with F2 and F4 were 0.945 and 1.355, respectively. The area under the curve of serum M2BPGi for prediction of significant fibrosis (F ≥ 4) using was comparable to that of APRI (0.892 vs. 0.873), while it was superior to that of other alternative markers, including FIB4 (0.818) and GPR (0.851). Compared with other non-invasive markers, M2BPGi had the greatest specificity for diagnosing cirrhosis and cirrhosis in hepatitis C patients.

Conclusions: Our results suggest that the level of serum M2BPGi would be a simple and reliable diagnostic tool for identifying liver fibrosis stage in Chinese patients with chronic hepatitis.

Keywords: Chronic hepatitis C, Liver fibrosis, Mac-2 Binding Protein Glycosylation isomer, Cirrhosis

Background

Hepatitis C virus (HCV) is a major cause of liver disease worldwide. HCV establishes persistent infection that often results in chronic hepatitis followed by liver fibrosis, cirrhosis, from which hepatocellular carcinoma arises. The stage of chronic liver disease is mainly evaluated based on the degree of liver fibrosis. Therefore, assessment of the degree of liver fibrosis is important in clinical practice. Liver biopsy is the gold standard method for evaluating the degree of liver fibrosis [1]. However, the invasiveness nature of liver biopsy makes it un-practical approach, especially for patients who require follow-up [2].

Recently, glycoprotein-based biomarkers (glyco-biomarker) have been emerged as novel disease biomarkers. Mac-2 Binding Protein Glycosylation isomer (M2BPGi), which is also named hyperglycosylated Wisteria floribunda agglutinin-positive Mac-2 binding protein (WFA+ -M2BP) is a new serological glyco-biomarker that has been recently developed for predicting the stage of liver fibrosis [3, 4]. This technical approach may be applicable to the development pipeline for a wide variety of glyco diagnostic tools.

* Correspondence: yupan20000@163.com; junqiniu@aliyun.com
†Equal contributors
[1]Department of Hepatology, First Hospital of Jilin University, Jilin University, Changchun 130021, China

Developed in France by Echosens, transient elastography (Fibro Scan®) is a novel, noninvasive technique that is used to assess the degree of liver fibrosis. The Vibration Controlled Transient Elastography™ system (VCTE™) implemented on the Fibro Scan®[5] is the most validated and commonly used elastography method worldwide and has been approved in China by the China Food and Drug Administration [6, 7]. Data suggest VCTE™ is reliable in diagnosing cirrhosis in patients with chronic liver disease [8], liver fibrosis in autoimmune hepatitis [9] advanced fibrosis in patients with alcoholic liver disease [10], significant fibrosis in patients with chronic hepatitis C [11], and in biliary diseases [12]. In recent years, the liver stiffness measurement (LSM) which is resulting from transient elastography has been applied to predict liver fibrosis in many hospitals in China [13, 14].

This study aimed to (1) identify optimal serum M2BPGi cut-off values for evaluating the stage of liver fibrosis in Chinese patients with chronic hepatitis C, (2) identify the factors independently associated with M2BPGi, and (3) compare the diagnostic value of M2BPGi versus the fibrosis biomarkers aspartate transaminase to platelet ratio index (APRI), fibrosis index based on four factors (FIB-4), and gamma-glutamyltrans peptidase to platelet ratio (GPR).

Methods

Patients

We retrospectively reviewed 1001 hepatitis C patients and 164 healthy controls who underwent Fibro Scan® testing and color Doppler ultrasound at The First Hospital of Jilin University (Changchun, China). Of these, 321 patients who had fatty liver, which might influence the value of the Fibro Scan®, were excluded from the study. The study was approved by the Ethics Committee at the First Hospital of Jilin University, Changchun, China and the written informed consent was obtained from each patient enrolled in this study.

LSM

Fibro Scan® (Echosens, France) was performed by skillful operator to assess LSM value. Ten LSM values were recoreded and the median value calculated by the statistics analyze system was called as the final score. According to Tsochatzis [15] et al, the liver stiffness cut-offs were staged on a scale of 0–4 according to Fibro Scan® given as 7.6 (range 5.1–10.1), 10.9 (8.0–15.4), and 15.3 (11.9–26.5) kPa for stages F2, F3, and F4 in hepatitis C patients respectively.

Direct measurement of serum M2BPGi

Serum M2BPGi levels were quantified by a lectin-antibody sandwich immunoassay using HISCL-5000 immunoanalyzer (Sysmex Co., Hyogo, Japan) [4, 16]. M2BPGi values conjugated to WFA were indexed with scored values using the following equation: Cutoff index = ([M2BPGi] sample – [M2BPGi] NC)/([M2BPGi] PC –[M2BPGi] NC), where [M2BPGi] sample is the M2BPGi level in the serum sample, PC is the positive control, and NC is negative control. The positive control was supplied as a calibration solution preliminarily standardized to yield a cutoff value of 1.0.

Surrogate serum markers

On the same day that Fibro Scan® examination was performed, blood specimens were obtained and subjected to hematological and biochemical examinations. Hyaluronic acid level, type 4 collagen (CIV) level, laminin (LN) level, platelet count, aspartate aminotransferase (AST) level and alanine aminotransferase (ALT) level were determined in the same laboratory. APRI, FIB-4, and GPR scores were calculated based on the following formulae:

$$\text{APRI} = ([\text{AST}/\text{ULN}*]/\text{platelet count}) \times 100;$$

$$\text{FIB-4} = (\text{age} \times \text{AST})/(\text{platelet count} \times \sqrt{\text{ALT}});$$

GPR = GGT/platelet count, where GGT is γ-glutamyltransferase.

Statistical analysis

Differences between continuous variables of paired samples were analyzed using Mann-Whitney U test. Receiver operating characteristic (ROC) curve and area under the curve (AUCs) were used to determine the optimal liver stiffness cutoffs for fibrosis staging. The optimal liver stiffness cutoffs were determined based on the optimal sensitivity, specificity, positive predictive value (PPV), and negative predictive value (NPV). Statistical analysis of the differences between the AUCs was based on the theory of generalized U-statistics. The P <0.05 was considered significant.

Results

Baseline clinical characteristics of patients

The baseline clinical characteristics of enrolled patients are shown in Table 1. The median age was 54.9 years with a male predominance (68.4%) in the hepatitis C group, while the median age was 56.5 years with a female predominance (54.7%) in the control group. Two hundred ninety-one patients were treated with interferon (IFN) + ribavirin (RBV). The median (interquartile range, IQR) values for the body mass index (BMI), APRI, FIB-4 index, AST/ALT ratio, and GPR were 23.4 (21.5–25.5), 0.48 (0.32–1.01), 2.81 (1.87–4.65), 1.44 (1.07–2.69), and 0.18 (0.09–0.47), respectively, in the hepatitis C-infected group. The fibrosis stage was < F2 (LSM < 7.6) for 437 cases (64.3%), F2 or F3

Table 1 Patients' clinical characteristics and laboratory data

Features	Cases ($n = 680$)	Healthy ($n = 164$)	P value
Male/Female, n	465/215	76/88	
Age (years)	54.9 ± 11.0	56.8 ± 14.8	0.02
IFN therapy N (%)	291 (42.8%)	0 (0.00%)	
Habitual alcohol intake N (%)	275 (40.4%)		
Body mass index	23.6 ± 3.1	24.0 ± 3.1	0.114
Platelet count (×10^9/l)	166.7 ± 74.8	228.3 ± 45.1	<0.001
AST (15–46 IU/l)	49.2 ± 39.9	26.4 ± 10.2	<0.001
ALT (0–40 IU/l)	37.7 ± 43.8	23.7 ± 15.1	0.011
GGT (12–73 IU/l)	63.7 ± 105.3	27.2 ± 27.7	<0.001
AFP (0–6.2 IU/l)	7.46 ± 33.9		
HCV genotype N (%)			
1b	126 (18.5%)		
2a	94 (13.8%)		
1b/2a	2 (0.3%)		
Unknown	459 (67.4%)		
Fibrosis markers			
APRI	1.06 ± 2.72	0.30 ± 0.13	<0.001
FIB4	4.84 ± 12.05	1.33 ± 0.55	<0.001
AST/ALT ratio	2.62 ± 2.80	1.45 ± 1.43	<0.001
GPR	0.58 ± 1.21	0.12 ± 0.12	<0.001
M2BPGi	1.57 ± 2.28	0.38 ± 0.23	<0.001
Fibrosis stage (0 ~ 1/2 ~ 3/4)	437/175/68	155/9/0	

($7.6 \leq LSM < 15.3$) for 175 cases (25.7%), and F4 ($LSM > 15.3$) for 68 cases (10.0%). BMI, APRI, FIB-4 index, AST/ALT ratio, GPR, and M2BPGi level differed significantly between hepatitis C patients and healthy controls.

Correlation between M2BPGi and LSM in patients with HCV infection

Among chronic hepatitis C patients, the median level of serum M2BPGi was positively associated with fibrosis stage as 0.88 (<F2), 1.70 (F2/F3), and 5.68 (F4). As the median serum M2BPGi level was 0.38 in healthy controls, there was also a significant difference between healthy controls and hepatitis C patients ($P < 0.001$). Figure 1a shows a box-plot of liver fibrosis stage (LSM) vs. M2BPGi level. Moreover, significant differences were noted for M2BPGi level among the fibrosis stages. The differences were significant ($P < 0.001$) between healthy controls and chronic hepatitis C patients and between F2/3 and F4 stages ($P < 0.001$). Using Spearman rank correlation analysis, a positive correlation between LSM and M2BPGi level (rho = 0.504, $P < 0.001$) was observed (Fig. 1b).

Variables associated with LSM obtained by Fibro Scan®

Correlation between LSM and baseline demographic (age and gender), hematological and biochemical characteristics (platelet count, total protein, albumin, ALT, AST, alkaline phosphatase, γ-glutamyltransferase, bilirubin, FIB-4 index, APRI, AST/ALT ratio, and GPR) was also examined (Table 2). LSM was significantly correlated with ALT (rho = 403, $P < 0.001$), AST (rho = 0.499, $P < 0.001$), alkaline phosphatase (ALP; rho = 0.309, $P < 0.001$), GGT (rho = 0.432, $P < 0.001$), total bilirubin (rho = 0.274, $P < 0.001$), FIB-4 (rho = 0.412, $P < 0.001$), APRI (rho = 0.536, $P < 0.001$), and all histological results and was inversely correlated with platelet count (rho = -0.386, $P < 0.001$) and AST/ALT ratio (rho = -0.141, $P < 0.001$). Gender, age, cigarette smoking, platelet count, total protein, albumin, liver function markers (AST, ALT, ALP, GGT, TB, HA, LN, α-fetoprotein) and M2BPGi level were associated with LSM in univariate analysis. Subsequently these factors were entered in logistic regression multivariable analysis. This analysis identified platelet count (effect size = -0.07, $P \leq 0.05$),total protein level (effect size = -0.08, $P \leq 0.05$), ALP (effect size = 0.116, $P \leq 0.05$), GGT (effect size = 0.13, $P < 0.001$), total bilirubin (effect size = 0.111, $P = 0.001$), HA (effect size = 0.137, $P < 0.001$),

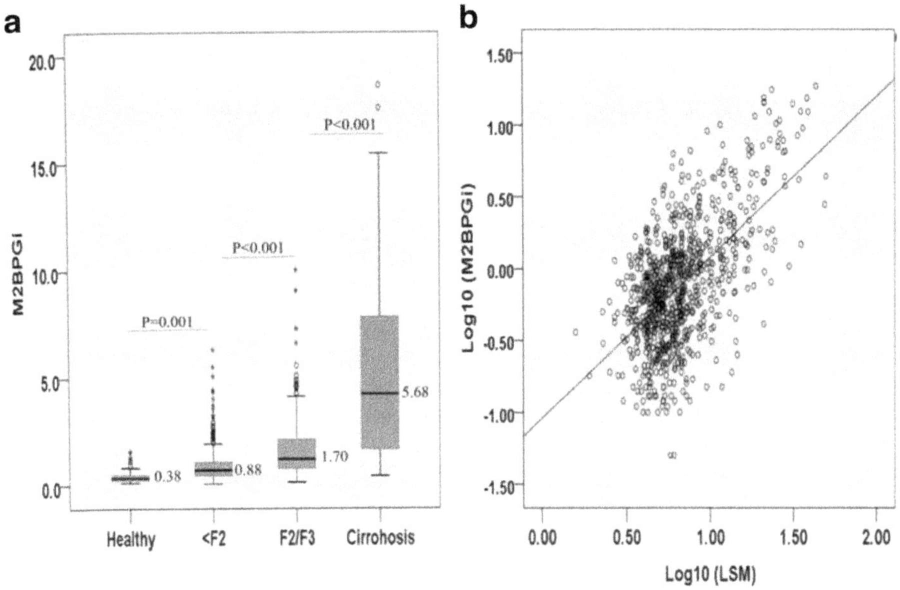

Fig. 1 a The serum Wisteria floribunda agglutinin-positive Mac-2 binding protein (M2BPGi) values for each fibrosis stage. The *top* and *bottom* of each *box* represent the first and third quartiles, respectively, with the height of the box representing the interquartile range, covering 50% of the values. The line across each box represents the median. The whiskers show the highest and lowest values. **b** Correlation of log10 (M2BPGi) values with log10 (LSM)

CIV (effect size = 0.099, P ≤ 0.05), AFP (effect size = 0.069, P ≤ 0.05), and M2BPGi (effect size = 0.275, $P < 0.001$) levels as independent factors that were significantly associated with LSM (Table 2). Notably, serum level of M2BPGi was the most significant factor associated with LSM.

Table 2 Variables associated with the LSM according to liner regression analyses

Characteristic	Correlation analysis		liner regression analysis	
	rho	*P* value	Effect size	*P* value
Age	0.188	<0.001	0.015	0.606
Gender	−0.099	0.01	−0.026	0.404
BMI	0.038	0.318	-	-
Laboratory findings				
Platelet count	−0.386	<0.001	−0.07	0.02
Total protein	0.194	<0.001	−0.08	0.032
Albumin	−0.18	<0.001	−0.071	0.073
ALT	0.403	<0.001	0.017	0.732
AST	0.499	<0.001	0.008	0.893
ALP	0.309	<0.001	0.116	0.001
GGT	0.432	<0.001	0.13	<0.001
Total Billirubin	0.274	<0.001	0.111	0.001
HA	0.338	<0.001	0.137	<0.001
LN	0.234	<0.001	0.03	0.38
CIV	0.34	<0.001	0.099	0.003
AFP	0.379	<0.001	0.069	0.033
Fibrosis markers				
FIB-4 indext	0.412	<0.001	-	-
APRI	0.536	<0.001	-	-
AST/ALT ratio	−0.141	<0.001	-	-
GPR	0.487	<0.001	-	-
M2BPGi	0.504	<0.001	0.275	<0.001

Comparison of AUCs and cut-off values for fibrosis markers

ROC analyses were carried out to evaluate the diagnostic accuracy of serum M2BPGi, FIB-4 index, APRI, and GPR for fibrosis stage in chronic hepatitis C. The calculated AUC, optimal cut-off value, sensitivity, specificity, PPV, and NPV for each fibrosis stage are listed in Table 3. The AUCs were 0.774 and 0.892 for ≥ F2 and F4, respectively. The optimal cut-off values predicted fibrosis stages ≥ F2 and F4 were 0.945 and 1.355, respectively.

The ROC curves for M2BPGi, FIB-4 index, APRI, and GPR for predicting severe fibrosis (≥F2) and cirrhosis (F4) are shown in Fig. 2a–b. The AUC of M2BPGi for predicting significant fibrosis (≥F2) was significantly greater than those for the FIB-4 index (AUC = 0.702, $P < 0.001$), and similar to those for GPR (AUC = 0.764, $P > 0.05$) and APRI (AUC = 0.787, $P > 0.05$). For estimating cirrhosis, the AUC for M2BPGi level (AUC = 0.892) was superior to those for the FIB-4 (AUC = 0.818, $P < 0.05$), but the differences were not significant and were comparable to that or the APRI (AUC = 0.873, $P = 0.598$) and GPR

Table 3 Diagnostic performance of M2BPGi in 680 patients with chronic hepatitis C

Fibrosis stage		Cutoff	AUC	Sensitivity	Specificity	*P* value
≥F2	M2BPGi	0.945	0.774 (0.736, 0.812)	0.745	0.694	Reference
	APRI	0.635	0.787 (0.750, 0.824)	0.708	0.799	>0.05
	FIB4	3.145	0.702 (0.661, 0.743)	0.650	0.686	<0.001
	GPR	0.221	0.764 (0.726, 0.801)	0.704	0.716	>0.05
≥F4	M2BPGi	1.355	0.892 (0.851, 0.933)	0.868	0.786	Reference
(Cirrhosis)	APRI	0.885	0.873 (0.835, 0.910)	0.838	0.783	>0.05
	FIB4	4.395	0.818 (0.768, 0.868)	0.750	0.775	<0.05
	GPR	0.291	0.851 (0.808, 0.894)	0.882	0.691	>0.05

(AUC = 0.851, *P* = 0.352). Overall, serum M2BPGi showed high reliability for the diagnosis of significant fibrosis and cirrhosis.

Discussion

Early detection and intervention are critical for successes in disease curability. In chronic hepatitis C infection, it is quite critical to screen the patients for the status of liver fibrosis because those with advance fibrosis are at greater risk of developing severe complications [17–19]. Although a liver biopsy is the gold standard for staging of liver fibrosis, its invasive nature restricts its application in the clinic, especially in follow up cases. Therefore, the field of non-invasive approaches for liver staging has been recently evolved [20–23]. In the present study, we found that the serum M2BPGi levels as a simple and reliable glyco-biomarker diagnostic tool for staging of liver fibrosis in chronic hepatitis C patients (Fig. 2). The glycan-based immunoassay was previously developed as a simple system for automatically detecting unique fibrosis-related glyco-alterations [24–27]. To the best of our knowledge, the present study is the first study to evaluate the efficiency of serum M2BPGi in prediction of liver fibrosis stage in a large population of Chinese patients with HCV infection.

This study clearly demonstrated that the M2BPGi level in chronic hepatitis C patients increased with the progression of liver fibrosis stage (Fig. 2). This result came in a good agreement with previous studies [28–30]. Moreover, M2BPGi concentrations could also distinguish between healthy controls and hepatitis C patients, and this result suggests that alterations in serum M2BPGi may forecast liver disease. We also showed that M2BPGi level is an independent factor significantly associated with liver fibrosis in hepatitis C patients. Several other variables have been proposed to contribute to liver fibrosis, such as platelet count, total protein, ALP, GGT, total billirubin, HA, CIV, and AFP in our study (Table 2).

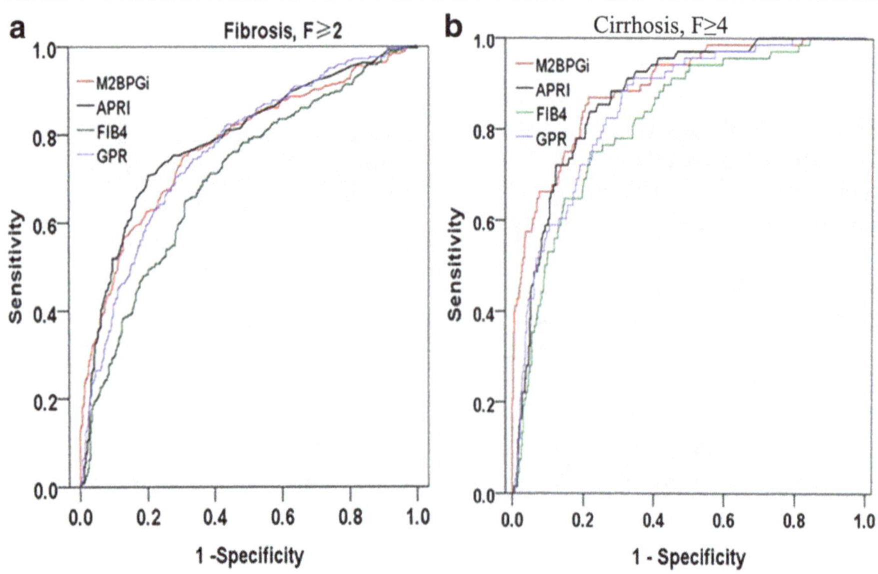

Fig. 2 The diagnostic capabilities of the M2BPGi values for assessing the stage of liver fibrosis. The AUCs for serum M2BPGi in diagnosing liver fibrosis were as follows: **a** 0.774 for stage ≥ F2; **b** 0.892 for stage ≥ F4

Interestingly, among nine variables, including M2BPGi level, platelet count, total protein, ALP, GGT, total billirubin, HA, CIV, and AFP, M2BPGi level was the most significant serum marker associated with LSM.

Studies have showed that several risk scores such as the APRI, FIB-4, and GPR, which are calculated using the above variables, appeared to be a good surrogate marker for predicting fibrosis stages. Additionally, our results also showed that the M2BPGi level was strongly associated with other noninvasive fibrosis markers. As the AUCs of previously reported fibrosis markers (APRI, FIB-4, and GPR) increased by the progression of liver fibrosis stage, the AUC of M2BPGi increased accordingly as well. It worth to note that serum level of M2BPGi showed higher efficiency in predicting liver fibrosis grade F ≥ 2 than other surrogate markers, such as the FIB-4 and GDR (Table 3). Taken together, this suggests that the M2BPGi assay would be a good serological marker for predicting and differentiating liver fibrosis stags, especially the early and significant fibrosis stages.

On the other hand, M2BPGi level was also efficient in predicting cirrhosis (LSM > 15.3) with an AUC of 0.892 at a cut-off of 1.355, which is consistent with previous studies. In a study that included 106 Japanese patients with hepatitis C, cut-off values of M2BP for four fibrosis stages (F1–F4) ranged from 1.0 to 2.64 [31]. In another Japanese study performed on 137 primary biliary cirrhosis patients, performances were better than ours, with AUCs for significant fibrosis, severe fibrosis, and cirrhosis of 0.979, 0.933, and 0.965, respectively, and the cut off values for M2BPGi in fibrosis stages > F1, >F2, >F3, and > F4 were 0.7, 1.0, 1.4, and 2.0, respectively [14]. In our study, M2BPGi did not perform well for classifying patients at the extremes of significant and severe fibrosis (F2–F3). The reason may be coursed that Fibro Scan® is less accurate for detecting significant fibrosis (F2–F3) compared with Castera L [32].

The range of the M2BPGi serum thresholds observed in chronic hepatitis C patientswas different from those described in primary biliary cirrhosis (PBC) or non-alcoholic fatty liver disease [14, 33], typeIautoimmune hepatitis [34], and hepatitis B (Matsumoto and Umemura, personal communications). This difference might be contributed to the difference in patients' ethnicity or due to the fact that the majority of our cohort was asymptomatic and exhibited mild fibrosis.

There are two main strengths of this study. First, relatively large sample size ($n = 680$) with well characterized baseline clinical characteristics. Second, in this study, we excluded patients who had fatty liver disease, which may have affected the Fibro Scan® value. On the other hand, the present study also has several limitations. First, we estimated the fibrosis stage using LSM and APRI or FIB4 in this study, while liver biopsy was not considered which could be a source of bias.

Conclusions

Our study suggests that the level of serum M2BPGi would be a simple and reliable diagnostic tool for identifying liver fibrosis stage in Chinese patients with chronic hepatitis.

Abbreviations

ALT: Alanine aminotransferase; anti-HBc: Antibody to hepatitis B core antigen; anti-HBsAg: Antibody to HBsAg; APRI: Aspartate transaminase to platelet ratio index; AST: aspartate aminotransferase; CI: Confidence interval; CIV: Type 4 collagen; ELISA: Enzyme-linked immunosorbent assay; FIB4: Fibrosis index based on four factors; GPR: Gamma-glutamyltranspeptidase to platelet ratio; HA: Hyaluronic acid; HBsAg: Hepatitis B surface antigen; HBV: Hepatitis B virus; HCV: Hepatitis C virus; IQR: Inter-quartile range; LN: Laminin; LSM: Liver stiffness measurement; M2BPGi: Mac-2 Binding Protein Glycosylation isomer; OR: Odds ratio; PBC: Primary biliary cirrhosis; RNA: Ribonucleic acid; VCTE: Vibration Controlled Transient Elastography™ system; WFA + -M2BP: Wisteria floribunda agglutinin-positive human Mac-2-binding AFP (α-fetoprotein)

Acknowledgement

We thank Sysmex Company who provide M2BPGi testing reagent in our study.

Funding

This work was sponsored by the National Science and Technology Major Project (2014ZX10002002), the National Basic Research Program of China (973 Program) (2015CB554304), the National Natural Science Foundation of China under Grant nos. 81373057, 81301472 and 81301415, the Jilin Province Science and Technology Development Plan (20160520158JH), the Chinese foundation for hepatitis prevention and control–WBE liver fibrosis foundation (CFHPC20131053) and the Sysmex Company.

Authors' contributions

HX, WK, XC, XW, RW and XG performed the laboratory testing for HCV, HBV, HIV, and M2BPGi in this study. HW, LQ & YQ conducted Fibro Scan® test and collected information on demographic variables (age, gender, and race). LL conducted Fibro Scan® test and performed ultrasound examination. HX performed statistical analyses and drafted the manuscript. JN and YP participated in the design of the study and applied for the funding. All authors have read and approved the final manuscript.

Competing interest

Sysmex Company provided reagents and fund which were paid for sample management and test in this study. Sysmex Company did not involve in designing, samples collection, sample test, data analysis and paper writing in this study. We also declare that we have no financial and personal relationships with other people or organizations that can inappropriately influence our work.

Consent for publication

Not applicable.

Author details
[1]Department of Hepatology, First Hospital of Jilin University, Jilin University, Changchun 130021, China. [2]Ministry of Education Key Laboratory of Zoonosis, Changchun 130061, China. [3]Jilin Province Key Laboratory of Infectious Diseases, Laboratory of Molecular Virology, Changchun 130061, China. [4]Department of Pathology, First Hospital of Jilin University, Jilin University, Changchun 130021, China.

References

1. Bravo AA, Sheth SG, Chopra S. Liver biopsy. N Engl J Med. 2001;344(7):495–500.
2. Bedossa P, Dargere D, Paradis V. Sampling variability of liver fibrosis in chronic hepatitis C. Hepatology. 2003;38(6):1449–57.
3. Yamada N, Sanada Y, Tashiro M, Hirata Y, Okada N, Ihara Y, et al. Serum Mac-2 binding protein glycosylation isomer predicts grade F4 liver fibrosis in patients with biliary atresia. J Gastroenterol. 2017;52(2):245–52.
4. Kuno A, Ikehara Y, Tanaka Y, Ito K, Matsuda A, Sekiya S, et al. A serum "sweet-doughnut" protein facilitates fibrosis evaluation and therapy assessment in patients with viral hepatitis. Sci Rep. 2013;3:1065.
5. Sandrin L, Fourquet B, Hasquenoph JM, Yon S, Fournier C, Mal F, et al. Transient elastography: a new noninvasive method for assessment of hepatic fibrosis. Ultrasound Med Biol. 2003;29(12):1705–13.
6. Bonder A, Afdhal N. Utilization of FibroScan in clinical practice. Curr Gastroenterol Rep. 2014;16(2):372.
7. Tapper EB, Castera L, Afdhal NH. FibroScan (vibration-controlled transient elastography): where does it stand in the United States practice. Clin Gastroenterol Hepatol. 2015;13(1):27–36.
8. Ganne-Carrie N, Ziol M, de Ledinghen V, Douvin C, Marcellin P, Castera L, et al. Accuracy of liver stiffness measurement for the diagnosis of cirrhosis in patients with chronic liver diseases. Hepatology. 2006;44(6):1511–7.
9. Anastasiou OE, Büchter M, Baba HA, Korth J, Canbay A, Gerken G, Kahraman A. Performance and utility of transient elastography and non-invasive markers of liver fibrosis in patients with autoimmune hepatitis: a single centre experience. Hepat Mon. 2016;16(11):e40737.
10. Nguyen-Khac E, Chatelain D, Tramier B, Decrombecque C, Robert B, Joly JP, et al. Assessment of asymptomatic liver fibrosis in alcoholic patients using fibroscan: prospective comparison with seven non-invasive laboratory tests. Aliment Pharmacol Ther. 2008;28(10):1188–98.
11. Ziol M, Handra-Luca A, Kettaneh A, Christidis C, Mal F, Kazemi F, et al. Non-invasive assessment of liver fibrosis by stiffness measurement: a prospective multicentre study in patients with chronic hepatitis C. Hepatology. 2005;41:48–54.
12. Wong VW, Vergniol J, Wong GL, Foucher J, Chan HL, Le Bail B, et al. Diagnosis of fibrosis and cirrhosis using liver stiffness measurement in nonalcoholic fatty liver disease. Hepatology. 2010;51(2):454–62.
13. Zhang W, Wang L, Wang L, Li G, Huang A, Yin P, et al. Liver stiffness measurement, better than APRI, Fibro index, Fib-4, and NBI gastroscopy, predicts portal hypertension in patients with cirrhosis. Cell Biochem Biophys. 2015;71(2):865–73.
14. Shen QL, Chen YJ, Wang ZM, Zhang TC, Pang WB, Shu J, et al. Assessment of liver fibrosis by Fibroscan as compared to liver biopsy in biliary atresia. World J Gastroenterol. 2015;21(22):6931–6.
15. Tsochatzis EA, Gurusamy KS, Ntaoula S, Cholongitas E, Davidson BR, Burroughs AK. Elastography for the diagnosis of severity of fibrosis in chronic liver disease: a meta-analysis of diagnostic accuracy. J Hepatol. 2011; 54(4):650–9.
16. Umemura T, Joshita S, Sekiguchi T, Usami Y, Shibata S, Kimura T, et al. Serum Wisteria floribunda agglutinin-positive mac-2-binding protein level predicts liver fibrosis and prognosis in primary biliary cirrhosis. Am J Gastroenterol. 2015;110(6):857–64.
17. Adams LA, Lymp JF, St Sauver J, Sanderson SO, Lindor KD, Feldstein A, et al. The natural history of nonalcoholic fatty liver disease: a population based cohort study. Gastroenterology. 1992;129:113–21.
18. Yasui K, Hashimoto E, Komorizono Y, Koike K, Arii S, Imai Y, et al. Characteristics of patients with nonalcoholic steatohepatitis who develop hepatocellular carcinoma. Clin Gastroenterol Hepatol. 2011;9:428–33.
19. Angulo P, Hui JM, Marchesini G, Bugianesi E, George J, Farrell GC, et al. The NAFLD fibrosis score: a noninvasive system that identifies liver fibrosis in patients with NAFLD. Hepatology. 2007;45:846–54.
20. Yoneda M, Mawatari H, Fujita K, Yonemitsu K, Kato S, Takahashi H, et al. Type IV collagen 7 s domain is an independent clinical marker of the severity of fibrosis in patients with nonalcoholic steatohepatitis before the cirrhotic stage. J Gastroenterol. 2007;42:375–81.
21. Vallet-Pichard A, Mallet V, Nalpas B, Verkarre V, Nalpas A, Dhalluin-Venier V, et al. FIB-4: an inexpensive and accurate marker of fibrosis in HCV infection. Comparison with liver biopsy and fibrotest. Hepatology. 2007;46(1):32–6.
22. Guha IN, Parkes J, Roderick P, Chattopadhyay D, Cross R, Harris S, et al. Noninvasive markers of fibrosis in nonalcoholic fatty liver disease: validating the European Liver Fibrosis Panel and exploring simple markers. Hepatology. 2008;47:455–60.
23. Ochi H, Hirooka M, Koizumi Y, Miyake T, Tokumoto Y, Soga Y, et al. Real-time tissue elastography for evaluation of hepatic fibrosis and portal hypertension in nonalcoholic fatty liver diseases. Hepatology. 2012;56:1271–8.
24. Ito K, Kuno A, Ikehara Y, Sugiyama M, Saito H, Aoki Y, et al. LecT-Hepa, a glyco-marker derived from multiple lectins, as a predictor of liver fibrosis in chronic hepatitis C patients. Hepatology. 2012;56:1448–56.
25. Kuno A, Sato T, Shimazaki H, Unno S, Saitou K, Kiyohara K, et al. Reconstruction of a robust glycodiagnostic agent supported by multiple lectin-assisted glycan profiling. Proteomics Clin Appl. 2013;7(9-10):642–7.
26. Kuno A, Ikehara Y, Tanaka Y, Angata T, Unno S, Sogabe M, et al. Multilectin assay for detecting fibrosis-specific glyco-alteration by means of lectin microarray. Clin Chem. 2011;57(1):48–56.
27. Kuno A, Ikehara Y, Tanaka Y, Saito K, Ito K, Tsuruno C, et al. LecT-Hepa: a triplex lectin-antibody sandwich immunoassay for estimating the progression dynamics of liver fibrosis assisted by a bedside clinical chemistry analyzer and an automated pretreatment machine. Clin Chim Acta. 2011;412:1767–72.
28. Ura K, Furusyo N, Ogawa E, Hayashi T, Mukae H, Shimizu M, et al. Serum WFA+ -M2BP is a non-invasive liver fibrosis marker that can predict the efficacy of direct-acting anti-viral-based triple therapy for chronic hepatitis C. Aliment Pharmacol Ther. 2015;43:114–24.
29. Toyoda H, Kumada T, Tada T, Kaneoka Y, Maeda A, Korenaga M, et al. Serum WFA+ -M2BP levels as a prognostic factor in patients with early hepatocellular carcinoma undergoing curative resection. Liver Int. 2015;36: 293–301.
30. Yamasaki K, Tateyama M, Abiru S, Komori A, Nagaoka S, Saeki A, et al. Elevated serum levels of Wisteria floribunda agglutinin-positive human Mac-2 binding protein predict the development of hepatocellular carcinoma in hepatitis C patients. Hepatology. 2014;60(5):1563–70.
31. Toshima T, Shirabe K, Ikegami T, Yoshizumi T, Kuno A, Togayachi A, et al. A novel serum marker, glycosylated Wisteria floribunda agglutinin-positive Mac-2 binding protein (WFA (+)-M2BP), for assessing liver fibrosis. J Gastroenterol. 2015;50(1):76–84.
32. Castera L. Noninvasive methods to assess liver disease in patients with hepatitis B or C. Gastroenterology. 2012;142:1293–302.
33. Abe M, Miyake T, Kuno A, Imai Y, Sawai Y, Hino K, et al. Association between Wisteria floribunda agglutinin-positive Mac-2 binding protein and the fibrosis stage of non-alcoholic fatty liver disease. J Gastroenterol. 2015; 50(7):776–84.
34. Nishikawa H, Enomoto H, Iwata Y, Hasegawa K, Nakano C, Takata R, et al. Clinical significance of serum Wisteria floribunda agglutinin positive Mac-2-binding protein level and high-sensitivity C-reactive protein concentration in autoimmune hepatitis. Hepatol Res. 2016;46(7):613–21.

9

Add-on neurological benefits of antiviral therapy in HCV patients with chronic kidney disease

Ming-Shyan Lin[1], Tien-Hsing Chen[2], Wey-Yil Lin[3], Chi-Hung Liu[3], Yung-Yu Hsieh[4], Wen-Nan Chiu[5], Chih-Hsiang Chang[6], Mei-Yen Chen[7,8], Chang-Min Chung[9,10*] and Yu-Sheng Lin[9,10*]

Abstract

Background: Hepatitis C virus (HCV)-infected patients with chronic kidney disease (CKD) have rarely been studied because they rarely accept interferon-based therapy (IBT) and have been difficult to follow up. We investigated long-term outcomes of IBT on the population.

Methods: This population-based cohort study used the Taiwan National Health Insurance Research Database as its data source. HCV patients diagnosed with CKD between Jan. 1, 2003, and Dec. 31, 2013, were selected. They were then divided into two groups based on whether they had undergone IBT. All-cause mortality, acute myocardial infarction (AMI), ischemic stroke (IS), hemorrhagic stroke, and new-onset dialysis were evaluated using a Cox proportional hazard regression analysis after propensity score matching.

Results: We enrolled 9872 HCV patients with CKD: 1684 patients in the treated cohort and 8188 patients in the untreated cohort. The annual incidence of all-cause mortality (19.00 vs. 42.89 events per 1000 person-years; $p < 0.001$) and the incidences of hemorrhagic stroke (1.21 vs. 4.19 events per 1000 person-years; $p = 0.006$) were lower in the treated cohort. New-onset dialysis was also lower in the treated cohort (aHR: 0.31; 95% CI: 0.20–0.48; $p < 0.001$).

Conclusion: Antiviral therapy might provide protective benefits on all-cause mortality, hemorrhagic stroke, and new-onset dialysis in HCV-infected patients with CKD.

Keywords: Chronic kidney disease, Hepatitis C virus, Hemorrhagic stroke, Pegylated interferon

Background

Hepatitis C virus (HCV), which has a 2.8 ~ 3.0% prevalence worldwide, is strongly associated with major liver decompensation [1]. Chronic hepatitis C viral infection (CHC) is also strongly associated with end-stage renal disease (ESRD) [2] via extrahepatic metabovascular and immunological complications such as vasculitis, cryoglobulinemia, and glomerulonephritis [3]. The incidence of CHC is 10–50% in dialysis patients and kidney transplantation (KT) recipients [4, 5]. Although chronic kidney disease (CKD) poses a risk of cardiovascular disease and a higher mortality rate [6], HCV comorbid with CKD threatens even worse survival because of more comorbidities, more cardiovascular events, drug intolerance, and limited therapeutic responses.

Pegylated interferon-based therapy (IBT), a combination of pegylated interferon plus ribavirin, protected HCV patients against liver cirrhosis and hepatocellular carcinoma (HCC) [7], and successful viral eradication also reduced cardiovascular events and late dialysis in HCV patients without CKD [8, 9]. Additionally, IBT had satisfactory improvement of proteinuria and renal function in more than half HCV patients with cryoglobulinemic glomerulonephritis [10]. One meta-analysis also reported more than one half of dialysis patients with CHC had virological response to IBT [11]. Therefore,

* Correspondence: cmchung02@gmail.com; dissertlin@gmail.com
[9]School of Traditional Chinese Medicine, College of Medicine, Chang Gung University, Taoyuan County, Taiwan

Kidney Disease Improving Global Outcomes (KDIGO) guidelines [12] recommended that antiviral therapy should be individual and mandated for most CKD patients with chronic HCV. Moreover, the efficacy of IBT in HCV patients with comorbid CKD and on hemodialysis remains challenging because of drug intolerance, anemia, and potential infection from adverse toxic effects [13]. Despite the big advances of new directacting antiviral (DAA) agents for HCV patients with advanced renal impairment [14], interferon-free therapy is still dependent upon specific genotypes or subtypes, the stage of CKD or dialysis, and the reactivation of a hepatitis B virus coinfection [15]. Moreover, DAAs might be unavailable in some parts of the world because of high price.

Our review of the literature revealed no studies on the effect of IBT on hepatic and extrahepatic complications in HCV patients with CKD and on dialysis. Thus, we investigated the benefits of IBT on all-cause mortality and extra-hepatic outcomes in HCV patients with comorbid CKD.

Methods

Data source

The data source for this population-based longitudinal cohort study is the Taiwan National Health Insurance Research Database (NHIRD), which has been prospectively recording claim data of all forms of healthcare service in Taiwan since 1995 [16]. Because the NHI program is single-player and compulsory for citizens and legal residents, it covers almost all 23 million residents in Taiwan. By the end of 2014, > 99.6% of the population of Taiwan was enrolled in the NHI, and the contract rate was >93% [17]. In the NHIRD, disease is coded according to the International Classification of Diseases, Revision 9, Clinical Modification (ICD-9-CM). Patient information in the NHIRD is de-identified. The study protocol was approved by the Chang-Gung Memorial Hospital Research Ethics Committee (Institutional Review Board number: 103-6439B).

Patients with specific diagnosis codes (one inpatient or two outpatient codes) for HCV (070.41, 070.44, 070.51, 070.54, 070.70, 070.71, V02.62) recorded between 1 January 2003 and 31 December 2013 were identified.

Eligibility criteria and identification of study cohorts

First, we excluded HCV-infected patients without a claims-based diagnosis of CKD (Additional file 1) including dialysis (ICD-9-CM code 585) and registered in the Catastrophic Illness Patient Database (CIPD). Second, we excluded patients <20 years old and >80 years, co-infected with hepatitis B virus (HBV) or comorbidities possibly associated with interferon intolerance: stroke, myocardial infarction, heart failure, hepatic decompensation (esophageal or gastric varices, hepatic encephalopathy, hepatorenal syndrome, portal hypertension, and ascites), hepatic surgery or liver transplantation, all malignancies, catastrophic illness for autoimmune disease, and severe psychosis/mental disorder (Additional file 1). Additionally, to reduce survival bias, all patients who had died, had clinical outcomes, or had been lost to follow-up within 6 months after the index date were excluded. We finally enrolled 9872 HCV-infected patients with CKD in the study.

Patients undergoing anti-viral pegylated interferon (Peg-IFN) treatment (n = 1684) were assigned to the IBT-treated cohort and patients, who had never undergone interferon or ribavirin treatment throughout the study period (n = 8188) were assigned to the IBT-untreated cohort. Each patient in the treated cohort was matched with one patient in the untreated cohort using the probability calculated by logistic regression based on the following confounding variables: gender, age, hospital levels, comorbidities, dialysis status, and medications (listed in Table 1). Figure 1 shows a detailed flowchart of the study. The index date was set as the date when HCV was first diagnosed in the untreated cohort and as the date when interferon was first prescribed in the treated cohort.

Definition of Comorbidities and drug exposure

The comorbidities were diagnosed and then recorded in NHIRD using ICD-9-CM codes. All of the comorbidities listed in this study were confirmed on at least two consecutive clinic visits or whenever the patient had been hospitalized before the index date. In addition, some comorbidities were also reconfirmed using long-term associated medications. The definitions of the comorbidities are listed in the Additional file 1. Personal socio-economic status was divided to five levels according to monthly income (<10,000, 10,000 ~ 19,999, 20,000 ~ 29,999, 30,000 ~ 39,999, ≥ 40,000 New Taiwan Dollar [NTD]). Based on Tzeng's classification [18], we modified the score and categorized all Taiwan areas into four levels (most to least urbanization). Drug information—drug names, date of prescription, and duration of use—was obtained from the outpatient pharmacy prescription database. Long-term drug use was defined as a prescription for at least 6 months after the index date.

The therapeutic duration of IBT generally ranged between 16 and 48 weeks [19] based on viral information (genotype and virological response) and the patient's ability to tolerate the treatment. According to the response-guided trial [20] and Taiwan Health insurance regulations, we will check early viral response (EVR) at week 12 and premature termination (before 16 weeks) usually results from either intolerance to side effects or failure of early virological response or death. Treated

Table 1 Characteristics of the study patients before and after propensity score matching

Variable	Before matching			After matching		
	Treated cohort (n = 1684)	Untreated cohort (n = 8188)	P-value	Treated cohort (n = 1531)	Untreated cohort (n = 1531)	P-value
Characteristic and comorbidity						
Gender			<0.001			0.476
Male	1090 (64.7)	4359 (53.2)		978 (63.9)	959 (62.6)	
Female	594 (35.3)	3829 (46.8)		553 (36.1)	572 (37.4)	
Age in years	57.7 ± 10.2	60.5 ± 11.8	<0.001	58.1 ± 10.2	58.4 ± 11.6	0.406
Age group			<0.001			0.603
20 ~ 40 years	97 (5.8)	468 (5.7)		88 (5.7)	88 (5.7)	
40 ~ 60 years	852 (50.6)	3225 (39.4)		747 (48.8)	720 (47.0)	
60 ~ 80 years	735 (43.6)	4495 (54.9)		696 (45.5)	723 (47.2)	
Income, NTD per month			<0.001			0.849
< 10,000	290 (17.2)	1980 (24.2)		282 (18.4)	302 (19.7)	
10,000 ~ 19,999	112 (6.7)	600 (7.3)		105 (6.9)	100 (6.5)	
20,000 ~ 29,999	768 (45.6)	3679 (44.9)		704 (46.0)	680 (44.4)	
30,000 ~ 39,999	199 (11.8)	678 (8.3)		168 (11.0)	168 (11.0)	
≥ 40,000	315 (18.7)	1251 (15.3)		272 (17.8)	281 (18.4)	
Urbanization level			0.249			0.713
1, most urbanized	382 (22.7)	1711 (20.9)		338 (22.1)	344 (22.5)	
2	481 (28.6)	2280 (27.8)		441 (28.8)	430 (28.1)	
3	537 (31.9)	2758 (33.7)		495 (32.3)	518 (33.8)	
4, least urbanized	284 (16.9)	1439 (17.6)		257 (16.8)	239 (15.6)	
Hospital levels			<0.001			0.942
Medical center	590 (35.0)	1779 (21.7)		528 (34.5)	523 (34.2)	
Region hospital	814 (48.3)	2706 (33.0)		725 (47.4)	731 (47.7)	
District hospital	174 (10.3)	1892 (23.1)		172 (11.2)	178 (11.6)	
Clinics	106 (6.3)	1811 (22.1)		106 (6.9)	99 (6.5)	
Medical history						
Diabetes mellitus	717 (42.6)	2913 (35.6)	<0.001	644 (42.1)	651 (42.5)	0.798
Hypertension	1004 (59.6)	4479 (54.7)	<0.001	915 (59.8)	914 (59.7)	0.971
Dyslipidemia	203 (12.1)	1179 (14.4)	0.012	191 (12.5)	191 (12.5)	1.000
Liver cirrhosis	187 (11.1)	566 (6.9)	<0.001	161 (10.5)	179 (11.7)	0.301
COPD	78 (4.6)	544 (6.6)	0.002	74 (4.8)	87 (5.7)	0.293
PAD	42 (2.5)	262 (3.2)	0.127	39 (2.5)	46 (3.0)	0.441
Thyroid disease	42 (2.5)	132 (1.6)	0.012	32 (2.1)	37 (2.4)	0.543
On dialysis	253 (15.0)	3102 (37.9)	<0.001	251 (16.4)	228 (14.9)	0.469
Medication						
Anti-platelet agents	251 (14.9)	1458 (17.8)	0.004	235 (15.3)	237 (15.5)	0.920
Oral hypoglycemia agents	592 (35.2)	2136 (26.1)	<0.001	529 (34.6)	535 (34.9)	0.820
Insulin	202 (12.0)	986 (12.0)	0.957	189 (12.3)	193 (12.6)	0.827
Statin	113 (6.7)	909 (11.1)	<0.001	111 (7.3)	116 (7.6)	0.730
NSAID	661 (39.3)	3502 (42.8)	0.008	609 (39.8)	597 (39.0)	0.657
COX-II inhibitors	90 (5.3)	767 (9.4)	<0.001	88 (5.7)	88 (5.7)	1.000
Beta blockers	416 (24.7)	2060 (25.2)	0.694	386 (25.2)	397 (25.9)	0.649

Table 1 Characteristics of the study patients before and after propensity score matching *(Continued)*

Diuretics	93 (5.5)	934 (11.4)	<0.001	93 (6.1)	100 (6.5)	0.603
Spironolactone	32 (1.9)	217 (2.7)	0.074	32 (2.1)	41 (2.7)	0.286
Steroid	156 (9.3)	897 (11.0)	0.041	149 (9.7)	151 (9.9)	0.903
Anti-HTN agent						
ACEi/ARB	652 (38.7)	2755 (33.6)	<0.001	600 (39.2)	593 (38.7)	0.795
CCB (Dihydropyridine CCB)	486 (28.9)	2659 (32.5)	0.004	447 (29.2)	436 (28.5)	0.661
Others (include alpha blocker)	106 (6.3)	645 (7.9)	0.026	101 (6.6)	103 (6.7)	0.885
Number of anti-HTN agents			0.260			0.979
0	808 (48.0)	4032 (49.2)		725 (47.4)	731 (47.7)	
1	546 (32.4)	2460 (30.0)		499 (32.6)	500 (32.7)	
2	292 (17.3)	1489 (18.2)		272 (17.8)	268 (17.5)	
≥ 3	38 (2.3)	207 (2.5)		35 (2.3)	32 (2.1)	
Follow-up (years)	3.6 ± 2.6	5.0 ± 3.0	<0.001	3.8 ± 2.7	3.6 ± 2.6	0.070

ACEi angiotensin converting enzyme inhibitor, *ARB* angiotensin receptor blocker, *CCB* calcium channel blockers, *COX-II* Cyclooxygenase II, *COPD* chronic obstructive pulmonary disease, *HTN* hypertension, *NSAID* non-steroidal anti-inflammatory drug, *NTD* New Taiwan Dollar, *PAD* peripheral arterial disease

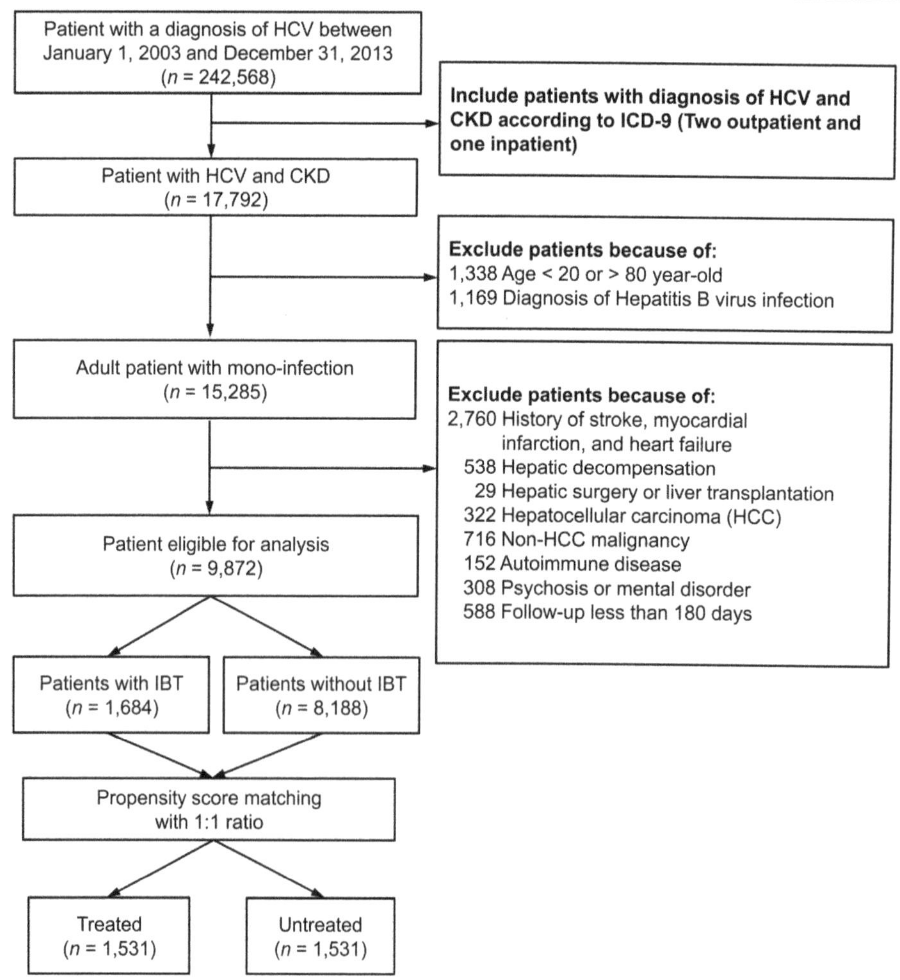

Fig. 1 Flowchart of using stepwise exclusion to identify and enroll patients

patients were consequently subgrouped based on whether or not their antiviral treatment was ≥16 weeks or <16 weeks. "Incompletely treated" cohort means "treated <16 weeks".

Definition and ascertainment of outcomes

Enrollees were observed until occurrence of the clinical outcomes, death, or 31 December 2013, whichever came first. The clinical outcomes were all-cause mortality, acute myocardial infarction, ischemic stroke, and hemorrhagic stroke, all of which were confirmed based on the primary diagnosis of the index hospitalization. These outcomes have been validated before and confirmed as highly accuracy [8, 9]. The other outcome was new-onset dialysis, which was defined as first-time and necessary maintenance dialysis by certification in the CIPD registry.

Statistical analysis

We performed propensity score matching (PSM) before comparing the treated cohort with the untreated cohort because there was substantial difference between the two cohorts that might confound the result [21]. Covariates to be calculated in the propensity score included index year (as the year of IBT) and variables listed in Table 1 (except for the follow up year). Propensity score indicates the predicted probability of the logistic regression and each patient in the treated cohort was matched with a corresponding patient in the untreated cohort. To warranty the quality of matching, the tolerance level on the maximum propensity score distance (caliper) was set as 0.2 × standard deviation of the propensity score under the greedy nearest neighbor matching algorithm.

We compared the patient's characteristics between groups (i.e. treated cohort vs. untreated cohort) using independent sample t-test for continuous variable or using chi-square test for categorical variable. The incidence of outcome (mortality, acute myocardial infarction, ischemic stroke, hemorrhagic stroke, and new onset dialysis) was estimated using incidence density as number of event per 1000 person-years since entry of index date. The time-to-event between the two cohorts was compared using a Cox proportional hazard analysis adjusted for the propensity score. In an additional subgroup analysis, we stratified the treated cohort into two groups (incompletely treated <16 weeks and treated ≥16 weeks) and compared the time-to-event between the groups using a log-rank test. Data analysis was performed with SAS Version 9.3 (SAS Institute, Cary, NC).

Results

Baseline characteristics of the study population

We identified 17,792 HCV-infected patients with CKD among the 242,568 patients diagnosed with HCV between January 1, 2003, and December 31, 2013. After patients who did not meet our inclusion criteria had been excluded, 1684 patients (mean age: 57.7 ± 10.2 years; men: 65%) were in the pre-PSM treated group, and 8188 (mean age: 60.5 ± 11.8 years; men: 53%) were in the pre-PSM untreated group (Table 1). Most patients also accepted antiviral therapy at medical center and regional hospital. Despite higher income status in pre-PSM treated group, the residential urbanization level was insignificantly different among both cohorts. The pre-PSM treated HCV patients had a higher prevalence of diabetes and hypertension and they tended to receive oral hypoglycemia agents and ACEi/ARB other than CCB. Only 15% of the patients in the pre-PSM treated cohort were on dialysis, but 38% in the pre-PSM untreated cohort were. The prevalence of liver cirrhosis without hepatic decompensation was higher in the pre-PSM treated than in untreated cohorts (11.1% vs. 6.9%, $P < 0.001$). Finally, after 1:1 PSM, the distribution of demographic factors, hospital levels, comorbidities, and associated medications were not significantly different between the two cohorts (Table 1).

Outcomes during the 10-year longterm follow up

Outcomes were assessed after 1:1 PSM, which yielded 1531 treated patients and 1531 untreated patients. The annual incidence of all-cause mortality was apparently higher in the untreated cohort (incidence density [ID], 42.89; 95% confidence interval [CI], 37.43–48.35) than in the treated cohort (ID: 19.00; 95% CI: 15.45–22.55), which was significantly different (adjusted hazard ratio [aHR], 0.45; 95% CI: 0.36–0.56, $P < 0.001$). The risk of secondary outcomes, including acute myocardial infarction and ischemic stroke, were comparable between the two cohorts. Noticeably, the ID of hemorrhagic stroke was 1.21 (95% CI: 0.31–2.11) in the treated cohort and 4.19 (95% CI: 2.48–5.91) in the untreated cohort, a significantly different risk reduction in the treated cohort (aHR: 0.31; 95% CI, 0.13–0.71, $P = 0.006$). The cumulative incidence between the two cohorts for all-cause mortality is plotted in Fig. 2a, and for hemorrhagic stroke in Fig. 2b.

An evaluation of the effect of dialysis on IBT showed that all-cause mortality reduction was less efficacy for HCV patients on dialysis than for HCV patients not on dialysis (aHR: 0.80 vs. 0.39; P for interaction = 0.018). The effect of IBT on the other three outcomes was comparable between the two cohorts (Additional file 2).

Effect of incomplete IBT on clinical outcomes

We stratified the treated cohort into two groups (incompletely treated <16 weeks and treated 16 ≥ weeks). The mortality rate was higher in the incompletely treated (<16 weeks) cohort than in the treated (≥16 weeks)

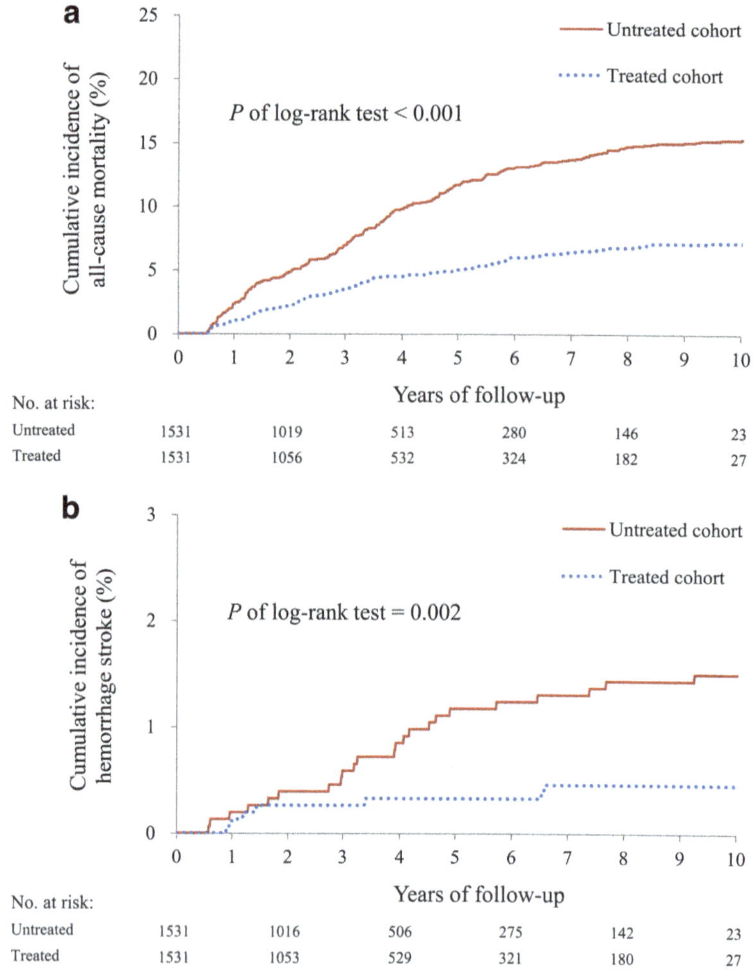

Fig. 2 a All-cause mortality survival curves in the treated and untreated cohorts; **b** incidence density of hemorrhagic stroke between the treated and untreated cohorts

cohort ($P < 0.001$), but it was comparable with the untreated cohort ($P = 0.118$) (Fig. 3a). The risk of hemorrhagic stroke in the incompletely treated cohort was comparable with the risks in the other two groups (Fig. 3b).

Patients in the incompletely treated cohort tended to be older, have a higher prevalence of liver cirrhosis and dialysis, took more beta blockers, number of anti-HTN agents and diuretics, including spironolactone, a potassium-sparing diuretic (Additional file 3).

Renoprotective effect in non-dialytic patients

After patients on dialysis before the index date had been excluded, antiviral therapy was associated with a lower risk of new-onset dialysis (aHR: 0.31; 95% CI: 0.20–0.48, $P < 0.001$) (Table 2 and Fig. 4a). Additionally, the incidence of new-onset dialysis in the incompletely treated (<16 weeks) cohort was greater than that in the treated (≥16 weeks) cohort ($P < 0.001$), but it was comparable with that of the untreated cohort ($P = 0.357$) (Fig. 4b).

Discussion

This is the first nationwide cohort study to investigate long-term outcomes of patients with HCV and comorbid CKD treated with IBT, which demonstrated significant benefits on all-cause mortality and new-onset dialysis compatible with previous non-CKD HCV analysis [8, 9]. We also found a markedly lower incidence for hemorrhagic stroke among treated patients regardless of dialysis, but not in untreated patients. Although many patients cannot tolerate IBT and stop the therapy, the survival benefit for treated HCV-infected patients with comorbid CKD is higher than that for untreated patients.

Survival benefits of IBT in HCV-infected patients with comorbid CKD

High mortality of chronic HCV infection is attributable not only to hepatic decompensation, liver cirrhosis, and hepatocellular carcinoma (HCC), but also to multiple extrahepatic complications, which can be ameliorated by using complete IBT in HCV-infected patients without

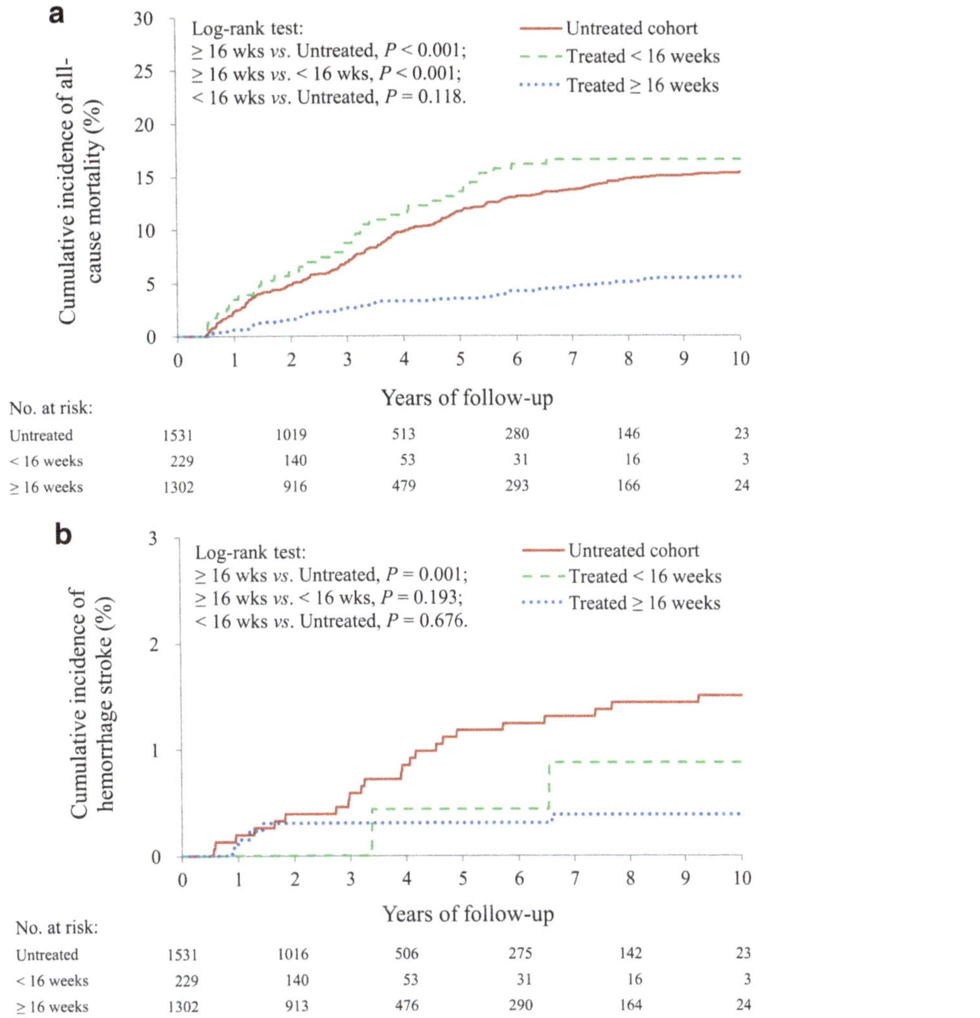

Fig. 3 a All-cause mortality survival curves in the "treated ≥16 weeks" and incompletely treated (<16 weeks) and untreated cohorts; **b** incidence density of hemorrhagic stroke in the three cohorts based on the duration of therapy

CKD [8, 9]. Because of the genotype distribution of 50% for HCV-1 and 45% for HCV-2 in Taiwan [19], sustained viral response (SVR) for HCV with comorbid CKD or dialysis was 50–64% [10, 11]. Hsu et al. [8] demonstrated a small reduction of cardiovascular events (<20%) in a treated cohort, which was comparable with the findings of a study on diabetes [9]. However, our study showed neural cardiovascular effects of antiviral therapy in HCV-infected patients with CKD, which might be related to drug intolerability, IBT inefficacy, and severe atherosclerosis in CKD patients, but not in patients without CKD.

IBT might reduce all-cause mortality because it ameliorates the hepatic complications of decompensation, liver cirrhosis, and HCC, or non-hepatic problems like a tendency to hemorrhage, immunocompromised sepsis, advanced renal impairment, hemodialysis, etc.

Cerebrovascular protection of IBT in patients with chronic HCV and CKD

Our study showed a significant reduction of hemorrhagic stroke (10-year hemorrhagic stroke incidence rate: untreated = 1.5% vs. treated = 0.46%), which is comparable to the findings of Arase et al. [22] on HCV clearance (10-year incidence rate in HCV non-clearance = 1.1% vs. clearance = 0.4%; P = 0.02). However, their study lacked renal function data before IBT and background matching between cohorts. Despite conventional factors like age, being male, smoking, hypertension, diabetes, and drinking alcohol [23], HCV contributed to hemorrhagic stroke [24, 25], liver cirrhosis [26–28], and unstable hemostasis [29]. Moreover, HCV was critically involved in systemic atherosclerosis, vascular remodeling, ectasia change, and microaneurysms, which manifested as cerebral microbleeds (CMBs) in the MRIs of patients with

Table 2 Event numbers and incidence density (ID) of the outcomes between the study cohorts

Variable	Treated cohort (*n* = 1531)	Untreated cohort (*n* = 1531)	*P*-value‡
All-cause mortality			
Follow-up (years), mean ± SD	3.78 ± 2.66	3.61 ± 2.57	
Event number, n (%)	110 (7.18)	237 (15.48)	
ID (95% CI)[a]	19.00 (15.45–22.55)	42.89 (37.43–48.35)	
Hazard ratio (95% CI)	0.45 (0.36–0.56)	Reference	<0.001
Acute myocardial infarction			
Follow-up (years), mean ± SD	3.77 ± 2.66	3.59 ± 2.56	
Event number, n (%)	12 (0.78)	13 (0.85)	
ID (95% CI)[a]	2.08 (0.90–3.26)	2.36 (1.08–3.65)	
Hazard ratio (95% CI)	0.92 (0.42–2.01)	Reference	0.826
Ischemic stroke			
Follow-up (years), mean ± SD	3.75 ± 2.64	3.58 ± 2.56	
Event number, n (%)	17 (1.11)	18 (1.18)	
ID (95% CI)[a]	2.96 (1.55–4.37)	3.28 (1.77–4.80)	
Hazard ratio (95% CI)	0.91 (0.47–1.76)	Reference	0.774
Hemorrhagic stroke			
Follow-up (years), mean ± SD	3.77 ± 2.66	3.58 ± 2.55	
Event number, n (%)	7 (0.46)	23 (1.50)	
ID (95% CI)[a]	1.21 (0.31–2.11)	4.19 (2.48–5.91)	
Hazard ratio (95% CI)	0.31 (0.13–0.71)	Reference	0.006
New onset dialysis (*n* = 2583)[b]			
Study number	1280	1303	
Follow-up (years), mean ± SD	3.93 ± 2.75	3.61 ± 2.61	
Event number, n (%)	27 (2.11)	79 (6.06)	
ID (95% CI)[a]	5.37 (3.34–7.39)	16.78 (13.08–20.48)	
Hazard ratio (95% CI)	0.31 (0.20–0.48)	Reference	<0.001

SD standard deviation, *CI* confidence interval
[a]Incidence density (ID): event numbers per 1000 person-years
[b]Patients who were under dialysis were excluded
‡Adjusted for propensity score

advanced hepatic fibrosis [30]. In addition to viral replication and HCV receptor expression in microvascular endothelium [31], neurological vasculitis was highly prevalent with mixed cryoglobulinemia in 25–60% of HCV-infected patients [32, 33]. Both consequences increased the risk of microvascular destruction and disturbance of the brain–blood-barrier related to spontaneous hemorrhagic events. Indeed, the protection of complete IBT against hemorrhagic stroke comes not only because it ameliorates advanced liver cirrhosis, but also because it attenuates extrahepatic immunological complications.

Both the brain and the kidneys are the end-organs for high blood pressure and autoregulation in hypertensive patients [34]. Thus, CKD might be another risk factor of hemorrhagic stroke because of an altered response to antiplatelet agents, platelet dysfunction, endothelial hyper-permeability [35], microvascular dysregulation [36], and occult CMBs [37], Our subgroup analysis showed that IBT promised a greater reduction of new-onset dialysis and constant protection against hemorrhagic stroke, regardless of whether the patient was on dialysis, and that antiviral therapy provided many benefits for the liver, kidney, and brain triangle.

Effect of incomplete IBT on clinical outcomes

According to a meta-analysis [11], the dropout rate in patients on dialysis was 18%. Our finding was 14.4% for incompletely treated patients. Both rates were higher than that of Hsu et al. [8, 9]: 10.4% in a general population without CKD. Hsu et al. showed that patients who underwent incomplete IBT were older, as were our patients, who also had more liver cirrhosis and more dialysis. Additionally, many incompletely treated patients had

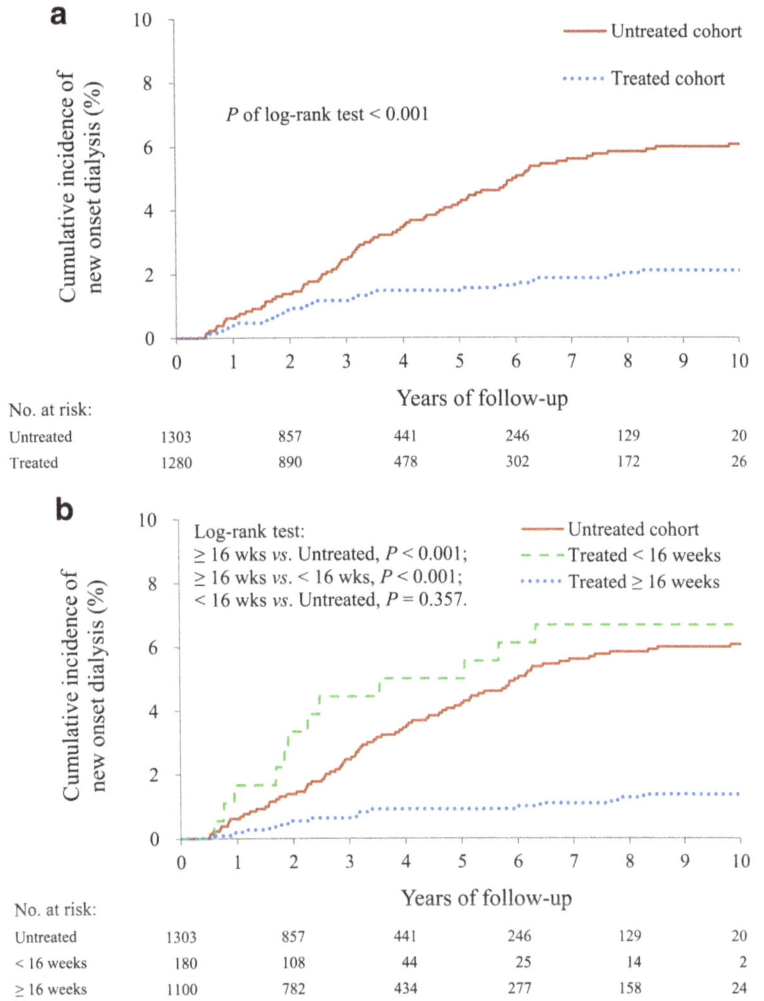

Fig. 4 a Incidence density of new-onset dialysis between the treated and untreated cohorts in CKD patients without dialysis; **b** the treated cohort was subgrouped by therapeutic duration

been prescribed diuretics because they had more fluid overloading or ascites due to hepatic decompensation. Despite the loss of benefits because of incomplete IBT, our analysis and other studies also found slightly higher mortality in patients treated for <16 weeks, possibly because they had more critical comorbidities, marked anemia, immunocompromised status, or malnutrition. In addition, interferon might cause adverse effects or complications, including heart failure and infection [38]. Because of high mortality in the incompletely treated group, identifying the precipitating factors before starting IBT is critical.

Limitations

This study has some limitations. First, details of the HCV genotype, IL-28B polymorphism, virus load, viral response, serum creatinine or eGFR, duration of renal impairment, duration of dialysis, platelet and coagulation function, echogenic study, degree of hepatic fibrosis, body weight, and personal lifestyles are not included in the Taiwan NHIRD. However, by carefully excluding confounding comorbidities and estimating associated variables, including medications, we obtained information that contributed to outcomes. Second, the misdiagnoses of CKD or cirrhosis might occur because of the ICD-9 codes used in several NHIRD-based nationwide cohort studies, but we used the standard methodology (1 inpatient or 2 outpatient diagnosis codes) to identify CKD patients in the NHIRD. Underdiagnosis of cirrhosis might also occur in CKD or dialysis population due to relatively low aminotransferase [39]. Moreover, our study tried to the gap of longterm outcomes in HCV-infected patients with CKD, which is difficult to do in clinical researched because of individual decision making unpredictable dose adjustments at various stages. Third, alcohol consumption might be involved in hemorrhagic stroke because of alcohol-induced hypertension and coagulation disorders, whether or not the patient has cirrhosis [23]. Moreover, we had carefully excluded alcohol-related liver cirrhosis the number of confounding factors as much as possible. Fourth, variable doses of ribavirin according to renal function, body weight or drug tolerance might influence effect of viral eradication, but all treated patients would receive guided interferon therapy. Fifth, the effects of events that occurred within the therapeutic course (<6 months) and their association with clinical benefits, adverse side effects of drugs, and underlying comorbidities were not clear. Therefore, we excluded patients who had died, or had a myocardial infarction, ischemic stroke, hemorrhagic stroke, new-onset dialysis, or who were lost to follow-up within 6 months, which is different from other studies [8, 9].

Conclusion

Despite neural effect on AMI and IS, our study showed that antiviral therapy might provide benefits on all-cause mortality, late dialysis, and hemorrhagic stroke in those HCV infected patients with CKD. In addition, DAA, as an agent with higher SVR and better tolerance, would enhance effective viral eradication and comprehensive cardiovascular protection for the difficultly treated population.

Additional files

Additional file 1: Appendix of ICD-9-CM codes. List of all ICD-9-CM codes used for diagnosis in the current study.

Additional file 2: Subgroup analyses of IBT efficacy. The effect of IBT on all outcomes was comparable between the two cohorts regarding dialysis.

Additional file 3: Characteristics comparison by different IBT courses. Characteristics differences of HCV-infected patients receiving IBT ≥ 16 or <16 weeks after propensity score matching.

Abbreviations

ACEi: Angiotensin converting enzyme inhibitor; aHR: Adjusted hazard ratio; ARB: Angiotensin receptor blocker; CI: Confidence intervals; CKD: Chronic kidney disease; COPD: Chronic obstructive pulmonary disease; COX-II: Cyclooxygenase-2; DM: Diabetes mellitus; ESRD: End-stage renal disease; HCV: Hepatitis C virus; HR: Hazard ratio; HTN: Hypertension; IBT: Interferon-based therapy; ICD-9-CM: International Classification of Diseases, Ninth Revision, Clinical Modification; NHI: National Health Insurance; NHIRD: National health Insurance Research Database; NSAID: Non-steroidal anti-inflammatory drug; PAD: Peripheral arterial disease; SD: Standard deviation

Acknowledgments

We thank Alfred Hsing-Fen Lin and Zoe Ya-Jhu Syu for the assistance with statistics.

Funding

This study was supported by grants from the Chang Gung Medical Research Fund of Chang Gung Memorial Hospital, Chiayi, Taiwan (CMRPGME0011).

Authors' contributions

All authors reviewed the manuscript and completed final approval. Study concept and design: MSL, THC, YSL, YYH, MSC; acquisition of data: MSL, CHL, CHC, WYL; analysis and interpretation of data: CHL, YYH, MSC, CHC, WYL, MYC, CMC, YSL; manuscript draft: MSL, YSL; critical revision of the manuscript for important intellectual content: MSL, THC, WYL, YSL.

Consent for publication

Not applicable.

Competing interests

The authors declare that they have no competing interests.

Author details

[1]Department of Cardiology, Department of Internal Medicine, Chang Gung Memorial Hospital, Yunlin, Taiwan. [2]Department of Cardiology, Department of Internal Medicine, Chang Gung Memorial Hospital, Chang Gung University College of Medicine, Keelung, Taiwan. [3]Stroke Center and Department of Neurology, Chang Gung Memorial Hospital, Linkou Medical Center, Chang Gung University College of Medicine, Taoyuan, Taiwan. [4]Department of Hepato-Gastroenterology, Chang Gung Memorial Hospital, Chiayi, Taiwan. [5]Department of Hepato-Gastroenterology, Chang Gung Memorial Hospital, Yunlin, Taiwan. [6]Department of Nephrology, Kidney research center, Chang Gung Memorial Hospital, Chang Gung University, College of medicine, Taoyuan, Taiwan. [7]College of Nursing, Chang Gung University of Science and Technology (CGUST), Taoyuan, Taiwan. [8]Department of Nursing, Chang Gung University, Taoyuan, Taiwan. [9]School of Traditional Chinese Medicine, College of Medicine, Chang Gung University, Taoyuan County, Taiwan. [10]Department of Cardiology, Chiayi Chang Gung Memorial Hospital, 6, Sec. West Chai-Pu Road, Pu-TZ City, Chai Yi Hsien 61363, Taiwan.

References

1. Gower E, Estes C, Blach S, et al. Global epidemiology and genotype distribution of the hepatitis C virus infection. J Hepatol. 2014;61(1 Suppl): S45–57.
2. Molnar MZ, Alhourani HM, Wall BM, et al. Association of hepatitis C viral infection with incidence and progression of chronic kidney disease in a large cohort of US veterans. Hepatology. 2015;61(5):1495–502.
3. Castillo I, Martinez-Ara J, Olea T, et al. High prevalence of occult hepatitis C virus infection in patients with primary and secondary glomerular nephropathies. Kidney Int. 2014;86(3):619–24.
4. Hinrichsen H, Leimenstoll G, Stegen G, et al. Prevalence and risk factors of hepatitis C virus infection in haemodialysis patients: a multicentre study in 2796 patients. Gut. 2002;51:429–33.
5. Su Y, Norris JL, Zang C, et al. Incidence of hepatitis C virus infection in patients on hemodialysis: a systematic review and meta-analysis. Hemodial Int. 2013;17:532–41.
6. Go AS, Chertow GM, Fan D, et al. Chronic kidney disease and the risks of death, cardiovascular events, and hospitalization. N Engl J Med. 2004; 351(13):1296–305.
7. Koh C, Heller T, Haynes-Williams V, et al. Long-term outcome of chronic hepatitis C after sustained virological response to interferon-based therapy. Aliment Pharmacol Ther. 2013;37:887–94.
8. Hsu YC, Ho HJ, Huang YT, et al. Association between antiviral treatment and extrahepatic outcomes in patients with hepatitis C virus infection. Gut. 2015; 64(3):495–503.
9. Hsu YC, Lin JT, Ho HJ, et al. Antiviral treatment for hepatitis C virus infection is associated with improved renal and cardiovascular outcomes in diabetic patients. Hepatology. 2014;59(4):1293–302.
10. Liu CH, Liu CJ, Huang CF, et al. Peginterferon alfa-2a with or without low-dose ribavirin for treatment-naive patients with hepatitis C virus genotype 2 receiving haemodialysis: a randomised trial. Gut. 2015;64:303–11.
11. Fabrizi F, Dixit V, Messa P, et al. Antiviral therapy (pegylated interferon and ribavirin) of hepatitis C in dialysis patients: meta-analysis of clinical studies. J Viral Hepat. 2014;21:681–9.
12. Kidney Disease: Improving Global Outcomes. KDIGO clinical practice guidelines for the prevention, diagnosis, evaluation, and treatment of hepatitis C in chronic kidney disease. Kidney Int Suppl. 2008;73(Suppl 109):S1–99.
13. Sulkowski MS, Cooper C, Hunyady B, et al. Management of adverse effects of peg-IFN and ribavirin therapy for hepatitis C. Nat Rev Gastroenterol Hepatol. 2011;8:212–3.

14. Roth D, Nelson DR, Bruchfeld A, et al. Grazoprevir plus elbasvir in treatment-naive and treatment-experienced patients with hepatitis C virus genotype 1 infection and stage 4–5 chronic kidney disease (the C-SURFER study): a combination phase 3 study. Lancet. 2015;386(10003):1537–45.
15. De Monte A, Courjon J, Anty R, et al. Direct-acting antiviral treatment in adults infected with hepatitis C virus: reactivation of hepatitis B virus coinfection as a further challenge. J Clin Virol. 2016;78:27–30.
16. Wu CY, Chen YJ, Ho HJ, et al. Association between nucleoside analogues and risk of hepatitis B virus-related hepatocellular carcinoma recurrence following liver resection. JAMA. 2012;308:1906–14.
17. National Health Insurance Administration MoHaW. 2014–2015 National Health Insurance Annual Report; 2014. p. 122. Accessed 29 Apr 2015.
18. Tzeng GH, Wu TY. Characteristics of urbanization levels in Taiwan districts. Geogr Res. 1986;12:287–323.
19. Yu ML, Chuang WL. Treatment of chronic hepatitis C in Asia: when east meets west. J Gastroenterol Hepatol. 2009;24(3):336–45.
20. Yu ML, Dai CY, Huang JF, et al. A randomised study of peginterferon and ribavirin for 16 versus 24 weeks in patients with genotype 2 chronic hepatitis C. Gut. 2007;56(4):553–9. Epub 2006 Sept 6.
21. d'Agostino RB. Tutorial in biostatistics: propensity score methods for bias reduction in the comparison of a treatment to a non-randomized control group. Stat Med. 1998;17(19):2265–81.
22. Arase Y, et al. Impact of virus clearance for the development of hemorrhagic stroke in chronic hepatitis C. J Med Virol. 2014;86(1):169–75.
23. Marques-Vidal P, Arveiler D, Evans A, et al. Different alcohol drinking and blood pressure relationships in France and Northern Ireland: the PRIME study. Hypertension. 2001;38:1361–6.
24. Karibe H, Niizuma H, Ohyama H, et al. Hepatitis C virus (HCV) infection as a risk factor for spontaneous intracerebral haemorrhage: hospital based case–control study. J Clin Neurosci. 2001;8:423–5.
25. Tseng CH, Muo CH, Hsu CY, et al. Increased risk of intracerebral hemorrhage among patients with hepatitis C virus infection. Medicine (Baltimore). 2015; 94(46):e2132.
26. Lai CH, Cheng PY, Chen YY. Liver cirrhosis and risk of intracerebral hemorrhage: a 9-year follow-up study. Stroke. 2011;42(9):2615–7.
27. Grønbaek H, Johnsen SP, Jepsen P, et al. Liver cirrhosis, other liver diseases, and risk of hospitalisation for intracerebral haemorrhage: a Danish population-based case–control study. BMC Gastroenterol. 2008;8:16.
28. Parikh NS, Navi BB, Kumar S, et al. Association between liver disease and intracranial hemorrhage. J Stroke Cerebrovasc Dis. 2016;25(3):543–8.
29. Tripodi A, Primignani M, Chantarangkul V, et al. The coagulopathy of cirrhosis assessed by thromboelastometry and its correlation with conventional coagulation parameters. Thromb Res. 2009;124(1):132–6.
30. Kim YD, Song D, Heo JH, et al. Relationship between cerebral microbleeds and liver stiffness determined by transient elastography. PLoS One. 2015; 10(9):e0139227.
31. Fletcher NF, Yang JP, Farquhar MJ, et al. Hepatitis C virus infection of neuroepithelioma cell lines. Gastroenterology. 2010;139(4):1365–74.
32. Casato M, Saadoun D, Marchetti A, et al. Central nervous system involvement in hepatitis C virus cryoglobulinemia vasculitis: a multicenter case–control study using magnetic resonance imaging and neuropsychological tests. J Rheumatol. 2005;32(3):484–8.
33. Erro Aguirre ME, Ayuso Blanco T, Tuñón Alvarez T, et al. Brain hemorrhage as a complication of chronic hepatitis C virus-related vasculitis. J Neurol. 2008;255(6):944–5.
34. Seliger SL, Longstreth WT Jr. Lessons about brain vascular disease from another pulsating organ, the kidney. [comment]. Stroke. 2008;39(1):5–6.
35. Jalal DI, Chonchol M, Targher G. Disorders of hemostasis associated with chronic kidney disease. Semin Thromb Hemost. 2010;36(1):34–40.
36. Toyoda K, Ninomiya T. Stroke and cerebrovascular diseases in patients with chronic kidney disease. Lancet Neurol. 2014;13:823–33.
37. Ovbiagele B, Wing JJ, Menon RS, et al. Association of chronic kidney disease with cerebral microbleeds in patients with primary intracerebral hemorrhage. Stroke. 2013;44(9):2409–13.
38. Aspinall RJ, Pockros PJ. The management of side-effects during therapy for hepatitis C. Aliment Pharmacol Ther. 2004;20(9):917–29.
39. Fabrizi F, Lunghi G, Finazzi S, et al. Decreased serum aminotransferase activity in patients with chronic renal failure: impact on the detection of viral hepatitis. Am J Kidney Dis. 2001;38(5):1009–15.

Addition of nucleoside analogues to peg-IFNα-2a enhances virological response in chronic hepatitis B patients without early response to peg-IFNα-2a

Yan Xu, Xu Wang, Zhenhua Liu, Changyu Zhou, Wenqian Qi, Jian Jiao, Fan Yu, Honghua Guo, Ping Zhao and Jiangbin Wang*

Abstract

Background: Current treatments for chronic hepatitis B (CHB) include pegylated interferon alpha (PEG-IFN-α) which is an immune modulator, and nucleos(t)ide analogs (NAs) which directly inhibit HBV DNA polymerase. With the limited efficacy of PEG-IFN-α and prolonged treatment periods associated with NAs, there is an urgent need for novel therapeutic strategies, especially for patients with a poor early response to anti-viral therapy.

Methods: In this study, 178 patients with chronic hepatitis B (n = 131) and compensated (n = 47) HBV-induced cirrhosis were enrolled, 120 patients with HBeAg (+). All the patients were treated for 12 weeks with PEG-IFN-α. Among them, a total of 138 patients with a poor virological response after 12 weeks were treated for an additional 48 weeks with Peg-IFNα-2a (control) (n = 43), with Peg-IFNα-2a + entecavir (ETV) (n = 49), or Peg-IFNα-2a + adefovir dipivoxil (ADV) (n = 46), and were followed for 48 weeks after therapy. Early virological response was defined as undetectable HBV DNA after anti-viral therapy for 12 weeks. Sustained virological response (SVR) was defined as no change in therapeutic effectiveness after 6 months follow-up, and no recurrence.Therapeutic efficacy was determined by evaluating HBV DNA levels, serum and liver HBsAg levels, liver function tests and liver histology.

Results: Patients in the Peg-IFNα-2a + ETV and Peg-IFNα-2a + ADV groups showed a significantly greater decrease in HBV DNA levels over time, and a significantly higher SVR compared to patients receiving Peg-INFα-2a monotherapy (both P values <0.05). Although patients receiving combination therapy had a significantly higher change in serum HBsAg levels compared to the monotherapy group, there was no significant difference in liver HBsAg levels between the three treatment groups.

Conclusion: This study demonstrated that in patients with a poor virological response after 12 weeks of treatment with Peg-IFNα-2a alone, addition of ADV or ETV significantly reduced HBV DNA levels, serum HBsAg levels, and increased SVR. Individualization of anti-viral therapy would ensure that only patients who do not respond to Peg-IFNα-2a would receive combination therapy. Our data have important implications for the treatment of CHB patients who fail to show an early response to Peg-IFNα-2a monotherapy.

Keywords: Chronic hepatitis B, Interferon, Nucleoside analog, Virological response, Combination therapy

* Correspondence: zrlwangjb@medmail.com.cn
Department of Gastroenterology, China-Japan Union Hospital, Jilin University, Changchun, Jilin Province 130033, China

Background

It is estimated that approximately 350 million people worldwide are chronically infected with the hepatitis B virus (HBV) [1], and a large percentage of these patients have been shown to be at increased risk of developing liver cirrhosis or hepatocellular carcinoma (HCC) [2, 3]. The primary therapeutic goals in patients with chronic hepatitis B (CHB) are clearance of the hepatitis B surface antigen (HBsAg) from the serum, which is associated with normalization of ALT and histological improvement of inflammation and fibrosis [4, 5].

Currently approved treatments for CHB include two categories of drugs: 1) immune modulators such as Peg-INFα-2a, and 2) nucleoside (lamivudine, entecavir and telbivudine) and nucleotide analogs (adefovir dipivoxil and tenofovir disoproxil fumarate), which suppress viral replication by selectively inhibiting the activity of HBV DNA polymerase. Although nucleos(t)ide analogues (NAs) are cheap and safe, their limited long-term efficacy result in prolonged treatment periods, particularly in patients with HBeAg-negative CHB. Extended use of NAs has been shown to be associated with the generation of drug-resistant mutations [6]. In contrast, the duration of interferon-based therapy is predetermined and finite. However, only 30% of HBeAg-negative CHB patients treated with Peg-INFα-2a achieve a sustained virologic response (SVR) off-treatment, and HBsAg seroconversion in seen in 3–4% of patients after 1 year of treatment [7]. Although it was recently shown that CHB patients treated with PEG-IFN had higher rates of HBeAg seroconversion and HBsAg seroclearance compared to those treated with entecavir (ETV) [8], interferons have been shown to be effective only in patients with low viral loads, when the ALT levels are >2–5 ULN, or in patients infected with HBV genotype A/B. Additionally, although the rate of HBV DNA loss with interferon-based therapy can range from 14%–58.6%, more than 50% of the patients show low levels of viral replication, especially those with a poor early response to Peg-IFN [9–12]. Other challenges with using interferon-based therapy include the need for parenteral administration, frequent clinical follow-ups and the side-effects.

There has been a recent focus on developing novel therapeutic strategies for patients with a poor response to Peg-INF-α-2a. Some studies have combined the immunomodulatory properties of Peg-IFN along with the direct anti-viral activity of NAs in an attempt to improve therapeutic efficacy in CHB patients. Patients treated with a combination of Peg-INFα and lamivudine (LAM) had a higher on-treatment virological response rate compared to patients treated with LAM monotherapy, but there was no improvement in post-therapy response rates [9, 10]. Similarly, although HBeAg-negative CHB patients treated with a combination of Peg-INF-α-2a and adefovir dipivoxil (ADV) had a more rapid on-treatment HBV DNA suppression compared to those treated with Peg-INF-α-2a monotherapy, this did not translate to higher rates of virological response after suspension of treatment [13]. A total of 17 CHB patients treated with a combination of Peg-INF-α-2a and ETV for 48 weeks and observed for an additional 24 weeks showed a significant decrease in serum HBV DNA [14].

The protocol of anti-viral therapy in these combination studies was not adjusted based on early response. Optimizing therapeutic regimens based on early virological response and individual characteristics would ensure that only patients who fail to achieve a good response with Peg-INF-α-2a monotherapy would receive combination therapy, thereby shortening the course of therapy, enhancing virological response, decreasing the economic burden and conserving medical resources [15, 16].

In this study, we aimed to investigate the influence of additional nucleoside analogues on the SVR and the improvement of liver histology in CHB patients who had a poor virological response to Peg-INFα-2a at the end of 12 weeks of therapy.

Methods

Patient recruitment

A total of 178 patients diagnosed with CHB were recruited from the Department of Gastroenterology at China–Japan Union Hospital between September 2005 and December 2010. CHB diagnosis was based on the "Guideline for the Prevention and Therapy of Chronic Hepatitis B in China" issued by the Infectious Diseases Branch of the Chinese Medical Association, Hepatological Diseases Branch of the Chinese Medical Association, and the Chinese Foundation for Hepatitis Prevention and Control [17]. The study was performed in accordance with Good Clinical Practice and the ethical principles of the Declaration of Helsinki (ChiCTR-OCC-12002196). The study protocol was approved by a central independent ethics committee of China-Japan Union Hospital of Jilin University. All patients provided written informed consent.

Inclusion criteria were 1) HBV DNA $\geq 10^4$copies/ml (HBV DNA ≥ 300 copies /ml in the case of CHB patients with hepatic cirrhosis), 2) ALT ≥ULN, but ≤10 × ULN (normal or increased ALT in the case of CHB patients with hepatic cirrhosis), 3) serum total bilirubin <2 × ULN, 4) liver histological examination showing Knodell HAI ≥4 or ≥ G2 inflammatory necrosis. Additionally, all study patients received anti-viral therapy with Peg-IFNα-2a. Exclusion criteria were 1) presence of decompensated cirrhosis, 2) history of mental illness, 3) presence of epilepsy, cancer or symptomatic heart diseases, 4) evidence of drug abuse or alcohol abuse, 5) concomitant infection with HCV, HDV or HIV. Breast-feeding and pregnant women were also excluded.

This study was approved by the Institutional Review Board of the hospital, and informed consent was obtained from all study participants.

Therapeutic protocol

All study patients received a subcutaneous injection of Peg-IFNα-2a (180 μg) once weekly for 12 weeks. The therapeutic protocol was then adjusted based on virological response. A total of 138 patients had a poor virological response after 12 weeks of anti-viral therapy with Peg-IFNα-2a. After fully communication with patients,According to patients' willingness,Study patients were divided into 3 groups: (1) Patients in Group 1 (control group; n = 43) were treated with Peg-IFNα-2a for 48 weeks and were followed for 48 weeks after therapy. (2) Patients in Group 2 (n = 49) were treated with and 0.5 mg of ETV once daily for 48 weeks and were followed for 48 weeks after therapy. (3) Patients in Group 3 (n = 46) were treated with Peg-IFNα-2a and 10 mg of ADV once daily for 48 weeks and were followed for 48 weeks after therapy. Liver histological examination was performed in 38 of these patients before therapy and after follow-up, in order to evaluate the improvement of liver histology.

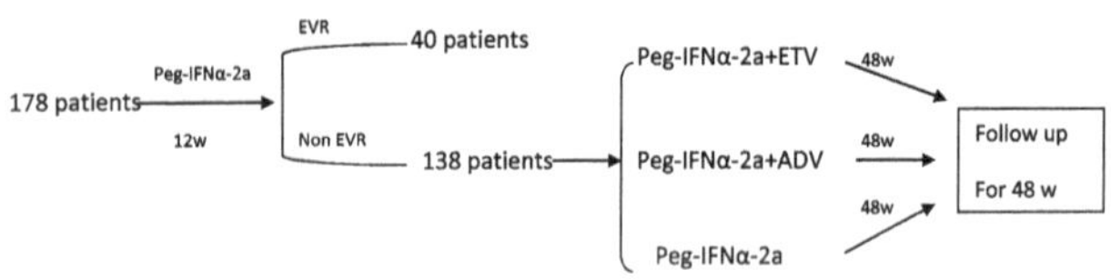

All study patients were subjected to a routine biochemical examination, routine urinalysis, and a routine blood test to evaluate thyroid function, and blood glucose levels. Patients were also evaluated for HBsAg levels, viral genotype. Routine blood tests were performed once weekly in the initial 4 weeks and thereafter once every 4 weeks. Biochemical examination and detection of HBV DNA and HBsAg levels were performed after 12 weeks of therapy, and once every 12 weeks thereafter. Patients receiving liver histological examination before therapy were evaluated for disease condition using the Knodell histology activity index (Knodell HAI) score, and were subjected to liver histological examination again after follow-up. Improvement in liver histology was defined as a reduction in Knodell score by ≥2 when compared to the baseline score, and no deterioration of hepatic fibrosis (deterioration of hepatic fibrosis is defined as an increase in Knodell fibrosis score by ≥1). Liver HBsAg levels were quantitated before and after anti-viral therapy in patients receiving liver histological examination.

Evaluation of biochemical and virological markers

Viral markers were detected by ELISA (Shanghai Kehua Biotech Co., Ltd). Serum HBsAg levels were semi-quantitatively evaluated with the ElecsysIIdetection system using the S-P method according to the manufacturer's instructions. Liver HBsAg expression was scored as 0, 1, 2, 3 and 4 based on cytoplasm and/or nuclear staining and as 25%, 25–50%, 50–75% and >75% based on the proportion of positive hepatocytes to total hepatocytes [18]. Liver function was detected with an automatic biochemical analyzer (Beckman, USA). HBV DNA levels in the serum and liver tissue were quantitated by real time fluorescence PCR using an RT-PCR kit (lower limit of detection is 300 copies/ml; COBAS TaqMan 48; Roche, Meylan, France). HBV genotypes were determined by PCR microplate hybridization ELISA (Guangzhou Lanxing Biotech Co., Ltd) according to the manufacturer's instructions.

Determination of therapeutic efficacy

Early virological response was defined as undetectable HBV DNA after anti-viral therapy for 12 weeks. After 12 weeks of therapy, patients were followed for 48 weeks. Sustained virological response (SVR) was defined as no change in therapeutic effectiveness after 6 months follow-up, and no recurrence. SVR was calculated as the ratio of patients with HBV DNA lower than the lower detection limit (<300copies/ml)to total patients.

Liver function was also re-examined regularly. However, it is important to note that patients treated with IFN and those with hepatic cirrhosis exhibit a transient increase in transaminases during anti-viral therapy with IFN. In addition, hepatic cirrhosis patients may occasionally exhibit a slight increase in transaminases although HBV DNA levels may be very low.

Assessment of safety

Side effects such as fever, muscle ache, fatigue and leukopenia were evaluated. The dose of Peg-IFNα-2a dose was decreased when neutrophil counts reached $\leq 0.75 \times 10^9$/L or platelet counts reached $<50 \times 10^9$/L; anti-viral therapy was stopped when the neutrophil count reduced to $\leq 0.5 \times 10^9$/L or platelet count reduced to$<30 \times 10^9$/L.

Determination of HBeAg conversion rate

HBeAg seroconversion rate was calculated as the ratio of HBeAg-positive patients who were HBeAb-positive after anti-viral therapy to the total number of HBeAg-positive patients.

Statistical analysis

Patients' demographic and baseline characteristic data were presented as mean ± standard deviations (SD) and median (IQR: 1st and 3rd quartiles) for continuous data with and without normal distribution; categorical data were presented as n (%). Differences among three groups were compared using one-way ANOVA and the Kruskall-

Wallis test for continuous data with and without normal distribution, respectively; the Pearson Chi-square test was used for categorical ones.

The changes in HBV DNA levels after 4 wks, 12 wks, 24 wks, 36 wks, and 48 wks of treatment, and after 48 wks follow-up as compared with baseline HBV DNA levels were presented as mean ± SD at each time point for a given treatment group. Differences in HBV DNA levels over time were compared between the treatment groups using repeated measurement ANOVA test with post-hoc Bonferroni pair-wise comparisons.

The HBV DNA SVR and HBsAg conversion rate were represented as percentage of rate for each group, and the change in HBsAg levels was represented as mean with standard deviation (SD) for each group. Differences between the groups were compared using the Pearson Chi-square test for HBV DNA SVR and HBsAg conversion rate and one-way ANOVA with a post-hoc Bonferroni pair-wise comparisons for change in HBsAg levels.

The Knodell score (necroinflammatory score), Ishak score (fibrosis score) and improvement of liver histology among three groups were represented as median (IQR: 1st, 3rd quartiles) for Knodell score and Ishak score; and n (%) for improvement of liver histology. Differences between the groups were compared using the Kruskall-Wallis test for Knodell and Ishak scores. The improvement of liver histology was compared using Fisher's exact test since some cell numbers were less than 5.

The association of the change in HBsAg levels with each treatment and the association of improvement rate with the change in HBsAg levels were evaluated. The change in HBsAg levels was represented as mean ± SD for each group and compared using one-way ANOVA with post-hoc Bonferroni pair-wise comparisons. The improvement rate was represented as percentages of patients for a given change in HBsAg levels. Differences between multiple changes in HBsAg levels were compared by Pearson Chi-square test.

All statistical assessments were two-tailed and $P < 0.05$ was considered significant. An adjusted significance level of 0.0167 (0.05/3) was considered for the post-hoc pair-wise comparison, Bonferroni test. All statistical analyses were performed using the SPSS statistics software (SPSS Inc., Chicago, IL, USA).

Results

Demographics and clinical characteristics

After the first 12 weeks of Peg-IFNα-2a treatment, a total of 43 study patients (24 males and 19 females) received Peg-IFNα-2a. Forty nine patients (35 males and 14 females) received Peg-IFNα-2a + ETV, and 46 patients (31 males and 15 females) received Peg-IFNα-2a + ADV. The mean ages of patients in the Peg-IFNα-2a, Peg-IFNα-2a + ETV, and Peg-IFNα-2a + ADV groups were 34.9 years (SD = 10.9), 37.4 years (SD = 9.5), and 38.6 years (SD = 10.0) respectively. There was no significant difference in the demographic data and baseline characteristics between the three groups (Table 1; all P values >0.05).

Efficacy of additional nucleoside analogues in patients treated with peg-IFNα-2a

The temporal profiles of HBV DNA levels were evaluated before and after treatment (Fig. 1). Patients in the Peg-INFα-2a + ETV as well as the Peg-INFα-2a + ADV groups showed a significantly greater decrease in HBV DNA levels over time compared to the group treated with Peg-INFα-2a alone (both P values <0.0167). Notably, Peg-INFα-2a + ETV and Peg-INFα-2a + ADV had similar efficacies, resulting in overlapping profiles after week 12 of treatment, but none patient achieve HBsAg loss during or after therapy (Fig. 1).

There was a significant difference in SVR between the three treatment groups (Fig. 2a). Patients in the Peg-IFNα-2a + ETV and Peg-IFNα-2a + ADV groups had significantly higher SVRs(69.4%, and 71.7%) compared to the group treated with Peg-IFNα-2a alone (32.6%), both P values <0.001.

Table 1 Demographic and baseline characteristic data of study patients

Variables	Peg-IFNα-2a (n = 43)	Peg-IFNα-2a + ETV (n = 49)	Peg-IFNα-2a + ADV (n = 46)	P value
Age	34.86 ± 10.86	37.38 ± 9.51	38.63 ± 9.98	0.188
Sex, males (%)	24 (55.8%)	35 (71.4%)	31 (67.4%)	0.272
Baseline HBV DNA, (log_{10}copies/mL)	6.47 ± 1.16	6.48 ± 1.01	6.24 ± 1.14	0.513
Baseline ALT, U/L	102 (87, 159)	119 (85, 162)	105 (87.8, 197.8)	0.744
HBeAg status				0.905
positive	28 (65.1%)	33 (67.3%)	32 (69.6%)	
negative	15 (34.9%)	16 (32.7%)	14 (30.4%)	
Genotype				0.183
B	10 (23.8%)	14 (28.6%)	19 (41.3%)	
C	32 (76.2%)	35 (71.4%)	27 (58.7%)	

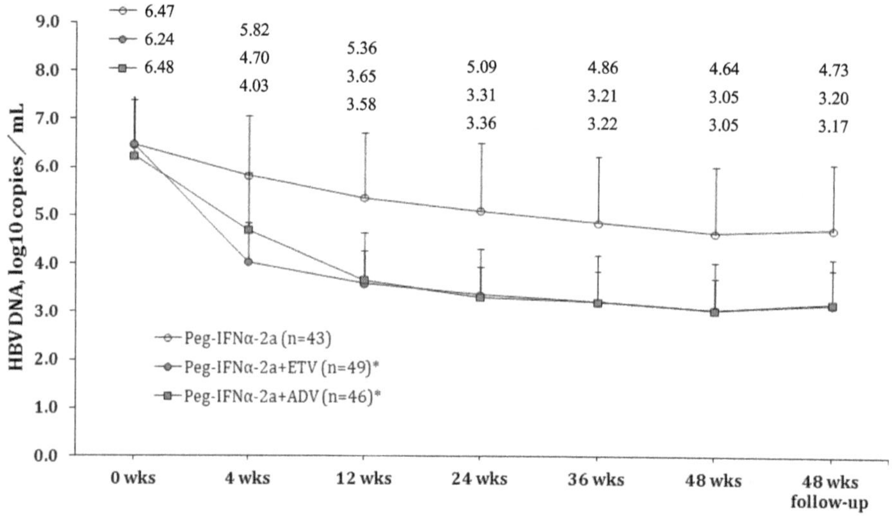

Fig. 1 Dispersion of HBV DNA before and after treatment for each group. Data were represented as mean ± standard deviation (SD) for patients in Peg-IFNα-2a group, Peg-IFNα-2a + ETV group, and Peg-IFNα-2a + ADV group at baseline (0 wks), 4 wks, 12 wks, 24 wks, 36 wks, 48 wks of therapy, and 48 wks follow-up. Abbreviations: wks, weeks; ETV, Entecavir, 0.5 mg; ADV, Adefovir 10 mg. *$P < 0.0167$, indicates a significant difference compared to the Peg-IFNα-2a group. There was no significant difference between the Peg-IFNα-2a + ETV and Peg-IFNα-2a + ADV groups

Patients in the Peg-IFNα-2a + ETV and Peg-IFNα-2a + ADV groups had higher HBeAg conversion rates compared to the group treated with Peg-IFNα-2a alone, although these differences were not significant (Peg-IFNα-2a vs. Peg-IFNα-2a + ETV: 14.3% vs. 24.2%, $P = 0.204$; Peg-IFNα-2a vs. Peg-IFNα-2a + ADV: 14.3% vs. 21.9%, $P = 0.339$) (Fig. 2b).

The changes in serum HBsAg levels compared to basal levels were evaluated at week 24 and week 48 of treatment and at 48 weeks after treatment. At each time point, patients in the Peg-IFNα-2a + ETV and Peg-IFNα-2a + ADV groups exhibited significantly higher reduction in HBsAg levels compared to patients treated with Peg-IFNα-2a alone (both P values <0.0167; Fig. 2c).

Thirty eight patients (11 in Peg-IFNα-2a group, 14 in Peg-IFNα-2a + ETV group, and 13 in Peg-IFNα-2a + ADV group) received liver histological examinations before therapy and after the 48 week follow-up period. (Liver histological examination was performed in a fraction of the study patients since not all study patients were willing to undergo this procedure). There was no significant difference in any of these indices between the three groups (All P >0.05). There was no significant difference in improvement of liver histology between the three groups (27.3%, 64.3% and 69.2% for Peg-IFNα-2a, Peg-IFNα-2a + ETV and Peg-IFNα-2a + ADV groups, respectively; $P > 0.05$) (Table 2).

The change in liver HBsAg levels was evaluated after 48 weeks of treatment in the 19 HBsAg-positive patients who received liver histological examination (5 in the Peg-IFNα-2a, 8 in Peg-IFNα-2a + ETV, and 6 in Peg-IFNα-2a + ADV. There was no significant difference ($P > 0.05$) in HBsAg levels between the three groups after 48 weeks of treatment (mean of 0.4 (SD = 0.55) for the Peg-IFNα-2a group, 1.4 (SD = 1.06) for the Peg-IFNα-2a + ETV group, and 1.8 (SD = 1.2) for the Peg-IFNα-2a + ADV group).

The rate of improvement versus the change in HBsAg levels was calculated in the 19 HBsAg-positive patients who received liver histological examination. The rate of improvement was 100% (3/3) in patients who had a change in HBsAg level = 3. The rate of improvement was 60% (3/5) in patients who had a change in HBsAg level = 2; 40% (2/5) in patients who had a change in HBsAg level = 1, and 50% (3/6) in patients who had a change in HBsAg level = 0. There was no significant association between rate of improvement versus the change in HBsAg levels ($P = 0.459$).

All study patients were monitored for adverse events. The most common adverse events reported were fatigue and muscle ache, fever, and thrombocytopenia (Table 3).

Discussion

In this study, patients who had a poor virological response after 12 weeks of Peg-IFNα-2a monotherapy were treated for an additional 48 weeks with a combination of Peg-IFNα-2a + ETV or Peg-IFNα-2a + ADV. Both regimens of combination therapy resulted in a significantly greater decrease in HBV DNA levels over time, and a significantly higher SVR compared to Peg-INFα-2a monotherapy. Although patients receiving combination therapy had a significantly higher change in serum HBsAg levels compared to the monotherapy group, there was no significant difference in liver HBsAg levels between the three treatment groups.

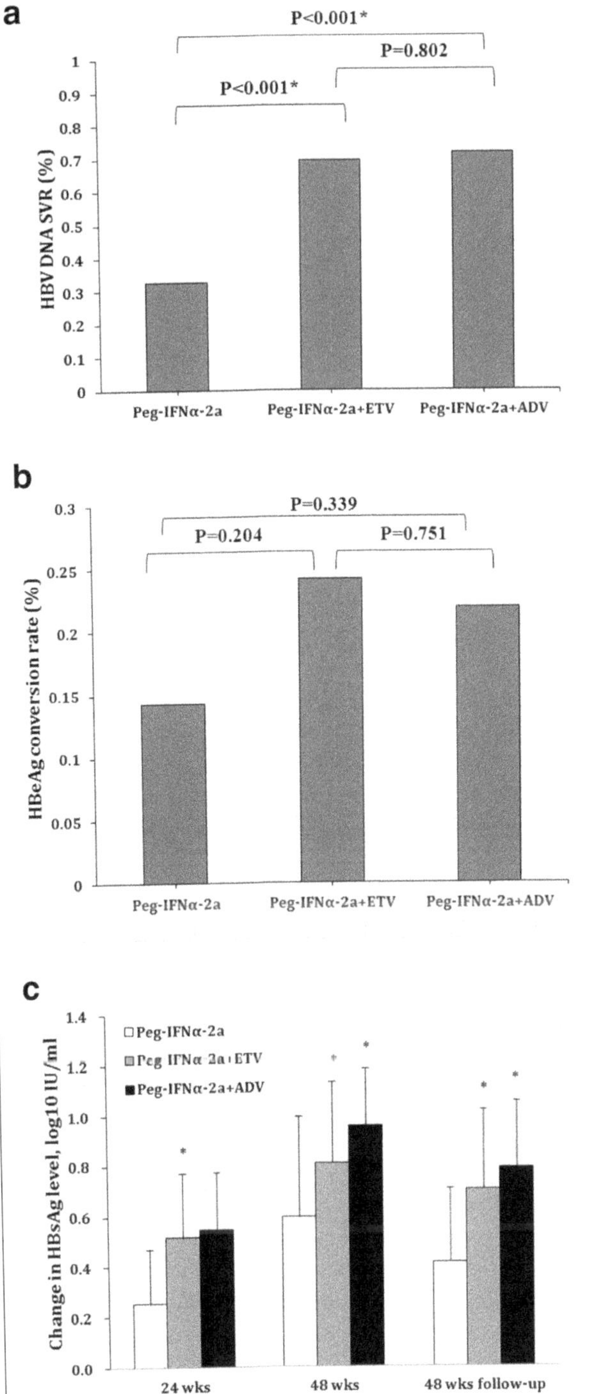

Fig. 2 Summary of HBV DNA SVR (**a**), HBeAg conversion rate (**b**), and change in serum HBsAg levels after treatments (**c**) by groups. The change in HBsAg levels after therapy was calculated as the difference between baseline HBsAg level and the HBsAg level at a specific time point. HBV DNA SVR was represented as percentage of rate and the change in HBsAg levels was represented as mean with standard deviation (SD).* $P < 0.001$, indicates a significant difference

A number of studies have investigated therapeutic strategies which combined the immunomodulatory effects of Peg-IFNα-2a along with the direct anti-viral activity of NAs for patients with a poor response to anti-viral therapy. The addition of LAM to Peg-IFN therapy failed to enhance therapeutic efficacy compared to monotherapy in early studies [9, 10, 19]. However, a recent meta-analysis suggested that a combination of PEG-IFN and LAM increased SVR [20]. A combination of Peg-IFN with ADV or ETV for 48 weeks had a significantly higher therapeutic efficacy in HBeAg-negative CHB patients compared to Peg-IFN monotherapy [14, 21]. A recent study showed the efficacy of a sequential treatment strategy where patients received 24 weeks of telbuvidine followed by 24 weeks of Peg-IFNα-2a [22]. It is important to note that these studies used combination therapy as the first-line therapy, whereby patients having the potential to achieve a virological response with Peg-IFN alone also received combination therapy. In the present study, 138 study patients were treated Peg-IFNα-2a for 12 weeks, and only 95 patients who had a poor virological response at the end of this period received combination therapy of Peg-IFNα-2a with either ETV or ADV for 48 weeks. The Peg-IFN-α2a + ETV and Peg-IFN-α2a + ADV groups showed a reduction in HBV DNA by 3.3 and 3.0 $\log_{10}$ copies/mL, respectively and the proportion of patients with undetectable HBV DNA was 69.4% and 71.7%, respectively, which were significantly higher than that in patients treated with Peg-IFNα-2a alone.

Anti-viral therapy with Peg-IFN was shown to improve liver histology in 38–48% of patients and significantly delay disease progression [23]. A meta-analysis of 26 prospective studies also revealed that reduction of HBV DNA levels after anti-viral therapy was positively related to improvement of liver histology [24]. In the present study, a significantly higher percentage of patients in the Peg-IFN-α2a + ADV and Peg-IFN-α2a + ETV groups showed an improvement in liver histology compared to the Peg-IFNα-2a monotherapy group (69.2% and 64.3% vs. 27.3%). These data suggested that in patients with an early poor virological response to Peg-IFN-α2a, addition of NAs could promote inhibition of viral replication, which is associated with SVR and improvement of liver histology. These findings have important implications for attenuation of hepatic inflammation and fibrosis and slowing the progression of hepatic cirrhosis in CHB patients.

Baseline and on-treatment HBsAg levels have been shown to be strong predictors of therapeutic efficacy, and patients with HBsAg levels >20,000 IU/ml after 24 weeks of Peg-IFNα-2a treatment failed to achieve a virologic response [25]. Reduction in HBsAg levels has been shown to be closely related to seroconversion of HBeAg and HBsAg, and a larger reduction in HBsAg levels during therapy is associated with a higher possibility of HBsAg

Table 2 Knodell and Ishak scores before and after anti-viral therapy and improvement of liver histology after anti-viral therapy in the three treatment groups (*N* = 38)

Variables	Peg-IFNα-2a (*n* = 11)	Peg-IFNα-2a + ETV (*n* = 14)	Peg-IFNα-2a + ADV (*n* = 13)	*P* value
Before anti-viral therapy				
Ishak score	3 (2, 3)	3 (2, 4)	4 (3, 4)	0.070
Knodell score	6 (5, 7)	6 (4.7, 7)	6 (5, 7.5)	0.154
After anti-viral therapy				
Ishak score	3 (2, 3)	2.5 (2, 3.3)a	3 (2.5, 3.5)a	0.613
Knodell score	4 (4, 5)b	4 (3, 5)b	4 (3, 6)b	0.573
Improvement of liver histology	3 (27.3%)	9 (64.3%)	9 (69.2%)	0.083

Data were represented as median (IQR: 1st, 3rd quartiles) for Knodell score and Ishak score; and n (%) for improvement of liver histology
Differences between groups were compared using the Kruskall-Wallis test for Knodell and Ishak scores; Differences between pre- and post-inflammation were compared using the Wilcoxon Sign-rank test because the Knodell score and Ishak score were ordinal data. The improvement of liver histology was compared using Fisher's exact test since some cell numbers were less than 5
There was no significant difference between the groups
ab $P < 0.05$, significant difference compared with pre-treated a (Ishak score) and b (Knodell score) for a given group

loss after long-term anti-viral therapy [26–29]. However, the association between serum HBsAg levels and liver histological score and HBV DNA levels remains unclear. One study reported that serum HBsAg levels were negatively associated with HBV DNA levels [30], while another study showed that 1) HBV DNA in the liver of CHB patients and HBV cccDNA before therapy were positively related to serum HBsAg, and 2) the reduction in serum HBsAg was positively associated with the reduction in HBV DNA in the liver and HBV cccDNA after combination therapy with LAM and Peg-IFN [31, 32]. In the present study, we showed that patients in the Peg-IFN-α-2a + ADV and Peg-IFN-α-2a + ETV groups had a more significant change in serum HBsAg levels compared to patients in the Peg-IFN-α-2a monotherapy group, as well as a higher rate of HBsAg seroconversion. Our data suggested that using combination therapy to achieve modulation of the immune response by Peg-IFNα-2a and inhibition of viral inhibition by Peg-IFNα-2a and NAs, significantly enhanced therapeutic efficacy which was reflected by a reduction in serum HBsAg. However, there was no correlation between change in liver HBsAg levels and rate of improvement in liver histology. The current study about the relation of serum HBsAg and liver histologic is not very clear, all the results are also different. This study not only observed the changes of serum HBsAg levels, also for the iver histologic HBsAg levels, designed to examine whether changes in the level of HBsAg can predict the effect. But because the patients with liver histological examination is less, the results found no significant differences.

We aimed to investigate the influence of additional nucleoside analogues on the SVR and the improvement of liver histology in CHB patients who had a poor virological response to Peg-INFα-2a at the end of 12 weeks of therapy. We can further observe the effect of sequential interferon therapy following nucleoside analogue for a long time .

Table 3 Summary of adverse events

Adverse events	Peg-IFNα-2a (*n* = 43)	Combination groups (*n* = 95)
Fatigue and muscle ache	36 (83.7%)	76 (80%)
Fever	30 (70%)	70 (73.7%)
Thrombocytopenia	22 (51.2%)	47 (49.5%)
Anemia	16 (37.2%)	36 (37.9%)
Neutropenia	14 (32.6%)	33 (34.7%)
Loss of appetite	15 (34.9%)	30 (31.6%)
Hair Loss	10 (23.3%)	24 (25.3%)
Abnormal blood glucose	2 (4.7%)	5 (5.3%)
Rash	2 (4.7%)	3 (3.2%)
Hypothyroidism	1 (2.3%)	1 (1.1)

Data were summarized as n (%) for given adverse events in each group

Conclusions

In summary, this study demonstrated that in patients with a poor virological response after 12 weeks of treatment with Peg-IFNα-2a alone, addition of ADV or ETV significantly reduced HBV DNA levels, serum HBsAg levels, and increased SVR. Individualization of anti-viral therapy would ensure that only patients who do not respond to Peg-IFNα-2a would receive combination therapy. Our data have important implications for the treatment of CHB patients who fail to show an early response to Peg-IFNα-2a monotherapy.

Abbreviations

ADV: adefovir dipivoxil; cccDNA: covalently closed circular HBV DNA; CHB: chronic hepatitis B; ETV: entecavir; HBV: hepatitis B virus; HCC: hepatocellular carcinoma; LAM: lamivudine; PEG-IFN-α-2a: pegylated interferon alpha 2a; SVR: sustained virologic response

Acknowledgements
Medica Communicus Zhuhai Ltd. provided writing assistance which was sponsored by Shanghai Roche Pharmaceuticals Ltd.

Authors' contribution
YX and JBW participated in the study design and coordination and the manuscript preparation. XW and ZHL performed the biochemical and virological assays. CYZ, JJ, FY, HHG, PZ participated in the implementation of the study. WQQ participated in study design and performed the statistical analysis. All authors read and approved the final manuscript.

Funding
This study was supported by a grant from the Key projects of Science and Technology Agency of Jilin province (grant no: 20,090,440).

Consent for publication
Not applicable.

Competing interests
Writing assistance was sponsored by Shanghai Roche Pharmaceuticals Ltd.

References

1. Liang TJ. Hepatitis B: the virus and disease. Hepatology. 2009;49(5 Suppl): S13–21.
2. Janssen HL, van Zonneveld M, Schalm SW. Hepatitis B. N Engl J Med. 2004; 350(26):2719–20.
3. Lai CL, Ratziu V, Yuen MF, Poynard T. Viral hepatitis B. Lancet. 2003; 362(9401):2089–94.
4. European Association For The Study Of The L. EASL clinical practice guidelines: management of chronic hepatitis B virus infection. J Hepatol. 2012;57(1):167–85.
5. Lok AS, McMahon BJ. Chronic hepatitis B: update 2009. Hepatology. 2009; 50(3):661–2.
6. Liaw YF, Chien RN, Yeh CT, Tsai SL, Chu CM. Acute exacerbation and hepatitis B virus clearance after emergence of YMDD motif mutation during lamivudine therapy. Hepatology. 1999;30(2):567–72.
7. Manesis EK, Hadziyannis SJ. Interferon alpha treatment and retreatment of hepatitis B e antigen-negative chronic hepatitis B. Gastroenterology. 2001; 121(1):101–9.
8. Sonneveld MJ, Zoutendijk R, Hansen BE, Janssen HL. Pegylated interferon results in higher serological, but not virological, response rates when compared to continuous entecavir. Antivir Ther. 2012;17(8):1605–8.
9. Lau GK, Piratvisuth T, Luo KX, Marcellin P, Thongsawat S, Cooksley G, et al. Peginterferon alfa-2a, lamivudine, and the combination for HBeAg-positive chronic hepatitis B. N Engl J Med. 2005;352(26):2682–95.
10. Marcellin P, Lau GK, Bonino F, Farci P, Hadziyannis S, Jin R, et al. Peginterferon alfa-2a alone, lamivudine alone, and the two in combination in patients with HBeAg-negative chronic hepatitis B. N Engl J Med. 2004; 351(12):1206–17. https://doi.org/10.1056/NEJMoa040431.
11. Karabay O, Tuna N, Esen S, Group P-HS. Comparative efficacy of pegylated interferons alpha-2a and 2b in the treatment of HBeAg-negative chronic hepatitis B infection. Eur J Gastroenterol Hepatol. 2012;24(11):1296–301.
12. Gulsun S, Tekin R, Bozkurt F. Treatment of chronic delta hepatitis: a nine-year retrospective analysis. Hepat Mon. 2011;11(9):731–5.
13. Piccolo P, Lenci I, Demelia L, Bandiera F, Piras MR, Antonucci G, et al. A randomized controlled trial of pegylated interferon-alpha2a plus adefovir dipivoxil for hepatitis B e antigen-negative chronic hepatitis B. Antivir Ther. 2009;14(8):1165–74.
14. Hagiwara S, Kudo M, Osaki Y, Matsuo H, Inuzuka T, Matsumoto A, et al. Impact of peginterferon alpha-2b and entecavir hydrate combination therapy on persistent viral suppression in patients with chronic hepatitis B. J Med Virol. 2013;85(6):987–95.
15. Fried MW, Piratvisuth T, Lau GK, Marcellin P, Chow WC, Cooksley G, et al. HBeAg and hepatitis B virus DNA as outcome predictors during therapy with peginterferon alfa-2a for HBeAg-positive chronic hepatitis B. Hepatology. 2008;47(2):428 34.
16. Zoulim F, Perrillo R. Hepatitis B: reflections on the current approach to antiviral therapy. J Hepatol. 2008;48(Suppl 1):S2–19.
17. Branch of Infectious Diseases and Parasitic Diseases of Chinese Medical Association BoHDoCMAaCFfHPaC. Chinese J Hepatol. 2008;8(6):6.
18. Lindh M, Savage K, Rees J, Garwood L, Horal P, Norkrans G, et al. HBeAg immunostaining of liver tissue in various stages of chronic hepatitis B. Liver. 1999;19(4):294–8.
19. Janssen HL, van Zonneveld M, Senturk H, Zeuzem S, Akarca US, Cakaloglu Y, et al. Pegylated interferon alfa-2b alone or in combination with lamivudine for HBeAg-positive chronic hepatitis B: a randomised trial. Lancet. 2005; 365(9454):123–9.
20. Shi Y, Wu YH, Shu ZY, Zhang WJ, Yang J, Chen Z. Interferon and lamivudine combination therapy versus lamivudine monotherapy for hepatitis B e antigen-negative hepatitis B treatment: a meta-analysis of randomized controlled trials. Hepatobiliary Pancreat Dis Int. 2010;9(5):462–72.
21. Piccolo P, De Melia, L, Bandiera F, et al. Peginterferon alpha-2a plus adefovir dipivoxil vs. peginterferon alpha-2a monotherapy for 48 weeks in HBeAg-negative chronic hepatitis B: final results of the PEG for B randomized multicenter trial. Digestive Disease Week. 2008;May 17–22(Abstract 256).
22. Piccolo P, Lenci I, di Paolo D, Demelia L, Sorbello O, Nosotti L, et al. A randomized controlled trial of sequential pegylated interferon-alpha and telbivudine or vice versa for 48 weeks in hepatitis B e antigen-negative chronic hepatitis B. Antivir Ther. 2013;18(1):57–64.
23. Cooksley WG, Piratvisuth T, Lee SD, Mahachai V, Chao YC, Tanwandee T, et al. Peginterferon alpha-2a (40 kDa): an advance in the treatment of hepatitis B e antigen-positive chronic hepatitis B. J Viral Hepat. 2003;10(4):298–305.
24. Mommeja-Marin H, Mondou E, Blum MR, Rousseau F. Serum HBV DNA as a marker of efficacy during therapy for chronic HBV infection: analysis and review of the literature. Hepatology. 2003;37(6):1309–19.
25. Sonneveld MJ, Hansen BE, Piratvisuth T, Jia JD, Zeuzem S, Gane E, et al. Response-guided peginterferon therapy in hepatitis B e antigen-positive chronic hepatitis B using serum hepatitis B surface antigen levels. Hepatology. 2013;58(3):872–80.
26. Moucari R, Korevaar A, Lada O, Martinot-Peignoux M, Boyer N, Mackiewicz V, et al. High rates of HBsAg seroconversion in HBeAg-positive chronic hepatitis B patients responding to interferon: a long-term follow-up study. J Hepatol. 2009;50(6):1084–92.
27. Brunetto MR, Moriconi F, Bonino F, Lau GK, Farci P, Yurdaydin C, et al. Hepatitis B virus surface antigen levels: a guide to sustained response to peginterferon alfa-2a in HBeAg-negative chronic hepatitis B. Hepatology. 2009;49(4):1141–50.
28. Manesis EK, Hadziyannis ES, Angelopoulou OP, Hadziyannis SJ. Prediction of treatment-related HBsAg loss in HBeAG-negative chronic hepatitis B: a clue from serum HBsAg levels. Antivir Ther. 2007;12(1):73–82.
29. Tangkijvanich P, Komolmit P, Mahachai V, Sa-nguanmoo P, Theamboonlers A, Poovorawan Y. Low pretreatment serum HBsAg level and viral mutations as predictors of response to PEG-interferon alpha-2b therapy in chronic hepatitis B. J Clin Virol. 2009;46(2):117–23.
30. Ozdil B, Cosar AM, Akkiz H, Sandikci MU, Kece C. Negative correlation between viral load and HBsAg levels in chronic HBV-infected patients. Arch Virol. 2009;154(9):1451–5.
31. Chan HL, Wong VW, Chim AM, Chan HY, Wong GL, Sung JJ. Serum HBsAg quantification to predict response to peginterferon therapy of e antigen positive chronic hepatitis B. Aliment Pharmacol Ther. 2010;32(11–12):1323–31.
32. Chan HL, Wong VW, Tse AM, Tse CH, Chim AM, Chan HY, et al. Serum hepatitis B surface antigen quantitation can reflect hepatitis B virus in the liver and predict treatment response. Clin Gastroenterol Hepatol. 2007;5(12): 1462–8.

Diminished accuracy of biomarkers of fibrosis in low replicative chronic hepatitis B

Faisal M. Sanai[1,8*], Taha Farah[8], Khalid Albeladi[8], Faisal Batwa[8], Yaser Dahlan[8], Mohammed A. Babatin[3], Hamad Al-Ashgar[4], Hadeel AlMana[5], Khaled S. Alsaad[6], Khalid AlSwat[1], Abdulrahman Aljumah[7,9], Ibrahim H. AlTraif[7,9], Bahaa E. Kailani[10] and Khalid I. Bzeizi[2]

Abstract

Background: We evaluated the diagnostic accuracy of aspartate aminotransferase (AST)-to-platelet ratio index (APRI), fibrosis-4 index (FIB-4), AST/alanine aminotransferase (ALT) ratio (AAR), and age-platelet index (API) for significant fibrosis (Metavir F2–4) in low-replicative (HBV DNA <20,000 IU/mL) chronic hepatitis B virus (HBV) patients.

Methods: The sensitivity, specificity, and area under the receiver-operating characteristic curve (AUROC) of HBeAg-negative, low-replicative (n = 213) and high-replicative (HBV DNA ≥20,000 IU/mL, n = 153) patients was assessed.

Results: Overall, 113 patients (30.9%) had F2–4 fibrosis. Of the low and high-replicative patients, 40 (18.8%) and 73 (47.7%) had F2–4, respectively (P < 0.0001). APRI ≥0.5 less frequently identified F2–4 fibrosis in low vs. high-replicative patients (48.7% vs. 69.6%, P = 0.032) and AAR identified it more frequently in low-replicative patients (37.5% vs. 19.4%, P = 0.037). FIB-4 and API were not different (P > 0.05) for identifying F2–4 fibrosis in low and high-replicative patients. Higher specificities were seen at the lowest cut-offs in low vs. high-replicative states for APRI (≥0.5, 98% vs. 68.9%), AAR (84.3% vs. 76.6%), FIB-4 (≥1.45, 97.5% vs. 87.8%) and API (>4, 94.8% vs. 93.8%). At ROC-defined thresholds, APRI (≥0.33), AAR (≥0.93), FIB-4 (≥0.70) and API (>2) showed greater AUROCs for F2–4 diagnosis in low replicative (0.80, 0.62, 0.81 and 0.71, respectively) vs. high-replicative patients (0.73, 0.52, 0.67 and 0.69, respectively).

Conclusion: All 4 biomarkers in both, low and high-replicative HBV demonstrate modest accuracy for fibrosis diagnosis at conventional cut-offs. Lowering the cut-offs may increase the diagnostic relevance of these biomarkers, particularly for APRI and FIB-4 in low-replicative disease.

Keywords: Hepatitis B, Fibrosis, Biomarkers, APRI

Background

Assessment of histological disease is of immense importance in managing chronic hepatitis B virus (HBV) patients. Treatment is strongly recommended in patients with significant fibrosis (for instance, METAVIR score F2–4). In the absence of liver biopsy, treatment decisions are based on the surrogate markers of histological disease, namely, elevated alanine aminotransferase (ALT) and high HBV DNA levels [1, 2].

Significant fibrosis in patients with low viremia may occur, with reports of progression to cirrhosis [3]. We have previously shown that F2–4 fibrosis occurs in about 18% of patients with HBV DNA <20,000 IU/mL [4]. Thus, since fibrosis occurs in a minority of patients with 'low' viremia levels, it becomes essential to identify its predictors, prior to undertaking liver biopsy. Furthermore, a single biopsy does not measure the dynamic nature of liver fibrosis [5].

* Correspondence: sanaifa@ngha.med.sa
[1]Liver Disease Research Center, King Saud University, Riyadh, Saudi Arabia
[8]Gastroenterology Unit, Department of Medicine, King Abdulaziz Medical City, PO Box: 9515, Jeddah 21423, Saudi Arabia

Of the several combined biomarkers of fibrosis, FIB-4 (based on age, ALT, aspartate aminotransferase [AST] and platelet count), AST-to-platelet ratio index (APRI), AST/ALT ratio (AAR), and age-platelet index (API) have been well studied. Studies have suggested that these markers may be useful for predicting fibrosis and cirrhosis [6]. However, most validations occurred under controlled conditions and have shown sensitivity and specificity at the extreme stages of liver fibrosis. Additionally, previous studies have not evaluated these combination biomarkers in the context of low HBV DNA levels.

In this study, we aimed to evaluate the diagnostic performance of serum biomarkers in identifying significant fibrosis in an unselected cohort of HBeAg-negative, low-replicative, chronic hepatitis B patients.

Methods

Study patients

Consecutive patients were included by a retrospective search of clinical records and hospital databases for the period between January 2006 and January 2012. All data was anonymized and de-identified prior to analysis. The patients were included from four centres in Saudi Arabia. The institutional review boards of all centres (Retrospective Research Committee, Institutional Review Board, King Abdullah International Medical Research Centre; Research Advisory Council, King Faisal Specialist Hospital and Research Centre; Research and Ethics Committee, Prince Sultan Military Medical City; Central Institutional Review Board; Ministry of Health) approved the study. Eligible patients for the analysis had detectable HBsAg >6 months prior to inclusion in the study. All patients were HBeAg-negative and were between 16 to 80 years of age.

The exclusion criteria were: (i) co-infection with hepatitis C, delta virus or HIV; (ii) superimposed with other liver diseases; (iii) hepatotoxic medications in the preceding 3 months; (iv) previous immunosuppressive or antiviral therapy; (v) decompensated cirrhosis with a Child-Pugh score > 6, or evidence of portal hypertension, variceal bleeding, laboratory findings of a platelet count <100 (10^9/L), an international normalized ratio ≥ 1.3; (vii) creatinine >135 µmol/L (viii) presence of hepato-biliary malignancy; (ix) alcohol consumption >20 g/day; and (x) organ transplantation.

Study design

A minimum of three recordings of liver biochemistry for patients with normal levels and two recordings for those with elevated levels were required. The median number of ALT tests performed pre liver biopsy was 5 (interquartile range [IQR] 4–8), and these were sampled over a median period of 21 months (IQR 8–46). Serum biochemical and haematological values prior to the liver biopsy were recorded. Routine liver biochemical tests were performed using commercially available autoanalysers and hepatitis serological markers were assayed using commercially available enzyme-linked immunoassays. Patients with HBV DNA <20,000 IU/mL were classified as low-replicative while those with HBV DNA ≥20,000 IU/mL were classified as high-replicative. A minimum of three HBV DNA recordings was required and the reference value utilized for analysis was based on the pre biopsy level. Serum HBV DNA level was expressed in IU/mL (1 IU/mL = 5.6 copies/mL) [7]. Quantitative HBV DNA levels were measured by a COBAS TaqMan System (Roche Diagnostics, Indianapolis, IN, USA), which has a lower detection limit of 15 IU/mL, or Abbott Real-Time HBV assay (Abbott Molecular, Inc., Des Plaines, IL, USA), with a lower detection limit of 10 IU/mL. The median duration between the first and pre liver biopsy HBV DNA was 12 months (IQR 6–20).

Measurement of noninvasive biomarkers

Patient data included age (at time of liver biopsy), ALT and AST levels (upper limit of normal [ULN] values that were specific to the laboratory performing the test) and platelet counts. APRI, FIB-4 and AST/ALT ratio were calculated based on laboratory results from sera collected within 3 months of the liver biopsy using the following formulas:

$$\text{FIB-4} = \frac{\text{Age (years)} \times \text{AST (U/L)}}{\text{Platelet count } (10^9/\text{L}) \times [\text{ALT (U/L)}]^{1/2}}$$

$$\text{AAR} = \text{AST/ALT}$$

$$\text{APRI} = \frac{\text{AST (/ULN)}}{\text{Platelet count } (10^9/\text{L})} \times 100$$

API: Age (years): < 30 = 0; 30–39 = 1; 40–49 = 2; 50–59 = 3; 60–69 = 4; ≥70 = 5. Platelet count: >225 = 0; 200–224 = 1; 175–199 = 2; 150–174 = 3; 125–149 = 4; <125 = 5. AP index is the sum of the above (possible value 0–10).

Liver histology

All patients included in this study had liver biopsies stained with hematoxylin and eosin for morphological evaluation and reticulin for the assessment of fibrosis. Only liver specimens with more than nine portal tracts were considered sufficient. All specimens were centrally assessed and scored according to the METAVIR scoring system [8] by two experienced hepatopathologists who were blinded to all clinical information. Fibrosis scores of F0–1 were defined as minimal/mild, F2–4 as significant.

Statistical analyses

Quantitative variables were expressed as the mean ± standard deviation, and categorical variables as frequencies and proportions. The unpaired student's t-test was used to compare between the means or log means of the variable if the variable was normally or not normally distributed, respectively. The Chi-square or Fishers' exact tests were used to compare frequencies and proportions in categorical variables, as appropriate. The sensitivity, specificity, positive likelihood ratio (LR+), and negative likelihood ratio (LR-) of points on curve were calculated to obtain the optimal cut-off point to discriminate F2–4 with noninvasive biomarkers. The area under receiver operating characteristics (AUROC) curve was used to assess the overall diagnostic value of the biomarkers at different cut-offs that predicted fibrosis. All of the tests of significance were 2-tailed and a P-value of <0.05 was considered statistically significant. Statistical Package for Social Sciences (*SPSS, version* 17.0; Chicago, IL, USA) and MedCalc (MedCalc Software, Inc., Mariakerke, Belgium) were used for data analysis.

Results

Baseline characteristics of patients

A total of 366 patients were included in this analysis and of these 213 (58.2%) had HBV DNA < 20,000 IU/mL, and 153 (41.8%) had HBV DNA ≥ 20,000 IU/mL. The mean age was 38.6 ± 11.8 years and males constituted 272 (74.3%). In the overall cohort, F2–4 fibrosis was seen in 113 (30.9%) patients of whom 20 (5.5%) had F4 fibrosis. Of the low-replicative (HBV DNA <20,000 IU/mL) and high-replicative (≥20,000 IU/mL) patients, 40 (18.8%) and 73 (47.7%) had F2–4, respectively ($P < 0.0001$, Table 1). Low replicative patients were more obese compared to high-replicative ones ($P = 0.002$) and more likely to have normal ALT (55.4% vs. 19.6%, $P < 0.0001$). Mean biomarker scores between low-replicative and high-replicative patients were not significantly different ($P > 0.05$), however the mean scores were significantly higher for all biomarkers for F2–4 (compared to F0–1, $P < 0.05$, data not shown). Furthermore, all four biomarkers more frequently identified F2–4 fibrosis in both, low and high-replicative patients ($P < 0.05$, Additional file 1: Table S1).

Overall, there was an association between fibrosis stage and APRI, FIB-4 and API ($P < 0.05$ for all). For each successive fibrosis stage from F0 to F4, significantly higher APRI, FIB-4 and API values were seen ($P < 0.0001$ for all, Table 2). There was no difference between successive fibrosis stages by AAR ($P = 0.445$).

Sensitivity and specificity of biomarkers in relation to HBV DNA levels

For high-replicative patients, an APRI ≥0.5 more frequently identified F2–4 fibrosis (69.6%) as compared to those with low-replication (48.7%, $P = 0.032$). Other APRI cut-offs were not significantly different between the two groups (Table 3). On the other hand, AAR >1.0 less frequently identified F2–4 fibrosis in high-replicative patients (19.4 vs. 37.5%, $P = 0.037$). None of the cut-offs for FIB-4 or API differentiated F2–4 vs. F0–1 fibrosis between low and high-replicative patients. The specificity for F2–4 fibrosis at the lowest cut-offs was consistently greater in low compared to high-replicative states for APRI (98.0% vs. 68.9%, respectively), AAR (84.3% vs. 76.6%, respectively), FIB-4 (97.5 vs. 87.8%, respectively) and API (94.8% vs. 93.8%, respectively). This pattern remained similar for higher cut-offs (Table 4).

Performance characteristics of biomarkers

The overall sensitivity, specificity, LR+, LR- and AUROCs of the four biomarkers at different cut-offs for the diagnosis of F2–4 fibrosis are shown in Additional file 2:

Table 1 Baseline Characteristics of patients in relation to HBV DNA levels

Parameters	HBV DNA < 20,000 IU/mL (*n* = 213)	HBV DNA > 20,000 IU/mL (*n* = 153)	*P* value
Age (years)	38.2 ± 11.7	39.1 ± 12.0	0.485
Male gender (%)	156 (73.2)	116 (75.8)	0.578
BMI (Kg/m^2)	29.5 ± 10.4	26.9 ± 4.9	0.002
Diabetes mellitus (%)	30 (14.1)	20 (13.1)	0.781
Hyperlipidemia (%)	41 (19.2)	31 (20.3)	0.810
HBV DNA Log$_{10}$	3.3 ± 0.7	6.1 ± 1.3	< 0.0001
Platelets (10^9)	255.3 ± 68.9	232.2 ± 61.8	0.001
Elevated AST (%)	41 (20.0)	80 (54.1)	< 0.0001
Normal ALT (%)	118 (55.4)	30 (19.6)	< 0.0001
Elevated ALT (%)	95 (44.6)	123 (80.4)	
Fibrosis (F2–4, %)	40 (18.8)	73 (47.7)	< 0.0001

Data expressed as mean ± standard deviation or n (%) as appropriate. n, number. *AST* aspartate aminotransferase, *ALT* alanine aminotransferase ratio, *BMI* body mass index, *HBV* hepatitis B virus

Table 2 Mean scores of the four biomarkers in increasing stages (Metavir) of liver fibrosis

Fibrosis Stage	APRI (95% CI)	*P* value	AAR (95% CI)	*P* value	FIB-4 (95% CI)	*P* value	API (95% CI)	*P* value
STAGE 0	0.32 (0.27–0.38)	< 0.0001	0.77 (0.31–0.42)	0.445	0.66 (0.54–0.78)	< 0.0001	1.58 (1.22–1.94)	< 0.0001
STAGE 1	0.38 (0.31–0.45)		0.65 (0.69–0.83)		0.71 (0.63–0.78)		1.74 (1.52–1.96)	
STAGE 2	0.71 (0.52–0.90)		0.68 (0.60–0.77)		1.08 (0.88–1.29)		2.59 (2.11–3.07)	
STAGE 3	0.88 (0.66–1.09)		0.86 (0.58–1.14)		1.66 (1.06–2.25)		3.56 (2.68–4.44)	
STAGE 4	1.13 (0.51–1.76)		0.96 (0.68–1.24)		2.52 (1.49–3.55)		5.10 (3.93–6.27)	

AST aspartate aminotransferase, *APRI* AST-to-platelet ratio index, *AAR* AST/alanine aminotransferase ratio, *API* age-platelet index

Table S2. APRI demonstrated similar AUROCs for low and high-replicative states at all cut-offs (Table 4). However, higher AUROCs for F2–4 diagnosis were observed for low- compared to high-replicative state with AAR (0.61 vs. 0.48), FIB-4 (0.67 vs. 0.59) and API (0.66 vs. 0.55). Additionally, the AUROCs were serially lower across all biomarkers for both low and high-replicative states with incremental increase in the cut-off levels.

Figure 1a depicts the ROC curve analysis for optimum cut-offs with the best compromise sensitivity-specificity for distinguishing F2–4 for the four biomarkers in low-replicative state. At the ROC-derived optimum cut-offs, the sensitivity for APRI (≥0.33) is 76.4% and the specificity is 74.4% (AUROC, 0.80; 95% CI: 0.73–0.85; $P < 0.0001$), for AAR (≥0.93) the sensitivity is 73.5% and the specificity 47.5% (AUROC, 0.62; 95% CI: 0.55–0.69; $P = 0.023$), for FIB-4 (≥0.70) the sensitivity is 72.9% and specificity is 76.9% (AUROC, 0.81; 95% CI: 0.75–0.86; $P < 0.0001$), and for API (>2) the sensitivity is 75.1% and specificity is 55.0% (AUROC, 0.71; 95% CI: 0.64–0.77; $P < 0.0001$). Figure 1b depicts the ROC curve analysis in high-replicative patients. In patients meeting these optimum cut-offs, the sensitivity for APRI (≥0.33) is 52.7% and the specificity is 87.0% (AUROC, 0.73; 95% CI: 0.65–0.80; $P < 0.0001$), for AAR (≥0.91) the sensitivity is 24.7% and the specificity 79.2% (AUROC, 0.52; 95% CI: 0.44–0.60; $P = 0.643$), for FIB-4 (≥0.70) the sensitivity is 58.1% and specificity is 66.7% (AUROC, 0.67; 95% CI: 0.59–0.75; $P = 0.0001$), and for API (>2) the sensitivity is 75.0% and specificity is 56.2% (AUROC, 0.69; 95% CI: 0.61–0.76; $P < 0.0001$).

Table 3 Diagnosis of significant fibrosis (F2–4) in low and high replication HBV patients based on the four biomarkers

Fibrosis Biomarker	Total (*n* – 113)	HBV DNA < 20,000 IU/mL (*n* = 40)	HBV DNA > 20,000 IU/mL (*n* = /3)	*P* value
AST-Platelet Ratio Index (APRI)				
≥0.5	67 (62.0)	19 (48.7)	48 (69.6)	0.032
≥0.7	46 (42.6)	13 (32.3)	33 (47.8)	0.143
≥1.0	26 (24.1)	7 (17.9)	19 (27.5)	0.263
≥1.5	11 (10.2)	2 (5.1)	9 (13.0)	0.191
AST/ALT Ratio (AAR)				
>1.0	29 (25.9)	15 (37.5)	14 (19.4)	0.037
FIB-4				
≥1.45	35 (32.4)	14 (35.9)	21 (30.4)	0.560
≥2.0	25 (23.1)	9 (23.1)	16 (23.2)	0.999
≥3.25	10 (9.3)	6 (15.4)	4 (5.8)	0.164
Age-Platelet Index (API)				
>4	34 (30.1)	15 (37.5)	19 (26.0)	0.204
>5	21 (8.6)	9 (22.5)	12 (6.4)	0.428
>6	12 (10.6)	6 (15.0)	6 (8.2)	0.263
>7	5 (4.4)	3 (7.5)	2 (2.7)	0.344

Data expressed as n (%). *N* number, *AST* aspartate aminotransferase, *ALT* alanine aminotransferase ratio

Table 4 Sensitivity, specificity and AUROCs of the four different biomarkers in patients with low and high-replicative HBV at different cutoff values in identifying significant fibrosis (F2–4)

Biomarker Cut-off	HBV DNA ≤ 20,000 IU/mL			HBV DNA ≥ 20,000 IU/mL		
	Sensitivity (%, 95% CI)	Specificity (%, 95% CI)	AUROC (%, 95% CI)	Sensitivity (%, 95% CI)	Specificity (%, 95% CI)	AUROC (%, 95% CI)
	AST-Platelet Ratio Index (APRI)			AST-Platelet Ratio Index (APRI)		
≥0.5	48.7 (32.4–65.2)	98.0 (91.2–99.5)	0.70 (0.63–0.77)	69.6 (57.3–80.1)	68.9 (57.1–79.2)	0.69 (0.61–0.77)
≥0.7	33.3 (19.1–50.2)	98.1 (94.5–99.6)	0.66 (0.59–0.72)	47.8 (35.7–60.2)	77.0 (65.8–86.0)	0.62 (0.54–0.70)
≥1.0	17.9 (7.5–33.5)[a]	99.4 (96.5–100.0)	0.59 (0.51–0.66)	27.5 (17.5–39.6)	91.9 (83.2–97.0)	0.60 (0.51–0.68)
≥1.5	5.1 (0.6–17.3)[a]	100.0 (97.7–100.0)	0.53 (0.45–0.60)	13.0 (6.1–23.3)[a]	95.9 (88.6–99.2)	0.54 (0.46–0.63)
	AST/ALT Ratio (AAR)			AST/ALT Ratio (AAR)		
>1.0	37.5 (22.7–54.2)	84.3 (77.9–89.5)	0.61 (0.54–0.68)	19.4 (11.1–30.5)	76.6 (65.6–85.5)	0.48 (0.40–0.56)
	FIB-4			FIB-4		
≥1.45	35.9 (21.2–52.8)	97.5 (93.7–99.3)	0.67 (0.60–0.73)	30.4 (19.9–42.7)	87.8 (78.2–94.3)	0.59 (0.51–0.67)
≥2.0	23.1 (11.1–39.3)	98.7 (95.5–99.9)	0.61 (0.54–0.68)	23.2 (13.9–34.9)	91.9 (83.2–97.0)	0.58 (0.49–0.66)
≥3.25	15.4 (5.9–30.5)[a]	100.0 (97.7–100.0)	0.58 (0.50–0.65)	5.8 (1.6–14.2)[a]	97.3 (90.6–99.7)	0.52 (0.43–0.60)
	Age-Platelet Index (API)			Age-Platelet Index (API)		
>4	37.5 (22.7–54.2)	94.8 (90.3–97.6)	0.66 (0.59–0.72)	15.6 (7.7–26.9)	93.8 (86.0–97.9)	0.55 (0.46–0.63)
>5	22.5 (10.8–38.5)	97.1 (93.4–99.1)	0.60 (0.53–0.66)	16.4 (8.8–26.9)	96.3 (89.4–99.2)	0.56 (0.48–0.64)
>6	15.0 (5.7–29.8)[a]	100.0 (97.9–100.0)	0.58 (0.51–0.64)	8.2 (3.0–17.0)[a]	98.8 (93.2–99.9)	0.53 (0.45–0.59)
>7	7.5 (1.6–20.4)[a]	100.0 (97.9–100.0)	0.54 (0.47–0.61)	2.7 (0.3–9.6)[a]	98.8 (93.2–99.9)	0.51 (0.43–0.59)

AST aspartate aminotransferase, *ALT* alanine aminotransferase ratio, *HBV* Hepatitis B virus, *AUROC* Area under the receiver-operating characteristic. [a]numbers low in cells, analysis to be interpreted with caution

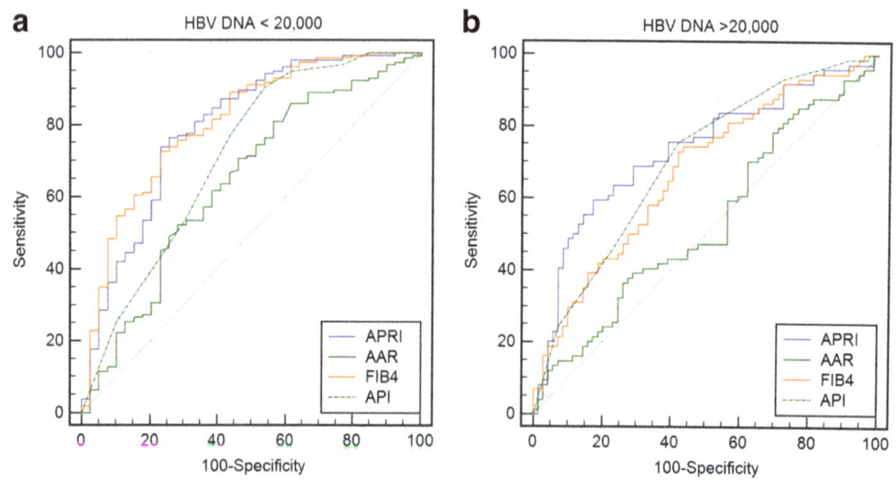

Fig. 1 **a** Receiver operating characteristics curve of the best compromise sensitivity-specificity of AST (aspartate aminotransferase)-platelet ratio index (APRI), AST/alanine aminotransferase ratio (AAR), FIB-4 index and age-platelet index (API) for identifying fibrosis score F2–4 in **low-replicative** HBV patients. In patients meeting these cut-offs, the sensitivity for APRI (≥0.33) is 76.4% and the specificity is 74.4% (AUROC, 0.80; 95% CI: 0.73–0.85; $P < 0.0001$), for AAR (≥0.93) the sensitivity is 73.5% and the specificity 47.5% (AUROC, 0.62; 95% CI: 0.55–0.69; $P = 0.023$), for FIB-4 (≥0.70) the sensitivity is 72.9% and specificity is 76.9% (AUROC, 0.81; 95% CI: 0.75–0.86; $P < 0.0001$), and for API (>2) the sensitivity is 75.1% and specificity is 55.0% (AUROC, 0.71; 95% CI: 0.64–0.77; $P < 0.0001$). **b** Receiver operating characteristics curve of the best compromise sensitivity-specificity of AST (aspartate aminotransferase)-platelet ratio index (APRI), AST/alanine aminotransferase ratio (AAR), FIB-4 index and age-platelet index (API) for identifying fibrosis score F2–4 in **high-replicative** HBV patients. In patients meeting these cut-offs, the sensitivity for APRI (≥0.33) is 52.7% and the specificity is 87.0% (AUROC, 0.73; 95% CI: 0.65–0.80; $P < 0.0001$), for AAR (≥0.91) the sensitivity is 24.7% and the specificity 79.2% (AUROC, 0.52; 95% CI: 0.44–0.60; $P = 0.643$), for FIB-4 (≥0.70) the sensitivity is 58.1% and specificity is 66.7% (AUROC, 0.67; 95% CI: 0.59–0.75; $P = 0.0001$), and for API (>2) the sensitivity is 75.0% and specificity is 56.2% (AUROC, 0.69; 95% CI: 0.61–0.76; $P < 0.0001$)

Discussion

Among the various markers available for evaluating HBV-related fibrosis, the ones utilized in this analysis are the most commonly studied, albeit not specifically in the context of low viremia levels. We have shown that APRI, FIB-4, AAR and API frequently identify F2–4 fibrosis, regardless of the HBV DNA levels. These findings are in concurrence with other studies dealing with chronic HBV in general that show a moderate utility in distinguishing F2–4 from F0–1 fibrosis. However, our analysis also demonstrates significant differences in the detection ability between patients with low and high-replicative states. Clearly, APRI seems to perform better in high-replicative patients (with only the cut-off ≥0.5 reaching statistical significance). However, the other biomarkers appear to perform better in patients with low-replicative states, detecting fibrosis more frequently than in those with high replication.

According to our analysis, at their lowest conventional cut-off points, the AUROCs of all the biomarkers were of low diagnostic value, with only APRI (AUROC 0.62) reaching statistical significance. At a cut-off point of 0.5, the higher sensitivity of APRI in high-replicative states was offset by a low specificity (69%), while those with low replication exhibited a high specificity of 98%. Similar results were seen in the sensitivity and specificity profile of the other biomarkers. However, despite these higher specificities, the overall accuracy of these biomarkers in diagnosing fibrosis remains poor in both groups of patients (<0.70 for all biomarkers at all conventional cut-offs), being far below the standard of diagnostic relevance (typically >0.80).

Interestingly, AAR appears better at distinguishing fibrosis in those with low replication. However, overall AAR only detects a quarter of the patients with F2–4 fibrosis with a diagnostic accuracy of 0.54. Thus, its poor performance as a predictor of fibrosis makes it unsuitable for use in clinical settings. Moreover, these observations can also be extended to FIB-4 and API where significant fibrosis was missed in more than two-thirds of the overall cohort of patients at their lowest cut-offs, thereby diminishing the clinical relevance of these findings. Nonetheless, when analysing patients at ROC-derived optimal cut-offs, all four biomarkers performed consistently better in the low-replicative state, suggesting greater diagnostic utility of these biomarkers in this category of patients. Our analysis shows that by lowering the cut-offs for APRI and FIB-4 a high diagnostic accuracy (>0.80) may be achieved in distinguishing F2–4 from F0–1 fibrosis in patients with low-replicative HBV.

The sensitivity levels of the biomarkers in identifying fibrosis in our study are somewhat lower (i.e. high number of patients with fibrosis incorrectly identified as being without) than that seen in other studies. In a recent meta-analysis [6], the summary sensitivities of APRI at cut-off levels of 0.5, 0.7, 1.0 and 1.5 in identifying F2–4 fibrosis were 70, 63.5, 40 and 34%, respectively, compared to the sensitivities in our analysis of 62, 43, 24 and 10%, respectively. Similar differences were also seen in the summary sensitivities of FIB-4. These differences must be seen in the context of the patient population being studied, where in previous studies the HBV population was mostly comprised of patients with high viral replication and elevated ALT levels. In contrast, our study population bears a close resemblance to real-life HBeAg-negative presentation, where a large number of patients had low replication and/or normal ALT. These consecutive patients also included those with 'high' replication and normal ALT, and 'low' replication with elevated ALT, eventually serving as a robust representative sample of HBeAg-negative patients. Thus, it is likely that the sensitivities and specificities shown in our analysis are closer to a real-life population, and the findings more representative.

The impact of elevated ALT and AST in our cohort could be more confounding than is apparent at face value. In most studies, patients with HBV who undergo liver biopsy are those that have high viral replication. However, in a more natural selection of HBV infected population, as in our cohort, liver enzyme elevation may be related to non-HBV factors such as steatosis, which in turn does not impact on development of fibrosis [4, 9, 10]. As such, this elevation of ALT and AST levels may cause an "artefactual" increase in APRI, FIB-4 and AAR thereby increasing the false-positive rate (i.e. high number of patients without fibrosis incorrectly identified as having disease).

Our analysis must be viewed in the context of its limitations. First, although we relied on pre-biopsy ALT and AST levels, it has been shown that HBV patients may show enzyme fluctuations [3, 11, 12], and consequently some of these patients could feasibly be underscored, having dropped or increased the enzyme levels at the time of biopsy. Similarly, HBV DNA levels may also fluctuate over time, although fluctuations at 20,000 IU/mL are uncommon [13, 14]. In order to correct for such aberrations we categorized patients on the basis of the HBV DNA level recordings falling predominantly within the high or low replicative state. Overall, despite guideline-stratified thresholds, it remains a questionable approach to divide patients arbitrarily into low and high replicative states given the nature of HBV DNA fluctuations. Second, test accuracy can be ascertained when there is no selection bias in evaluating the reported outcome. Our population of HBV patients does not essentially represent an unselected cohort, given the impracticality of performing a liver biopsy in all HBeAg-negative patients. It is feasible that a proportion of these patients may have been biopsied as a consequence of subtle hints for the presence of fibrosis, particularly since patients who are not biopsied tend to have lower ALT and HBV DNA levels, thus escaping the trigger for a liver biopsy [14]. Clearly, these results must be validated in larger, unselected and properly stratified HBV-infected populations before generalizing these results. Despite these limitations, our study with a substantially large number of patients with low viral replication, offers a leading insight into a poorly appreciated disease state.

Conclusion

In conclusion, our study shows a modest accuracy of commonly used biomarkers in the diagnosis of significant fibrosis. In low-replicative patients, at conventional cut-offs, APRI is less useful while AAR is more useful in detecting fibrosis as compared to high replication patients, although it detects only a small minority of patients with fibrosis. Lowering the cut-offs may increase the diagnostic relevance of these biomarkers, particularly for APRI and FIB-4 in low-replicative disease.

Abbreviations

AFP: α-fetoprotein; ALT: Alanine aminotransferase; AST: Aspartate aminotransferase; BMI: Body mass index; HBeAg: Hepatitis B envelope antigen; HBsAg: Hepatitis B surface antigen; HBV: Hepatitis B virus; ULN: Upper limit of normal

Acknowledgements

Not applicable

Funding

No current funding sources for this study.

Authors contributions

Drs. FMS, TF, MAB, BEK, KIB helped in study concept and design; HA1, KA1, KSA, HA2, FB, KA2, AA, IHA, MAB, KIB were responsible for acquisition of data; KA1, HA1, KA2, FB, FMS analysed and interpreted data; FMS, KA2, AA drafted the manuscript; All authors contributed to the critical revision of the manuscript for important intellectual content; FMS performed the statistical analysis. All authors read and approved the final manuscript.

Consent for publication

Not applicable

Competing interests

The authors declare that they have no competing interests.

Author details

[1]Liver Disease Research Center, King Saud University, Riyadh, Saudi Arabia. [2]Department of Gastroenterology, Prince Sultan Military Medical City, Riyadh, Saudi Arabia. [3]Division of Gastroenterology, Department of Medicine, King Fahad Hospital, Jeddah, Saudi Arabia. [4]Division of Gastroenterology, Department of Medicine, King Faisal Specialist Hospital & Research Center, Riyadh, Saudi Arabia. [5]Department of Pathology, King Faisal Specialist Hospital & Research Center, Riyadh, Saudi Arabia. [6]Department of Pathology, King Abdulaziz Medical City, Riyadh, Saudi Arabia. [7]Hepatobiliary Sciences & Liver Transplantation, King Abdulaziz Medical City, Riyadh, Saudi Arabia. [8]Gastroenterology Unit, Department of Medicine, King Abdulaziz Medical City, PO Box: 9515, Jeddah 21423, Saudi Arabia. [9]King Saud bin Abdulaziz University for Health Sciences, Riyadh, Saudi Arabia. [10]Gastroenterology Unit, Department of Medicine, King Fahad Armed Forces Hospital, Jeddah, Saudi Arabia.

References

1. European Association for the Study of the Liver. EASL clinical practice guidelines: management of chronic hepatitis B virus infection. J Hepatol. 2012;57:167–85.
2. Abaalkhail F, Elsiesy H, AlOmair A, Alghamdi MY, Alalwan A, AlMasri N. Et al; Saudi Association for the Study of liver diseases and transplantation (SASLT). SASLT practice guidelines for the management of hepatitis B virus. Saudi J Gastroenterol. 2014;20:5–25.
3. Iloeje UH, Yang HI, Su J, et al. Risk evaluation of viral load elevation and associated liver disease/cancer-in HBV (the REVEAL-HBV) study group. Predicting cirrhosis risk based on the level of circulating hepatitis B viral load. Gastroenterology. 2006;130:678–86.
4. Abdo AA, Bzeizi KI, Babatin MA, AlSohaibani F, AlMana H, Alsaad KO, et al. Predictors of significant fibrosis in chronic hepatitis B patients with low viremia. J Clin Gastroenterol. 2014;48(6):e50–6.
5. Bravo AA, Sheth SG, Chopra S. Liver biopsy. N Engl J Med. 2001;344:495–500.
6. Xiao G, Yang J, Yan L. Comparison of diagnostic accuracy of aspartate aminotransferase to platelet ratio index and fibrosis-4 index for detecting liver fibrosis in adult patients with chronic hepatitis B virus infection: a systemic review and meta-analysis. Hepatology. 2015;61(1):292–302.
7. Saldanha J, Gerlich W, Lelie N, et al. An international collaborative study to establish a World Health Organization international standard for hepatitis B virus DNA nucleic acid amplification techniques. Vox Sang. 2001;80:63–71.
8. Intraobserver and interobserver variations in liver biopsy interpretation in patients with chronic hepatitis C. The French METAVIR Cooperative Study Group. Hepatology 1994;20:15–20.
9. Yun JW, Cho YK, Park JH, et al. Hepatic steatosis and fibrosis in young men with treatment-naïve chronic hepatitis B. Liver Int. 2009;29(6):878–83.
10. Shi JP, Fan JG, Wu R, et al. Prevalence and risk factors of hepatic steatosis and its impact on liver injury in Chinese patients with chronic hepatitis B infection. J Gastroenterol Hepatol. 2008;23(9):1419–25.
11. Papatheodoridis GV, Manesis EK, Manolakopoulos S, et al. Is there a meaningful serum hepatitis B virus DNA cutoff level for therapeutic decisions in hepatitis B e antigen-negative chronic hepatitis B virus infection? Hepatology. 2008;48:1451–9.
12. Kumar M, Sarin SK, Hissar S, et al. Virologic and histologic features of chronic hepatitis B virus-infected asymptomatic patients with persistently normal ALT. Gastroenterology. 2008;134:1376–84.
13. Papatheodoridis GV, Chrysanthos N, Hadziyannis E, et al. Longitudinal changes in serum HBV DNA levels and predictors of progression during the natural course of HBeAg-negative chronic hepatitis B virus infection. J Viral Hepat. 2008;15:434–41.
14. Sanai FM, Babatin MA, Bzeizi KI, Alsohaibani F, Al-Hamoudi W, Alsaad KO, et al. Accuracy of international guidelines for identifying significant fibrosis in hepatitis B e antigen–negative patients with chronic hepatitis. Clin Gastroenterol Hepatol 2013;11:1493–99.e2.

12

Micro-costing analysis of guideline-based treatment by direct-acting agents: the real-life case of hepatitis C management in Brazil

Hugo Perazzo[1*], Marcelino Jose Jorge[2], Julio Castro Silva[3], Alexandre Monken Avellar[2], Patrícia Santos Silva[2], Carmen Romero[4], Valdilea Gonçalves Veloso[1], Ruben Mujica-Mota[5], Rob Anderson[5], Chris Hyde[5] and Rodolfo Castro[1,6]

Abstract

Background: Eradication of hepatitis C virus (HCV) using direct-acting agents (DAA) has been associated with a financial burden to health authorities worldwide. We aimed to evaluate the guideline-based treatment costs by DAAs from the perspective of the Brazilian Ministry of Health (BMoH).

Methods: The activity based costing method was used to estimate the cost for monitoring/treatment of genotype-1 (GT1) HCV patients by the following strategies: peg-interferon (PEG-IFN)/ribavirin (RBV) for 48 weeks, PEG-IFN/RBV plus boceprevir (BOC) or telaprevir (TEL) for 48 weeks, and sofosbuvir (SOF) plus daclastavir (DCV) or simeprevir (SIM) for 12 weeks. Costs were reported in United States Dollars without (US$) and with adjustment for purchasing power parity (PPP$). Drug costs were collected at the National Database of Health Prices and an overview of the literature was performed to assess effectiveness of SOF/DCV and SOF/SIM regimens in real-world cohorts.

Results: Treatment costs of GT1-HCV patients were PPP$ 43,176.28 (US$ 24,020.16) for PEG-IFN/RBV, PPP$ 71,196.03 (US$ 39,578.23) for PEG-IFN/RBV/BOC and PPP$ 86,250.33 (US$ 47,946.92) for PEG-IFN/RBV/TEL. Treatment by all-oral interferon-free regimens were the less expensive approach: PPP$ 19,761.72 (US$ 10,985.90) for SOF/DCV and PPP$ 21,590.91 (US$ 12,002.75) for SOF/SIM. The overview reported HCV eradication in up to 98% for SOF/DCV and 96% for SOF/SIM.

Conclusion: Strategies with all oral interferon-free might lead to lower costs for management of GT1-HCV patients compared to IFN-based regimens in Brazil. This occurred mainly because of high discounts over international DAA prices due to negotiation between BMoH and pharmaceutical industries.

Keywords: Chronic hepatitis C, Treatment, Micro-costing

Background

Chronic hepatitis C (CHC) remains a major public health issue that might lead to cirrhosis and its complications, such as portal hypertension and hepatocellular carcinoma [1]. Eradication of hepatitis C virus (HCV) has been associated with lower rates of liver-related complications [2]. Transient elastography (TE) by FibroScan® (EchoSens, Paris, France) is a validated method to liver fibrosis assessment [3] and seems to be cost-effective to diagnose cirrhosis compared to liver biopsy [4]. The high efficacy of direct-acting antiviral drugs (DAAs) has revolutionized the management of patients with CHC. High rates of sustained virological response (SVR), defined as undetectable serum HCV-RNA levels 12 weeks after completing treatment, has been obtained by DAA treatment in patients with advanced liver fibrosis or compensate cirrhosis [5].

* Correspondence: perazzohugo@gmail.com; hugo.perazzo@ini.fiocruz.br
[1]Fundação Oswaldo Cruz, FIOCRUZ, Instituto Nacional de Infectologia Evandro Chagas, INI, Laboratório de Pesquisa Clínica em DST e AIDS, LAPCLIN-AIDS, Rio de Janeiro, Brazil

However, the decrease of the burden of liver disease in CHC by DAA treatment might be associated with high costs to health authorities worldwide [6]. Public health strategies should be implemented to promote primary care access to interferon-free regimes, especially in low to middle-income countries with high prevalence of CHC.

Drug prices are very important in HCV management but they are clearly not the only costs to be considered in the analysis [7]. The decision to incorporate new drugs in guidelines for CHC management should take into account the cost and cost-effectiveness analysis. The evidence base from economic evaluations of new healthcare technologies has been limited by the quality of the available data, strengths and weaknesses of different methods used for cost determination and differences among public health systems worldwide [8]. In Brazil, it is estimated that 1.4 to 1.7 million of people are living with CHC [9], most of them genotype-1 (GT1) HCV [10] and up to 20% with advanced fibrosis or cirrhosis [11]. Recently, the Brazilian Ministry of Health (BMoH) has recommended the use of DAAs for CHC treatment due to high discounts given by pharmaceutical companies. Since July 2015, patients with advanced fibrosis (METAVIR $F \geq 3$) have free access to these drugs [12]. However, few studies have investigated the cost for CHC treatment with DAAs in a low to middle-income country. The aim of this study was to evaluate the guideline-based treatment costs by DAAs from the perspective of a public national reference healthcare institute in Brazil. In addition, we reviewed the literature for effectiveness of all-oral interferon-free regimens available in Brazil in real-life cohort studies.

Methods

Study design and setting

This cost-analysis study used cost data collected in a tertiary center for treatment of infectious diseases: National Institute of Infectious Diseases Evandro Chagas-Oswaldo Cruz Foundation (INI/FIOCRUZ) at Rio de Janeiro, Brazil. INI/FIOCRUZ has been playing an important role for the BMoH in development of public health policies and strategies for prevention and treatment of infectious diseases, including viral hepatitis. In the Brazilian Public Health System, known as *Sistema Único de Saúde* (SUS), individuals can have free access to HCV treatment whether confirmed presence of liver fibrosis. According to the recommendations for HCV treatment from the BMoH, treatment was delivery for free in patients with liver fibrosis stages $F \geq 2$ until 2012. However, from 2013 to nowadays, the threshold for free-treatment access has changed for fibrosis stages $F \geq 3$. This analysis simulated follow-up and antiviral regimens exclusively for treatment of GT1-HCV patients according to the recommendation of BMoH from 2011 to 2015.

Method for cost determination

The activity based costing (ABC) method was used for cost determination. This micro-costing method identifies different activities that the institution performs and includes the corresponding indirect costs (e.g. management costs) to estimate total cost of a procedure. ABC method recognizes the relationship between costs, activities (called cost drivers) and products (exams or medical visit) taking into account this relationship in the costing analysis [13]. Secondary data were obtained from: (i) public access production resources from the Department of Statistics; (ii) inventory of permanent material; (iii) records of expenditures with resources from the Financial Department for a one-year (2013) period (to correct the potential seasonal expenses due to diseases outbreaks in infectious diseases); and (iv) cost of 450 diagnostic tests and 100 sub-types of clinical procedures. Administrative costs were estimated through the determination of the proportional contribution of each activity to the pooled expenses and considered for all diagnostic tests and clinical procedures. Prices in national currency [Brazilian Real (BRL)] and inflated to average prices of July of 2015 in United States Dollars according to the World Bank, without (exchange rate = 3.11) and with adjustment for purchasing power parity (PPP adjustment rate = 1.73). We report these as the "nominal price" (US$) and the "PPP-adjusted price" (PPP$), respectively.

Costs of personnel, blood analysis tests and medical visits

Personnel costs for each procedure were calculated based on the annual salary payment of each employee and the working time spent in the specific activity. At INI/FIOCRUZ, salaries are determined according to employee's specialization (i.e., people with PhD degree have higher salaries compared to those without) for individuals working in similar activities. Regarding expenditures with blood analysis tests, we considered costs of materials needed to perform the test, such as kits and reagents. Methodology for cost determination of non-invasive methods for liver fibrosis assessment were detailed in the Supplementary Material. Briefly, the following aspects were taken into account to estimate the cost per unit of TE (i) the price and depreciation of the FibroScan® machine; (ii) annual maintenance by M probe calibration; (iii) salaries of personnel who perform the examination and (iv) indirect administrative costs. We reported the price of TE adjusted with the opportunity cost of using public resources for implementation of new technologies (cost of capital). Costs with specific material for liver biopsy [Menghini needle 16G (Biomedical, Florence,

Italy)] and histological analysis, as well as personnel costs and cost for a day-clinic hospitalization were considered for estimation of total cost to perform a liver biopsy. The market prices were considered for diagnostic tests not performed at INI/FIOCRUZ.

Cost of antiviral drugs for CHC treatment

Drug costs were collected in a web-based public domain site that describes the prices paid by the BMoH for all drugs incorporated in the Public Health System and purchased from the pharmaceutical industry (Database of Health Prices – "*Banco de Preços em Saúde*" - accessible at: http://www.saude.gov.br/bps). A weighted-mean price for each antiviral drug was estimated taking into account all drug payments made by the BMoH from January to December 2015. We then calculated the price for a single-dose of PEG-interferon α-2a 180 mcg (PEG-IFN) [Pegasys® - Roche] and a single capsule or tablet for ribavirin (RBV) [generic by BMoH], boceprevir (BOC) [Victrelis® – Merk], telaprevir (TEL) [Incivek® - Vertex Pharmaceuticals], sofosbuvir (SOF) [Sovaldi® – Gilead], daclastavir (DCV) [Daklinza® - Bristol-Myers Squibb] and simeprevir (SIM) Olysio® – Janssen Pharmaceuticals].

Strategies for treatment of GT1-HCV patients according to the BMoH guidelines

In the present study, we compared the strategies for HCV treatment of GT1 patients as recommended by the BMoH from 2011 to 2015. During this period, Brazilian guidelines for CHC treatment were published in 2011, 2013 and 2015. In 2011, GT1 patients should be treated by PEG-IFN plus RBV for 48 weeks and a liver biopsy with significant fibrosis (METAVIR F ≥ 2) was necessary for treatment access (regimen BMoH-2011) [14]. In 2013, presence of advanced fibrosis (liver biopsy METAVIR F ≥ 3 or TE ≥ 9.6 kPa) allowed the addition of first generation protease inhibitors [BOC for 44 weeks (regimen BMoH-2013A) or TEL for 12 weeks (regimen BMoH-2013B)] to PEG-IFN/RBV during 48 weeks [15]. More recently, in 2015, all-oral and interferon-free regimens [SOF plus DCV for 12 weeks (regimen BMoH-2015A) or SOF plus SIM for 12 weeks (regimen BMoH-2015B)] were recommended for GT1 HCV patients. Patients with decompensated cirrhosis, HIV co-infection or previous failure with PEG-IFN/RBV ± BOC or TEL might be treated by SOF/DCV 24 weeks. In addition, serological biomarkers or TE could replace liver biopsy for free-access to DAA treatment [12]. In all scenarios, liver fibrosis was staged for treatment access and patients were followed with blood tests and medical visits. Table 1 summarizes the strategies for treatment of GT1 HCV patients according to the BMoH guidelines from 2011 to 2015.

Literature review for efficacy of SOF/DCV and SOF/SIM regimens in real-life scenario

We systematically searched the references using the following predetermined inclusion criteria: cohort study that included GT1 HCV patients treated in real-life scenario by SOF/DCV or SOF/SIM ± RBV for 12 weeks. This search was performed in June 2017 at MEDLINE (PubMed) (1966–2017) using the following terms: ["sofosbuvir" OR "Sovaldi®" OR "GS-7977" OR "simeprevir" OR "Olysio®" OR"TMC-435" OR "daclastavir" OR "Daklinza®" OR "BMS-790052"] AND ["hepatitis C"] AND ["real-world" OR "real-life"] (Additional file 1: Table S1).

Results

Costs for liver fibrosis assessment

The estimated costs of TE with personnel, machine and administrative costs were PPP$ 40.08, 29.80 and 24.78, respectively. The nominal and PPP-adjusted costs of a single TE exam were PPP$ 95.32 (US$ 53.32). The adjustment using the opportunity cost lead to an increase in up 50% of TE price (Additional file 1: Table S2). Costs of APRI and FIB-4 were estimated at PPP$ 27.85 (US$ 15.48) and PPP$ 36.58 (US$ 20.33), respectively. Total cost for liver biopsy was PPP$ 834.41 (US$ 482.32) including material to perform liver biopsy and histological analysis [PPP$ 80.75 (US$ 46.68)], personnel costs [PPP$ 301.47 (US$ 174.26)] and cost for day-clinic hospitalization [PPP$ 452.19 (US$ 261.38)].

Costs for GT1 HCV treatment

The estimated price of GT1 HCV treatment drugs was an important source of variability in the total cost for HCV treatment. PEG-IFN α-2a 180 mcg cost PPP$ 648.00 (US$ 360.22) per weekly injection and RBV was the least expensive drug costing PPP$ 106.05 (US$ 58.80) per week. The regimen PEG-IFN (180 mcg SC weekly)/RBV (1250 mg PO daily if body weight ≥ 75 kg) cost PPP$ 754.05 or US$ 419.18 per week. Considering the first generation protease inhibitors (PI), TEL had a higher cost compared to BOC [PPP$ 87.01 (US$ 48.37) vs PPP$ 7.96 (US$ 4.42) per tablet). The weekly costs for treatment by BOC (800 mg PO q8hr) and TEL (750 mg PO q8hr) were PPP$ 668.64 and 3654.42, respectively. Thus, the weekly costs for PEG-IFN/first generation PI regimens ranges from PPP$ 1422.69 (with BOC) and 4408.47 (with TEL). Considering the DAAs, the NS5A inhibitor DCV 60 mg and the second generation PI SIM 150 mg cost PPP$ 388.78 (US$ 206.09) and PPP$ 541.24 (US$ 300.86) per week, respectively. In addition, SOF 400 mg, a NS5B polymerase inhibitor, had a PPP-adjusted and a nominal cost of PPP$ 1014.23 and US$ 563.78 weekly, respectively. The regimens SOF (400 mg PO daily)/DCV (60 mg PO daily) and SOF (400 mg PO daily)/SIM (150 mg PO daily) cost PPP$ 1403.01 and

Table 1 Description of strategies for treatment of genotype 1 chronic hepatitis C according to the Brazilian Ministry of Health from 2011 to 2015

Guideline	Fibrosis staging	Prerequisite for treatment	Drugs	Duration (weeks)	Doses	Interventions
BMoH-2011	Liver biopsy	METAVIR F ≥ 2	PEG-IFN α-2a 180 mcg [Pegasys® - Roche]	48	1 injection weekly	PEG-RBV for 48 weeks. Medical visit at screening, baseline, W2, W4 and every 4 weeks for W4 to W48. Response-guided therapy or stopping rules based on HCV-RNA at W4, W12 and W24. SVR at W72
			RBV 250 mg [BMoH generic]	48	5 capsules daily	
BMoH-2013A	TE	LSM ≥ 9.6 kPa	PEG-IFN α-2a 180 mcg [Pegasys® - Roche]	48	1 injection weekly	Leading-phase with PEG-RBV for 4 weeks and PEG-RBV/BOC for 44 weeks. Medical visit at screening, baseline, W2, W4, W5, W6 and W8, and every 4 weeks from W8 to W48. Response-guided therapy or stopping rules based on HCV-RNA on W4, W12 and W24. SVR at W72
			RBV 250 mg [BMoHgeneric]	48	5 capsules daily	
			BOC 200 mg [Victrelis® – Merk]	44	12 tablets daily	
BMoH-2013B	TE	LSM ≥ 9.6 kPa	PEG-IFN α-2a 180 mcg [Pegasys® - Roche]	48	1 injection weekly	PEG-RBV/TEL for 12 weeks and PEG-RBV for 36 weeks. Medical visit at at screening, baseline, W1, W2 and W4, then every 4 weeks from W4 to W48. Response-guided therapy or stopping rules based on HCV-RNA on W4, W12 and W24. SVR at W72
			RBV 250 mg [BMoH generic]	48	5 capsules daily	
			TEL 375 mg [Incivek ® - Vertex]	12	6 tablets daily	
BMoH-2015A	TE or APRI or FIB-4	LSM ≥ 9.6 kPa or APRI ≥1.5 or FIB-4 ≥ 3.25	SOF 400 mg [Sovaldi® – Gilead]	12	1 tablet daily	SOF/DCV for 12 weeks. Medical visits at screening, baseline, W2, W4, W8 and W12. No response-guided therapy or stopping rules. SVR at W24
			DCV 60 mg [Daklinza® - BMS]	12	1 tablet daily	
BMoH-2015B	TE or APRI or FIB-4	LSM ≥ 9.6 kPa or APRI ≥1.5 or FIB-4 ≥ 3.25	SOF 400 mg [Sovaldi® – Gilead]	12	1 tablet daily	SOF/SIM for 12 weeks or 24 weeks in presence of decompensated cirrhosis (Child-Pugh B/C). Medical visits at screening, baseline, W2, W4, W8 and W12. No response-guided therapy or stopping rules. SVR at W24
			SIM 150 mg [Olysio – Janssen®]	12	1 tablet daily	

APRI aspartate-to-platelet index, *BMoH* Brazilian Ministry of Health, *BOC* boceprevir, *DCV* daclastavir, *FIB-4* fibrosis-4 score, *kPa* kilopascal, *LSM* liver stiffness measurement, *PEG-IFN* peginterferon, *RBV* ribavirin, *SIM* simeprevir, *SOF* sofosbuvir, *SVR* sustained-virologic response, *TE* transient elastography, *TEL* telaprevir

US$ 1555.47 per week, respectively. Table 2 summarizes the nominal and PPP-adjusted costs per unit for tests, medical care and drugs used in GT1 HCV patient management.

According to the procedures recommended at the BMoH's guidelines, treatment with PEG-IFN/RBV/first generation PI [BMoH-2013A and B] was the most expensive approach. In those recommendations, patients were treated for 48 weeks by PEG-IFN/RBV and BOC for 44 weeks [total of PPP$ 71,196.03 (US$ 39,578.23) per patient] or TEL for 12 weeks [total of PPP$ 86,250.33 (US$ 47,946.92) per patient]. Treatments by new all-oral interferon-free regimens were the least expensive approach: the costs for SOF/DCV [BMoH-2015A] and SOF/SIM [BMoH-2015B] were PPP$ 19,761.72 (US$ 10,985.90) and PPP$ 21,590.91 (US$ 12,002.75), respectively (Table 3). In the presence of decompensated cirrhosis (Child-Pugh B/C), the necessity to treat with SOF/DCV for 24 weeks leads to an 84% increase in total costs [PPP$ 36,597.71 (US$ 20,345.04)]. In all scenarios, the drug costs were responsible by approximatively 90% of total cost for treat patients with CHC. The cost with medical visits and blood analysis tests fell by up to 40% in treatment with DAAs [guidelines BoMH-2015A/B] compared to regimens that used PEG-IFN [guidelines BMoH 2011 and 2013A/B].

Literature overview for efficacy of SOF/DCV and SOF/SIM regimens

Out of 150 identified articles, 25 references were eligible and 14 real-life cohort studies that reported the efficacy of SOF/DCV ($n = 2$) or SOF/SIM ± RBV ($n = 12$) in GT1

Table 2 Cost per unit and number of procedures for monitoring and injections/tablets for treatment of genotype 1 chronic hepatitis C according to different regimens recommended by the BMoH from 2011 to 2015

	Cost per unit		PEG-RBV	PEG-RBV/BOC	PEG-RBV/TEL	SOF/DCV	SOF/SIM
	US$	PPP$	n	n	n	n	n
Transient elastography	53.35	95.32	–	1	1	1	1
Liver biopsy	482.32	834.41	1	–	–	–	–
Blood analysis tests							
WBC. RBC and platelet	10.62	19.11	15	17	16	6	6
Fasting glucose	4.86	8.75	6	6	6	6	6
BUN/creatinine	4.84	8.70	15	16	15	6	6
ALT	4.85	8.73	15	16	15	6	6
AST	4.86	8.74	15	16	15	6	6
Alkaline phosphatases	4.77	8.58	6	6	6	6	6
GGT	4.83	8.69	6	6	6	6	6
Total bilirubin	4.84	8.71	6	6	6	6	6
Albumin	5.07	9.12	6	6	6	6	6
INR	6.68	12.02	6	13	14	6	6
HCV genotype	156.33	281.22	1	1	1	1	1
HCV-RNA	87.05	156.60	8	7	7	2	2
TSH	26.26	47.23	6	6	6	–	–
Beta-hCG	45.52	81.88	4	4	4	4	4
Medical follow-up							
GP's medical visit	54.54	98.11	1	1	1	1	1
Specialist's medical visit	62.92	113.19	14	14	14	5	5
Blood sample collection	37.83	68.06	15	15	15	6	6
Nursing consultation	31.83	57.26	5	5	5	4	4
Drugs							
PEG-IFN α-2a 180 mcg – SC injection	360.22	648.00	48	48	48	–	–
Ribavirin 250 mg – PO capsule	1.68	3.03	1680	1680	1680	–	–
Boceprevir 200 mg – PO tablet	4.42	7.96	–	3612	–	–	–
Telaprevir 375 mg – PO tablet	48.37	87.01	–	–	504	–	–
Sofosbuvir 400 mg – PO tablet	80.54	144.89	–	–	–	84	84
Daclastavir 60 mg – PO tablet	30.87	55.54	–	–	–	84	–
Simeprevir 150 mg - PO tablet	42.98	77.32	–	–	–	–	84

Costs in United States Dollars (US$) and with purchasing power parity (PPP$) on July 2015. Drug costs estimated as the weighted-mean price (http://www.saude.gov.br/bps)

BOC boceprevir, *DCV* daclastavir, *PEG-IFN* peginterferon, *RBV* ribavirin, *SIM* simeprevir, *SOF* sofosbuvir, *TEL* telaprevir, *WBC* white blood cell, *RBC* red blood cell, *BUN* blood urea nitrogen, *ALT* alanine aminotransferase, *AST* aspartate aminotransferase, *AP* alkaline phosphatases, *GGT* gamma-glutamyl transpeptidase, *INR* international normalized ratio, *TSH* thyroid-stimulating hormone, *hCG* human chorionic gonadotropin, *GP* general practicioner

Treatment regimens according to BMoH guidelines: PEG-RBV 48w [BMoH-2011]; PEG-RBV (48w)/BOC 44w [BMoH-2013A]; PEG-RBV (48w)/TEL (12w) [BMoH-2013B]; SOF/DCV 12w [BMoH-2015A] and SOF/SIM 12w [BMoH-2015B]

HCV patients were included (Fig. 1). Overall, SVR rates for SOF/DCV ± RBV and SOF/SIM ± RBV during 12 weeks ranged from 83 to 98% [16, 17] and from 75 to 96% [18–29], respectively. SVR rates were lower in presence of cirrhosis compared to non-cirrhotic patients (87% vs 98% with SOF/DCV [17] and 81% vs 91% with SOF/SIM [26]. Higher SVR rates can be achieved in cirrhotic patients when extending SOF/DCV for 24 weeks [17] or adding RBV to SIM/SOF [24]. Pol et al. reported lower SVR rates in GT1a patients compared to GT1b (89% vs 95% with SOF/DCV 12 weeks) that might be not significant when extending treatment for 24 weeks (95% for both) [17]. Similar results were observed in patients treated by SOF/SIM 12 weeks (83% for GT1a vs 90% for GT1b) [26]. Table 4 summarizes SVR rates from real-life cohort studies that analysed the efficacy of SOF/DCV and SOF/SIM regimens in GT1 patients stratified by GT1 subtype and presence or absence of cirrhosis or previous treatment.

Table 3 Monitoring and drugs costs (US$ and PPP-adjusted US$) for treatment of genotype-1 patient with chronic hepatitis C according to different regimens recommended by the BMoH from 2011 to 2015

	PEG-RBV		PEG-RBV/BOC		PEG-RBV/TEL		SOF/DCV		SOF/SIM	
	US$	PPP$	US$	PPP$	US$	PPP$	US$	PPP$	US$	PPP$
TE	–	–	53.35	95.32	53.35	95.32	53.35	95.32	53.35	95.32
Liver biopsy	482.32	834.41	–	–	–	–	–	–	–	–
Total	482.32	834.41	53.35	95.32	53.35	95.32	53.35	95.32	53.35	95.32
Blood analysis tests										
WBC. RBC and platelet	159.39	286.72	180.64	324.95	170.02	305.84	63.76	114.69	63.76	114.69
Fasting glucose	29.20	52.52	29.20	52.52	29.20	52.52	29.20	52.52	29.20	52.52
BUN/creatinine	72.58	130.56	77.41	139.26	72.58	130.56	29.03	52.22	29.03	52.22
ALT	72.78	130.92	77.63	139.65	72.78	130.92	29.11	52.37	29.11	52.37
AST	72.91	131.16	77.78	139.91	72.91	131.16	29.17	52.47	29.17	52.47
AP	28.61	51.46	28.61	51.46	28.61	51.46	28.61	51.46	28.61	51.46
GGT	28.99	52.15	28.99	52.15	28.99	52.15	28.99	52.15	28.99	52.15
Total bilirubin	29.04	52.24	29.04	52.24	29.04	52.24	29.04	52.24	29.04	52.24
Albumin	30.44	54.75	30.44	54.75	30.44	54.75	30.44	54.75	30.44	54.75
INR	40.10	72.14	86.89	156.30	93.57	168.32	40.10	72.14	40.10	72.14
HCV genotype	156.33	281.22	156.33	281.22	156.33	281.22	156.33	281.22	156.33	281.22
HCV-RNA	696.43	1252.80	609.38	1096.20	609.38	1096.20	174.11	313.20	174.11	313.20
TSH	157.55	283.41	157.55	283.41	157.55	283.41		–		–
Beta-hCG	182.07	327.53	182.07	327.53	182.07	327.53	182.07	327.53	182.07	327.53
Total	1756.41	3159.58	1751.94	3151.54	1733.45	3118.27	849.94	1528.95	849.94	1528.95
Medical follow-up										
GP's medical visit	54.54	98.11	54.54	98.11	54.54	98.11	54.54	98.11	54.54	98.11
Specialist's visit	880.95	1584.73	880.95	1584.73	880.95	1584.73	314.62	565.97	314.62	565.97
Blood sample	567.52	1020.90	567.52	1020.90	567.52	1020.90	227.01	408.36	227.01	408.36
Nursing consultation	159.15	286.29	159.15	286.29	159.15	286.29	127.32	229.03	127.32	229.03
Total	1662.15	2990.02	1662.15	2990.02	1662.15	2990.02	723.49	1301.47	723.49	1301.47
Drugs										
PEG-IFN 180 mcg	17,290.59	31,103.78	17,290.59	31,103.78	17,290.59	31,103.78	–	–	–	–
Ribavirin 250 mg	2828.69	5088.49	2828.69	5088.49	2828.69	5088.49	–	–	–	–
Boceprevir 200 mg	–	–	15,991.51	28,766.88	–	–	–	–	–	–
Telaprevir 375 mg	–	–	–	–	24,378.69	43,854.45	–	–	–	–
Sofosbuvir 400 mg	–	–	–	–	–	–	6765.68	12,170.68	6765.68	12,170.68
Daclastavir 60 mg	–	–	–	–	–	–	2593.44	4665.30	–	–
Simeprevir 150 mg	–	–	–	–	–	–	–	–	3610.29	6494.49
Total	20,119.28	36,192.27	36,110.79	64,959.15	44,497.97	80,046.72	9359.12	16,835.98	10,375.97	18,665.17
TOTAL COST	24,020.16	43,176.28	39,578.23	71,196.03	47,946.92	86,250.33	10,985.90	19,761.72	12,002.75	21,590.91

Costs in United States Dollars (US$) and with purchasing power parity (PPP$) on July 2015. Drug costs estimated as the weighted-mean price (http://www.saude.gov.br/bps)

PEG-IFN peginterferon, *WBC* white blood cell, *RBC* red blood cell, *BUN* blood urea nitrogen, *ALT* alanine aminotransferase, *AST* aspartate aminotransferase, *AP* alkaline phosphatases, *GGT* gamma-glutamyl transpeptidase, *INR* international normalized ratio, *TSH* thyroid-stimulating hormone, *hCG* human chorionic gonadotropin, *GP* general practicioner

Treatment regimens according to BMoH guidelines: PEG-RBV 48w [BMoH-2011]; PEG-RBV (48w)/BOC 44w [BMoH-2013A]; PEG-RBV (48w)/TEL (12w) [BMoH-2013B]; SOF/DCV 12w [BMoH-2015A] and SOF/SIM 12w [BMoH-2015B]

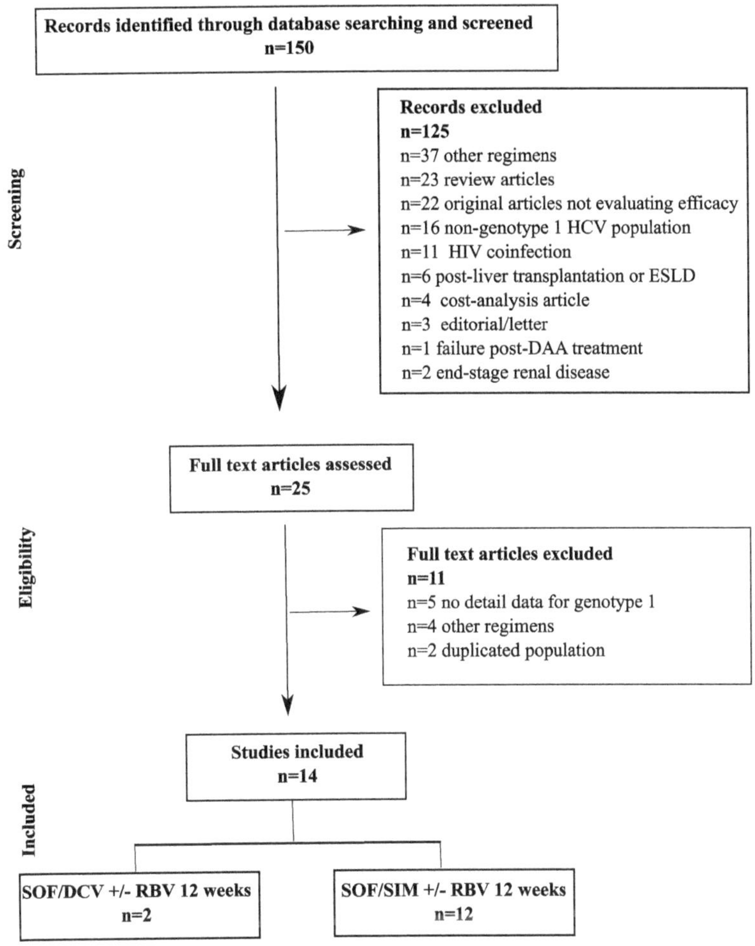

Fig. 1 Flow-chart of study selection for the literature overview

Discussion

The present study highlighted that GT1 HCV treatment by effective DAAs might be less expensive than interferon-based regimens in a low-to-middle income country, mainly due to price negotiation between health authorities and pharmaceutical companies and lower costs with monitoring in the all-oral interferon-free treatments.

The cost of TE was increased due to the very high interest rates used in Brazil [30, 31] and higher expenses with personnel at INI/FIOCRUZ. TE could be less costly in countries with lower opportunity cost of public funds and in those where nurses perform the exams. Liver fibrosis staging by TE seems to be cost-effective compared to liver biopsy and it was priced from US$ 21 to US$ 73 in the United Kingdom and up to US$ 145 in the United States [4].

HCV eradication has been associated with a financial burden, especially due to high DAAs costs which are extremely variable worldwide [6]. An analysis of for a 12-week SOF course price (PPP-adjusted) in 30 countries described that Poland (PPP$ 101,063.00), Turkey (PPP$ 91,339) and United States (PPP$ 64,680) were the top three ranking countries with the most expensive prices. On the other hand, India (PPP$ 1861), Mongolia (PPP$ 2604) and Egypt (PPP$ 3117) were the countries with the least expensive price for SOF-therapy [32]. In 36 clinical sites in USA, real-world costs for PEG-IFN/RBV/BOC 48 weeks, PEG-IFN/TEL 48 weeks and SOF/SIM 12 weeks were US$ 57,960; US$ 113,400; US$ 180,600; respectively. In addition, the mean cost per SVR in all-oral interferon-free was higher in patients with advanced fibrosis (US$ 167,467 for F3F4 vs 116,579 for F0F1F2) [33]. However, both studies only included cost of HCV medications, not adjunctive medications, hospital costs, or projected medical costs. Data from Europe and Canada reported a total cost [mean (95%CI)] of €14,559 (13,323–15,836) per patient and €38,514 (35,244–41,892) per SVR for IFN-based regimens considering treatment, monitoring and complications [34]. The price disparities among countries might be explained partly by the pharmaceutical price-setting

Table 4 Real-life cohort studies that evaluated efficacy (SVR12) of Sofosbuvir/Daclastavir (SOF/DCV) or Sofosbuvir/Simeprevir (SOF/SIM) regimens for treatment of HCV mono-infected genotype-1 patients

Authors	Year	Local	Regimen	Overall		Non-cirrhosis		Cirrhosis		Naive		Experimented		GT 1a		GT 1b	
				n	SVR	n	SVR	n	SVR	n	SVR	n	SVR	n	SVR	n	SVR
Sofosbuvir (400 mg)/Daclastavir (60 mg) regimen studies																	
Pol et al. [17]	2017	France	SOF/DCV 12w	160	92%	66	98%	94	87%	64	88%	96	95%	73	95%	83	89%
			SOF/DCV 24w	439	95%	97	97%	342	94%	48	85%	391	96%	210	95%	209	95%
Welzel et al. [16]	2016	Europe	SOF/DCV ± RBV 12w	319	98%	–	–	–	–	–	–	–	–	151	99%	155	97%
Sofosbuvir (400 mg)/Simeprevir (150 mg) regimen studies																	
Marino et al. [[28]	2017	Spain	SOF/SIM ± RBV 12w	835	92%	–	–	835	92%	–	–	–	–	–	–	–	–
Ramos et al. [29]	2017	Spain	SOF/SIM 12w	179	93%	–	–	–	–	–	–	–	–	–	–	–	–
Chang et al. [27]	2017	USA	SOF/SIM 12w	21	91%	–	–	–	–	–	–	–	–	–	–	–	–
Sulkowski et al. [26]	2016	USA	SOF/SIM 12w	639	85%	272	91%	367	81%	65	–	–	–	371	83%	185	90%
Lutchtman et al. [25]	2016	USA	SOF/SIM 12w	148	82%	43	88%	193	78%	62	87%	86	78%	94	79%	42	93%
Pellicelli et al. [24]	2016	Italy	SOF/SIM/RBV 12w	270	96%	–	–	270	96%	–	–	–	–	–	–	–	–
Roytman et al. [23]	2016	USA	SOF/SIM 12w	138	89%	43	93%	95	87%	76	87%	55	92%	–	–	–	–
Thornton et al. [22]	2016	USA	SOF/SIM 12w	114	89%	–	–	–	–	–	–	–	–	–	–	–	–
Jayasekera et al. [19]	2016	USA	SOF/SIM 12w	35	86%	13	92%	22	82%	7	86%	28	86%	–	–	–	–
Pillail et al. [20]	2016	USA	SOF/SIM ± RBV 12w	113	84%	23	91%	90	82%	57	89%	56	79%	–	–	–	–
Barron et al. [21]	2016	USA	SOF/SIM ± RBV 12w	35	83%	–	–	–	–	–	–	–	–	–	–	–	–
Backus et al. [18]	2015	USA	SOF/SIM 12w	1130	75%	664	81%	462	68%	699	78%	431	71%	632	73%	366	80%

DCV daclastavir, *GT* genotype, *SIM* simeprevir, *SOF* sofosbuvir, *SVR* sustained virological response, *w* week

policies used in different countries and negotiation between health authorities and pharmaceutical companies. Some countries set prices according to explicit cost-effectiveness thresholds based on gross domestic product (GDP) per capita resulting in high prices without consideration of budget impact [35]. Therefore, DAA treatment costs are lower in Brazil compared to others countries mainly due to intense negotiation of BMoH with pharmaceutical companies resulting in more than 90% discount over international prices for SOF, DCV and SIM [9].

In the present study, the reduced price for DAAs and shorten treatment duration might explain the lower total cost for HCV eradication with all-oral interferon-free compared to IFN-based regimens. Weekly prices for PEG-IFN (US$ 360 or PPP$ 648), BOC (US$ 371 or PPP$ 672) and TEL (US$ 2030 or PPP$ 3654) were relatively high and longer duration treatment with IFN-regimens led to higher costs with monitoring and medical visits (mean cost of PPP$ 6133.15 for IFN-based vs PPP$ 2830.42 for interferon-free regimens). In addition, adverse events are more frequent in IFN-based regimens than DAA treatment leading to higher costs. Previous studies reported that extra medical visits and drugs used for adverse events treatment, such as epoetin-α or filgrastim, lead to an increase in costs for treatment with IFN-based regimens with first generation PI (BOC/TEL) [36]. Costs per SVR might have 2-fold increase for patients with thrombocytopenia compared to those with normal platelet count when treated by IFN-based regimens [€50,907 (95% CI, 44,151–59,612) vs €26,105 (23,068–29,296)] [34].

Data from real-world cohort studies have been showing higher SVR rates by 12-week course of SOF/DCV (up to 92%) [17] and SOF/SIM regimens (up to 85%) [26] compared to IFN-based regimens (up to 40% in cirrhotic patients treated by PEG-IFN/RBV/BOC or TEL) [37]. However, presence of cirrhosis and GT subtype 1a might lead to lower SVR rates (Table 4). The extension of SOF/DCV for 24 weeks might be used to achieve higher SVR rates in cirrhotic patients [17]. In GT1 HCV infected patients, treatment using DAAs has been considered as cost-effective [38] and further analysis are needed to evaluate whether this approach is cost-saving [39]. In addition, treatment by SOF/DCV or SOF/SIM result in less medical visits and blood analysis tests for monitoring, lower rates of adverse events, no need of subcutaneous injection and lower intake of tablets/day compared to IFN-regimens. However, presence of decompensated cirrhosis highly increase the cost of treatment [from PPP$ 19,761.72to 36, 597.71 (from US$ 10,985.9 to 20,345.04] due to extension of SOF/DCV regimen for 24 weeks. Despite, the lack of cost-effectiveness studies in Brazil, given the fact that DAA-regimens are more effective compared to IFN-regimens and total cost for HCV treatment with all-oral interferon-free drugs is lower than IFN-based regimens, we could hypothesize that treatment with DAAs might be dominant in this country. Considering local costs and SVR rates reported in international real-life cohorts, the cost per SVR in Brazil could range from 20 to 30 thousand PPP$. Early viral kinetics might be used to individualize duration of DAA therapy decreasing costs by up to 20% [40]. On the other hand, treatment of patients with advanced fibrosis/compensated cirrhosis for 12 weeks, as recommended by the BMoH guideline, might lead to relative high rates of DAA failure or resistance and increased future costs for re-treatment. The addition of RBV (1250 mg PO daily) to SOF/SIM or SOF/DCV does not highly increase the cost of treatment due to local generic production and low price (US$ 706 or PPP$ 1273 per patient per 12 week duration). In Brazil, the prevalence of GT 1b seems to slightly higher than 1a (55% vs 45%) [41]. Considering our HCV prevalence and costs described in the present study, the financial burden could be up to PPP$ 21 billion (or US$ 12 billion) to treat all GT1 HCV infected people independently of fibrosis stage in Brazil. This amount represents approximately 13% of the general government expenditure on health in Brazil during 2014 [Health expenditure series. World Health Organization, available at: http://apps.who.int/nha/database/Select/Indicators/en; accessed at March 2017].

The main limitations of the present study are the lack of primary data on patient's follow-up and costs of treatment for non-GT1 patients and new generation of interferon-free regimens. Presence of adverse events might lead to increased costs for medical care and low treatment adherence might result in higher costs and higher costs per SVR than our estimates, due to non-response/relapse. However, primary data on DAA-treatment remain scarce in Brazil because the strategy from BMoH for universal access to SOF, DCV and SIM has been recently implemented. We estimated the costs of an ideal follow-up for standard treatment of GT1, the most prevalent genotype, HCV patients according to recent BMoH's recommendations. We are aware that treatment with fixed dose one-tablet daily of SOF/ledispavir (400/90 mg) or SOF/velpatasvir (400/100 mg) for 12 weeks has been recommended as first-line therapies for GT1 patients with or without cirrhosis [42]. These patients can also be treated with the fixed-dose combination of ombitasvir (12.5 mg), paritaprevir (75 mg) and ritonavir (50 mg) in one single tablet and dasabuvir (250 mg) [PTV/r/OMV + DSV regimen] or the fixed dose combination of grazoprevir (100 mg) and elbasvir (50 mg) in a single tablet once-daily [42]. However, these drug combinations are not currently available in Brazil for cost estimation. Another major limitation might be the fact that we evaluated the costs for HCV treatment in a short-term horizon and without prospective follow-up to evaluate whether DAAs treatment are cost-saving compared to PEG-IFN regimens.

The main strengths of this analysis are the PPP-adjustment for costs, the estimation of "real-price" for HCV-drugs and those related to monitoring/medical care accounting for the economic costs of public funds in medical investments. PPP adjustment is essential to allow comparison of prices of goods and services across countries. For high-income countries, PPP adjustment results in lower prices. In contrast, countries with weaker purchasing power, such as Brazil, have a significant increase in prices with PPP adjustment [43]. In the present study, the PPP-adjustment led to an increase in 1.8 fold in US$ costs. The cost for each drug were defined as the weighted-mean price of all HCV-drugs bought by the BMoH in 2015 and registered in web-based and open-access platform. In addition, we analysed micro-costs of all procedures recommended pre, during and post-HCV treatment to allow the estimation of medical care financial burden beyond drug costs.

Conclusions

In conclusion, therapies with all-oral interferon-free, such as SOF/DCV and SOF/SIM for 12 weeks, have a high efficacy and need shorter treatment duration leading to lower costs for monitoring and medical care compared to IFN-based regimens in Brazil where DAAs had more than 90% discount over international prices. HCV treatment by IFN-free regimens will probably be associated with high financial impact worldwide. However, reduced DAA prices due to negotiation between health authorities and pharmaceutical companies can turn HCV treatment into an accessible strategy to HCV eradication.

Abbreviations

ABC: Activity based costing; ALT: Alanine aminotransferase; APRI: Aspartate-to-platelet ratio index; AST: Aspartate aminotransferase; BMoH: Brazilian Ministry of Health; BOC: Boceprevir; BRL: Brazilian Real; CHC: Chronic hepatitis C; DAA: Direct-acting antiviral drugs; DCV: Daclastavir; FIB-4: Fibrosis-4 score; GDP: Gross domestic product; GT1: Genotype 1; HCV: Hepatitis C virus; PEG-IFN: PEG-interferon; PPP$: Purchasing power parity Dollars; RBV: Ribavirin; SELIC: Special System for Settlement and Custody; SIM: Simeprevir; SOF: Sofosbuvir; SUS: *Sistema Único de Saúde*; SVR: Sustained virological response; TE: Transient elastography; TEL: Telaprevir; US$: United States Dollars

Acknowledgements

Not applicable.

Funding

This work was supported by funding from Newton Fund RCUK-CONFAP Research Partnerships call, project "Brazil-UK collaboration in Health Technology Assessment of diagnostic strategies for infectious diseases" from Fundação

Carlos Chagas Filho de Amparo à Pesquisa do Estado do Rio de Janeiro (FAPERJ) under grant E-26/170.021/2015 [Brazil for RC] and Medical Research Council (MRC) grant reference MR/M026515/1 [UK for CH]. The funders had no role in study design, data collection and analysis, decision to publish, or preparation of the manuscript.

Authors' contributions

HP: study concept and design; interpretation of data; drafting and critical revision of the manuscript. MJJ: study concept and design; acquisition of data; analysis and interpretation of data; statistical analysis and critical revision of the manuscript. JCS, AMA, PSS: acquisition of data; analysis and interpretation of data; statistical analysis and critical revision of the manuscript. CR, VGV, RMM, RA: interpretation of data and critical revision of the manuscript. CH and RC: study concept and design; study supervision, interpretation of data and critical revision of the manuscript. All authors read and approved the final manuscript.

Consent for publication

Not applicable.

Competing interests

The authors declare that they have no competing interests.

Author details

[1]Fundação Oswaldo Cruz, FIOCRUZ, Instituto Nacional de Infectologia Evandro Chagas, INI, Laboratório de Pesquisa Clínica em DST e AIDS, LAPCLIN-AIDS, Rio de Janeiro, Brazil. [2]Fundação Oswaldo Cruz, FIOCRUZ, Instituto Nacional de Infectologia Evandro Chagas, INI, Laboratório de Pesquisa em Economia das Organizações de Saúde, LAPECOS, Rio de Janeiro, Brazil. [3]Fundação Oswaldo Cruz, FIOCRUZ, Instituto Nacional de Infectologia Evandro Chagas, INI, Plataforma de Pesquisa Clínica, Rio de Janeiro, Brazil. [4]Fundação Oswaldo Cruz, FIOCRUZ, Centro de Desenvolvimento Tecnológico em Saúde, CDTS, Rio de Janeiro, Brazil. [5]University of Exeter Medical School, UEMS, Evidence Synthesis & Modelling for Health Improvement, ESMI, Exeter, UK. [6]Universidade Federal do Estado do Rio de Janeiro, UNIRIO, Instituto de Saúde Coletiva, ISC, Rio de Janeiro, Brazil.

References

1. Westbrook RH, Dusheiko G. Natural history of hepatitis C. J Hepatol. 2014; 61(1 Suppl):S58–68.
2. Nahon P, Bourcier V, Layese R, Audureau E, Cagnot C, Marcellin P, Guyader D, Fontaine H, Larrey D, De Ledinghen V, et al. Eradication of hepatitis C virus infection in patients with cirrhosis reduces risk of liver and non-liver complications. Gastroenterology. 2017;152(1):142–56.
3. Bota S, Herkner H, Sporea I, Salzl P, Sirli R, Neghina AM, Peck-Radosavljevic M. Meta-analysis: ARFI elastography versus transient elastography for the evaluation of liver fibrosis. Liver Int. 2013;33(8):1138–47.
4. van Katwyk S, Coyle D, Cooper C, Pussegoda K, Cameron C, Skidmore B, Brener S, Moher D, Thavorn K. Transient elastography for the diagnosis of liver fibrosis: a systematic review of economic evaluations. Liver Int. 2017;37(6):851–61.
5. Flisiak R, Pogorzelska J, Flisiak-Jackiewicz M. Hepatitis C: efficacy and safety in real life. Liver Int. 2017;1:26–32.
6. Ward T, Gordon J, Bennett H, Webster S, Sugrue D, Jones B, Brenner M, McEwan P. Tackling the burden of the hepatitis C virus in the UK: characterizing and assessing the clinical and economic consequences. Public Health. 2016;141:42–51.
7. Linas BP. Understanding cost and value in hepatitis C therapy. Top Antivir Med. 2016;24(2):93–7.
8. Jacobs JC, Barnett PG. Emergent challenges in determining costs for economic evaluations. PharmacoEconomics. 2017;35(2):129–39.
9. Mesquita F, Santos ME, Benzaken A, Correa RG, Cattapan E, Sereno LS, Naveira MC. The Brazilian comprehensive response to hepatitis C: from strategic thinking to access to interferon-free therapy. BMC Public Health. 2016;16(1):1132.
10. Vigani AG, Pavan MH, Tozzo R, Goncales ES, Feltrin A, Fais VC, Lazarini MS, Goncales NS, Goncales FL Jr. Comparative study of patients with chronic hepatitis C virus infection due to genotypes 1 and 3 referred for treatment in southeast Brazil. BMC Infect Dis. 2008;8:164.
11. Fernandes FF, Ferraz ML, Andrade LE, Dellavance A, Terra C, Pereira G, Pereira JL, Campos F, Figueiredo F, Perez RM. Enhanced liver fibrosis panel as a predictor of liver fibrosis in chronic hepatitis C patients. J Clin Gastroenterol. 2015;49(3):235–41.
12. Brasil. Guideline for management and treatment of chronic hepatitis C and its co-infections [Protocolo Clinico e Diretrizes Terapêuticas para Tratamento da Hepatite viral Crônica C e co-infecções]. Brasilia: Brazilian Ministry of Health [Ministerio da Saude do Brasil]; 2015. http://portalarquivos.saude.gov.br/images/pdf/2015/julho/29/PCDT-FINAL-HEPATITE-C-FINAL-01.pdf [Accessed on 27 Mar 2017]
13. Udpa S. Activity-based costing for hospitals. Health Care Manag Rev. 1996; 21(3):83–96.
14. Brasil. Guideline for management and treatment of chronic hepatitis C and its co-infections [Protocolo Clinico e Diretrizes Terapêuticas para Tratamento da Hepatite viral Crônica C e co-infecções]. Brasilia: Brazilian Ministry of Health [Ministerio da Saude do Brasil]; 2011. http://bvsms.saude.gov.br/bvs/publicacoes/protocolos_diretrizes_hepatite_viral_c_coinfeccoes.pdf [Accessed on 27 Mar 2017]
15. Brasil. Guideline for management and treatment of chronic hepatitis C and its co-infections [Protocolo Clinico e Diretrizes Terapêuticas para Tratamento da Hepatite viral Crônica C e co-infecções]. Brasilia: Brazilian Ministry of Health [Ministerio da Saude do Brasil]; 2013. http://www.funed.mg.gov.br/wp-content/uploads/2011/07/suplemento_1_protocolo_hep_c.pdf [Accessed on 27 Mar 2017]
16. Welzel TM, Petersen J, Herzer K, Ferenci P, Gschwantler M, Wedemeyer H, Berg T, Spengler U, Weiland O, van der Valk M, et al. Daclatasvir plus sofosbuvir, with or without ribavirin, achieved high sustained virological response rates in patients with HCV infection and advanced liver disease in a real-world cohort. Gut. 2016;65(11):1861–70.
17. Pol S, Bourliere M, Lucier S, Hezode C, Dorival C, Larrey D, Bronowicki JP, Ledinghen VD, Zoulim F, Tran A, et al. Safety and efficacy of daclatasvir-sofosbuvir in HCV genotype 1-mono-infected patients. J Hepatol. 2017;66(1):39–47.
18. Backus LI, Belperio PS, Shahoumian TA, Loomis TP, Mole LA. Effectiveness of sofosbuvir-based regimens in genotype 1 and 2 hepatitis C virus infection in 4026 U.S. veterans. Aliment Pharmacol Ther. 2015;42(5):559–73.
19. Jayasekera CR, Perumpail RB, Chao DT, Pham EA, Aggarwal A, Wong RJ, Ahmed A. Task-shifting: an approach to decentralized hepatitis C treatment in medically underserved areas. Dig Dis Sci. 2015;60(12):3552–7.
20. Pillai AA, Wedd J, Norvell JP, Parekh S, Cheng N, Young N, Spivey JR, Ford R. Simeprevir and Sofosbuvir (SMV-SOF) for 12 weeks for the treatment of chronic hepatitis C genotype 1 infection: a real world (transplant) Hepatology practice experience. Am J Gastroenterol. 2016;111(2):250–60.
21. Barron J, Xie Y, Wu SJ, White J, Singer J, Tulsi B, Rosenberg A. Treatment of chronic hepatitis C infection with Sofosbuvir-based regimens in a commercially insured patient population. Am Health Drug Benefits. 2016;9(6):327–35.
22. Thornton K, Deming P, Manch RA, Moore A, Kohli A, Gish R, Sussman NL, Khaderi S, Scott J, Mera J, et al. Is response guided therapy dead? Low cure rates in patients with detectable hepatitis C virus at week 4 of treatment. Hepatol Int. 2016;10(4):624–31.
23. Roytman M, Ramkissoon R, Wu C, Hong L, Trujillo R, Huddleston L, Poerzgen P, Seto T, Wong L, Tsai N. Examining the clinical course of genotype 1 chronic hepatitis C patients treated with the cosmos regimen: including patients with advanced liver disease and east Asian ancestry. Hepatol Int. 2016;10(4):616–23.
24. Pellicelli AM, Pace Palitti V, Vignally P, Ceccherini-Silberstein F, Siciliano M, Giannelli V, Moretti A, Tarquini P, Scifo G, Messina V, et al. Efficacy and safety of sofosbuvir/simeprevir plus flat dose ribavirin in genotype 1 elderly cirrhotic patients: a real-life study. Liver Int. 2017;37(5):653–61.
25. Lutchman G, Nguyen NH, Chang CY, Ahmed A, Daugherty T, Garcia G, Kumari R, Gupta S, Doshi D, Nguyen MH. Effectiveness and tolerability of simeprevir and sofosbuvir in nontransplant and post-liver transplant patients with hepatitis C genotype 1. Aliment Pharmacol Ther. 2016;44(7): 738–46.
26. Sulkowski MS, Vargas HE, Di Bisceglie AM, Kuo A, Reddy KR, Lim JK, Morelli G, Darling JM, Feld JJ, Brown RS, et al. Effectiveness of Simeprevir plus

Sofosbuvir, with or without Ribavirin, in real-world patients with HCV genotype 1 infection. Gastroenterology. 2016;150(2):419–29.
27. Chang CY, Nguyen P, Le A, Zhao C, Ahmed A, Daugherty T, Garcia G, Lutchman G, Kumari R, Nguyen MH. Real-world experience with interferon-free, direct acting antiviral therapies in Asian Americans with chronic hepatitis C and advanced liver disease. Medicine (Baltimore). 2017;96(6): e6128.
28. Marino Z, Pascasio-Acevedo JM, Gallego A, Diago M, Baliellas C, Morillas R, Prieto M, Moreno JM, Sanchez-Antolin G, Vergara M et al. High efficacy of Sofosbuvir plus Simeprevir in a large cohort of Spanish cirrhotic patients infected with genotypes 1 and 4. Liver Int. 2017. doi: https://doi.org/10.1111/liv.13470. [Epub ahead of print].
29. Ramos H, Linares P, Badia E, Martin I, Gomez J, Almohalla C, Jorquera F, Calvo S, Garcia I, Conde P, et al. Interferon-free treatments in patients with hepatitis C genotype 1–4 infections in a real-world setting. World J Gastrointest Pharmacol Ther. 2017;8(2):137–46.
30. de Lucinda CR, Vieira RL. Interest rates and informational issues in the credit market: experimental evidence from Brazil. World Dev. 2014;59:47–58.
31. Modenesi AD, Modenesi RL. Development conventions: theory and the case of Brazil in the latter half of the twentieth century. J Post Keynesian Econ. 2015;38(1):131–61.
32. Iyengar S, Tay-Teo K, Vogler S, Beyer P, Wiktor S, de Joncheere K, Hill S. Prices, costs, and affordability of new medicines for hepatitis C in 30 countries: an economic analysis. PLoS Med. 2016;13(5):e1002032.
33. Bach TA, Zaiken K. Real-world drug costs of treating hepatitis C genotypes 1–4 with direct-acting Antivirals: initiating treatment at fibrosis 0–2 and 3–4. J Manag Care Spec Pharm. 2016;22(12):1437–45.
34. Maan R, Zaim R, van der Meer AJ, Feld JJ, Wedemeyer H, Dufour JF, Lammert F, Manns MP, Zeuzem S, Hansen BE, et al. Real-world medical costs of antiviral therapy among patients with chronic HCV infection and advanced hepatic fibrosis. J Gastroenterol Hepatol. 2016;31(11):1851–9.
35. Jakubiak-Lasocka J, Jakubczyk M. Cost-effectiveness versus cost-utility analyses: what are the motives behind using each and how do their results differ?—a polish example. Value Health Reg Issues. 2014;4:66–74.
36. Davitkov P, Chandar AK, Hirsch A, Compan A, Silveira MG, Anthony DD, Smith S, Gideon C, Bonomo RA, Falck-Ytter Y. Treatment selection choices should not be based on benefits or costs alone: a head-to-head randomized controlled trial of antiviral drugs for hepatitis C. PLoS One. 2016;11(10):e0163945.
37. Hezode C, Fontaine H, Dorival C, Zoulim F, Larrey D, Canva V, De Ledinghen V, Poynard T, Samuel D, Bourliere M, et al. Effectiveness of telaprevir or boceprevir in treatment-experienced patients with HCV genotype 1 infection and cirrhosis. Gastroenterology. 2014;147(1):132–42.
38. Younossi ZM, Park H, Dieterich D, Saab S, Ahmed A, Gordon SC. The value of cure associated with treating treatment-naive chronic hepatitis C genotype 1: Are the new all-oral regimens good value to society? Liver Int. 2016. doi:https://doi.org/10.1111/liv.13298. [Epub ahead of print].
39. Chhatwal J, He T, Hur C, Lopez-Olivo MA. Direct-Acting Antiviral Agents for Patients With Hepatitis C Virus Genotype 1 Infection Are Cost-Saving. Clin Gastroenterol Hepatol 2016. doi: https://doi.org/10.1016/j.cgh.2016.09.015. [Epub ahead of print].
40. Dahari H, Canini L, Graw F, Uprichard SL, Araujo ES, Penaranda G, Coquet E, Chiche L, Riso A, Renou C, et al. HCV kinetic and modeling analyses indicate similar time to cure among sofosbuvir combination regimens with daclatasvir, simeprevir or ledipasvir. J Hepatol. 2016;64(6):1232–9.
41. Peres-da-Silva A, Brandao-Mello CE, Lampe E: Prevalence of sofosbuvir resistance-associated variants in Brazilian and worldwide NS5B sequences of genotype-1 HCV. Antivir Ther. 2017. doi: https://doi.org/10.3851/IMP3131. [Epub ahead of print].
42. EASL. Recommendations on treatment of hepatitis C 2016. J Hepatol. 2017; 66(1):153–94.
43. Purchasing power parity vs market exchange rate. http://www.dawn.com/news/1214055. Accessed on 27 Mar 2017.

13

Hepatitis C virus eradication improves immediate and delayed episodic memory in patients treated with interferon and ribavirin

Mary Ellen Dias Barbosa[1,2,4*], Ana Luiza Zaninotto[1], Daniel Ferraz de Campos Mazo[2,3], Mario Guimarães Pessoa[2], Cláudia Pinto Marques Souza de Oliveira[2], Flair José Carrilho[2] and Alberto Queiroz Farias[2]

Abstract

Background: Chronic hepatitis C virus (HCV) infection is associated with impairment of cognitive function and mood disorders. Our aim was to evaluate the impact of sustained virological response (SVR) on cognitive function and mood disorders.

Method: A prospective exploratory one arm study was conducted. Adult clinically compensated HVC patients were consecutively recruited before treatment with interferon and ribavirin for 24 to 48 weeks, according to HCV genotype. Clinical, neurocognitive and mood assessments using the PRIME-MD and BDI instruments were performed at baseline, right after half of the expected treatment has been reached and 6 months after the end of antiviral treatment. Exclusion criteria were the use of illicit psychotropic substances, mental confusion, hepatic encephalopathy, hepatocellular carcinoma, severe anemia, untreated hypothyroidism, Addison syndrome and major depression before treatment.

Results: Thirty six patients were enrolled and 21 completed HCV treatment ($n = 16$ with SVR and $n = 5$ without). Regardless of the viral clearance at the end of treatment, there was a significant improvement in the immediate verbal episodic memory ($p = 0.010$), delayed verbal episodic memory ($p = 0.007$), selective attention ($p < 0.001$) and phonemic fluency ($p = 0.043$). Patients with SVR displayed significant improvement in immediate ($p = 0.045$) and delayed verbal episodic memory ($p = 0.040$) compared to baseline. The baseline frequency of depression was 9.5%, which rose to 52.4% during treatment, and returned to 9.5% 6 months after the end of treatment, without significant difference between patients with and without SVR. Depressive symptoms were observed in 19.1% before treatment, 62% during ($p = 0.016$) and 28.6% 6 months after the end of treatment ($p = 0.719$).

Conclusions: Eradication of HCV infection improved cognitive performance but did not affect the frequency of depressive symptoms at least in the short range.

Keywords: Cognition, Memory, Attention, Neuropsychology, Hepatitis C, Depression

* Correspondence: mary.dias@gmail.com
[1]Division of Psychology, Clinics Hospital, University of Sao Paulo School of Medicine, Avenida Dr. Eneas Carvalho de Aguiar, 255, São Paulo 05403-900, Brazil
[2]Division of Clinical Gastroenterology and Hepatology, Clinics Hospital, Department of Gastroenterology, University of São Paulo School of Medicine, Avenida Dr. Eneas Carvalho de Aguiar, 255, sala 9159, São Paulo 05403-900, Brazil

Background

Hepatitis C virus (HCV) infection is a global public health problem. It is estimated that between 130 and 185 million people are infected worldwide [1]. Roughly 85% of patients infected go on to develop chronic hepatitis and 20 to 40% develop end-stage liver disease (i.e. cirrhosis) within 10 to 20 years [2]. In addition to liver disease, HCV is related to a series of extrahepatic manifestations, with a negative impact on the physical and mental health of infected individuals [3]. Patients with advanced cirrhosis commonly display hepatic encephalopathy, with characteristic neuropsychological, behavioral and neurological changes. However, in recent years a number of studies have established that up to a third of patients without cirrhosis also develop a neuropsychiatric syndrome characterized by impairment of cognitive function and symptoms related to depression [4–6]. These abnormalities were shown by neuropsychological tests, magnetic resonance spectroscopy and other neuroimaging modalities and various inventories of depression [4, 7, 8]. The main cognitive abnormalities include impairment of attention span, concentration and psychomotor skills. Depressive symptoms are found in roughly 40% of patients and reach a prevalence of 20% to 40% during antiviral treatment, particularly with interferon, with detrimental effects on both quality of life and compliance with treatment [4, 9].

Various lines of evidence suggest the cognitive dysfunction and depressive symptoms are related to the release of pro-inflammatory cytokines caused by infection of the central nervous system by HCV. HCV replicates itself in mononuclear peripheral blood cells and in bone marrow, which are precursors to the microglial cells in the brain. It is in this way HCV is introduced to the central nervous system via a "Trojan horse" mechanism [4, 10, 11]. However, no clear correlation between HCV viral load and cognitive impairment could be demonstrated [12]. Despite HCV infection itself within the brain causing local inflammation and neurocognitive disturbances, another hypothesis suggest these disturbances, including depression, could be in part a result of elevated systemic cytokine levels due to chronic HCV activation of the immune system [13–15]. Putative inflammatory cytokines are interleukin-1, 4, and 6, tumor necrosis factor-α and interferon-α, that can cross the blood-brain barrier and impact brain functioning [14, 15].

Despite various rigorous studies having demonstrated that HCV infection is associated with a decline in neurocognitive function and depressive symptoms, data are scarce as to whether or not these changes are irreversible in patients who have eliminated HCV after successful treatment [4, 6, 8]. Therefore, we conducted the present study with the aim of evaluating the impact of sustained virological response (SVR), i.e. viral clearance, in improving neurocognitive function and mood disorders in patients infected with HCV.

Methods

Subjects

The participants were selected from a teaching hospital and national centre of reference for Hepatology (Hepatology Outpatient Center at the Department of Gastroenterology, Clinics Hospital, University of São Paulo School of Medicine, Brazil) between 2011 and 2013. The inclusion criteria were: outpatients between the ages of 18 and 70, eligible for antiviral treatment of chronic HCV infection. The exclusion criteria were: use of psychotropic substances, mental confusion evaluated by the Mini-Mental State Examination with a score < 24 points [16], overt hepatic encephalopathy identified under West Haven criteria [17], minimal/subclinical hepatic encephalopathy shown by the Inhibitory Control Test [18], hepatocellular carcinoma, severe anemia, untreated hypothyroidism, Addison syndrome and major depression before treatment. Alcohol intake was assessed in all patients by the Alcohol Use Disorders Identification Test –AUDIT [19].

Study design

A prospective exploratory one arm study was conducted in which the patients were assessed before the beginning, right after half of the expected treatment has been reached and 6 months after completion of antiviral therapy. All study participants underwent psychometric testing under the supervision of a psychologist and a neuropsychologist.

All patients were submitted to clinical assessment and blood tests for liver enzymes, hemoglobin, thyroid stimulating hormone, HCV genotype and viral load. HIV and hepatitis B co-infection were excluded using the appropriate serological tests. HCV-RNA was detected with real time polymerase chain reaction with kits purchased from Abbott Molecular (Illinois, USA). This assay achieves an inter-assay standard deviation of less than or equal to 0.25 log IU/mL of HCV RNA for samples containing HCV concentrations from 100 to 100 million IU/mL. The inter-assay SD at 5.97 and at 1.96 log IU/mL were of 0.04 and 0.09, respectively. Limits of detection were 12 to 100.000.000 IU/mL. Liver biopsy was carried out on all patients, with the exception of 3 ($n = 2$, hemophilia; $n = 1$ severe thrombocytopenia). The liver biopsies were carried out with a 14-G Tru-Cut™ needle (Medical Technology, Gainsville, FL, USA). Liver histology was examined by an experienced liver pathologist from the Department of Pathology of University of São Paulo School of Medicine. The classification score used for analysis of the biopsies was the METAVIR score: F0 - no fibrosis;

F1 - portal fibrosis without septa; F2 - portal fibrosis and few septa extending into lobules; F3 - numerous septa extending to adjacent portal tracts or terminal hepatic venules and F4 - cirrhosis [20].

The antiviral therapy consisted of subcutaneous injections of interferon administered weekly and ribavirin administered daily and adjusted to the weight of the patient over a period of 24 weeks (genotypes 2 and 3) or for 48 weeks (genotypes 1 and 5), according to scientific recommendations of HCV treatment at the time the study was performed [21]. SVR was defined as a negative HCV RNA polymerase chain reaction assay 24 weeks after cessation of hepatitis C treatment. Patients without early virological response were defined as those with absence of at least 2 log reduction in HCV RNA at 12 weeks of treatment initiation.

Neuropsychological assessment

Executive functions

Victoria Stroop test [22, 23] Selective Attention and inhibition - Consisting of three cards: first (color identification), second (identification of colored words) and third (color interference). On each card, the subject is encouraged to give the name of the color of the ink as quickly as possible. The score is calculated by the time spent on each card.

Trail Making Test A and B (TMT form A and B) [22, 24, 25] Sustained (TMT form A) and Alternated Attention (TMT form B). Consist of 25 circles distributed over a sheet of paper. In Form A, the circles are numbered 1–25, In Part B, the circles include both numbers (1–13) and letters (A – L); as in Part A, the patient draws lines to connect the circles in an ascending pattern, but with the added task of alternating between the numbers and letters (i.e., 1-A-2-B-3-C, etc.). The test is stopped if the patient has not completed both parts after 5 min have elapsed. The score is calculated by the time spent on each trial.

Phonemic Fluency – (COWAT FAS) [22] Assessed by asking the patient to say as many words as possible that begin with the letters F, then the letter A, then the letter S over the course of 1 min. Proper nouns, such as of people or places, are not permitted, nor are conjugations of verbs. The score is given as the sum of the correctly spoken words.

Semantic fluency [22] Assessed by asking the patient to recite the names of as many animals as possible in 1 min. For the scoring, words belonging to a larger category are not considered if the patient has already used words from the subcategory. Each word is afforded a score of 1.

Episodic verbal memory and learning

Hopkins Verbal Learning Test - Revised- HVLT-R [26] Verbal Learning and Long-term episodic memory. After the examiner reads the list of 12 words, the patient is asked to repeat as many words as possible, in any order (immediate recall). This process is repeated twice more and after 25 min a delayed recall is sought. Recognition is also required. Each right word scores 1 point.

Working memory

Forward and backward digit span [27] To assess the work memory, increasing sequences of digits are orally presented at a rate of one per second. At the end of each sequence, the subjects must repeat them in direct order (forward) and inverse order (backward). The score represents the number of digits counted in the largest correctly repeated sequence forward and backward.

Estimated Intelligence Quotient (IQ)

Vocabulary and reasoning matrices Subtest of Wechsler Adult Intelligent Scale (WAIS III) [27]. In the vocabulary assessment, 33 words are orally presented and the patient should define or explain their meanings. Six consecutive words incorrectly defined mark the end of the test. Each word receives a score of 0, 1 or 2. The subtest Reasoning Matrix consists of a logical sequence of figures presented incompletely and with a progressive difficulty which the patient chooses between six others, to complete a logical sequence. Eight consecutive incorrect responses end the test. The sum of the subtest scores gives an estimate of intellectual quotient.

Evaluation of depression and depressive symptoms

Primary Care Evaluation of Mental Disorders – PRIME – MD [28, 29] The module of major depression of the structured interview PRIME-MD, which is based on the diagnostic criteria of DSM-IV [30] was used because it is considered the gold standard of psychopathological disturbance assessment.

Beck Depression Inventory – BDI [31] The self-evaluation inventory numerically demonstrates descriptive items, attitudes and depressive symptoms to assess different conditions found in the general population. It was used in this study for the evaluation of depressive symptoms. The cutoff scores recommended for evaluation (by the non-professional population) were: 0–9 absence of depressive symptoms or minimal symptoms; 10–16 mild symptoms; 17–29 moderate symptoms; 30–63 severe symptoms.

Statistical analysis

Fisher exact test was used for comparison of patients with and without SVR. Student t and Mann –Whitney tests were used for continuous variables. Results were expressed as mean, standard deviation, percentage and Z-score. *Z*-score was used only for the neuropsychological tests and was obtained via the conversion of the points of the neuropsychological tests through the mean and standard deviation from the normative population. Values of z-score ≤ -1.50 were considered impairment. Covariate analysis was used to assess years of education and time as potential confounders. All data were analyzed as complete protocol. The R program version 3.12.1 (R Core Team, Auckland, New Zealand, 2014) was used for calculations. *P* value < 0.05 was considered statistically significant. A statistical review of the study was performed by a biomedical statistician.

Results

Patients

Seventy eight patients were consecutively recruited at the Hepatology Outpatient Center at the Department of Gastroenterology. Forty two patients of these were excluded (see Fig. 1). The remaining 36 comprise the present series, as shown in Fig. 1.

Baseline characteristics of included patients are provided in Table 1. Most of the patients were female in the middle age, with HCV genotype 1 and absence of advanced liver fibrosis. During the antiviral treatment, patients maintained appropriate levels of hemoglobin. Twenty one patients completed antiviral treatment. None of the participants displayed problematic alcohol intake, mental confusion or hepatic encephalopathy at inclusion, during and after treatment. Twenty three (63.9%) patients had other illnesses or associated conditions, i.e. arterial hypertension, $n = 15$ (65.2%); diabetes mellitus, $n = 5$ (21.7%); arthrosis/osteoporosis, $n = 5$ (21.7%); cardiopathy, $n = 4$ (17.4%); well-controlled hypothyroidism, $n = 3$ (13%); hemophilia, $n = 2$ (8.7%); nephrotic syndrome, $n = 2$ (8.7%) and miscellaneous, $n = 5$ (21.7%).

Neuropsychological assessment

Nineteen patients had the three neuropsychological assessments (before, during and after HCV treatment). Comparing before and during treatment (right after half of the expected treatment has been reached, at week 12 or 24), baseline z-score for selective attention was -2.10 ± 1.28 and improved to -1.04 ± 0.93 during antiviral therapy ($p = 0.004$). No improvement in other neurocognitive domains was observed during interferon-based therapy, as shown in Table 2.

Regardless of the viral clearance, there was significant improvement in the domains of immediate verbal episodic memory, delayed verbal episodic memory, selective attention and phonemic verbal fluency ($p < 0.05$) after the end of treatment (Table 3).

Of the 19 patients who completed HCV treatment, 15 patients had SVR. This subgroup of patients with SVR presented significant improvement in the domains of immediate verbal episodic memory ($p = 0.045$) and delayed verbal episodic memory ($p = 0.040$) when compared with the group without SVR, as shown in Table 4.

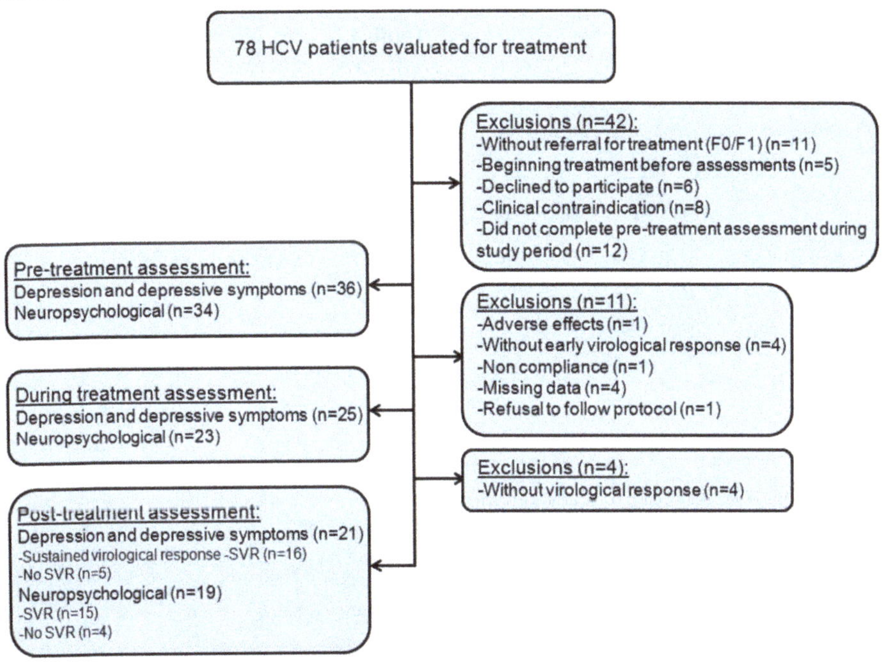

Fig. 1 Study flow chart

Table 1 Baseline characteristics

Characteristics	Patients (*n* = 36)
Age in years ± SD (range)	49.5 ± 12.04 (29–69)
Female (%)	20 (55.6)
Education level (%)	
University	7 (19.4)
High school	12 (33.3)
Primary school	17 (19.4)
Occupation (%)	
Employed	23 (63.9)
Unemployed	7 (19.4)
Retired	6 (16.7)
HCV genotype (%)	
Genotype 1	27 (75.0)
Genotype 3	7 (19.4)
Other genotypes	2 (5.6)
Histological stage (%)	
F1/F2	26 (72.2)
F3	4 (19.0)
F4	6 (8.8)

Table 3 Neuropsychological domains in patients before and after antiviral treatment, regardless of the viral clearance

Domain	Baseline (*n* = 19)	6 months after treatment (*n* = 19)	*p*-value
	M ± SD*	M ± SD*	
Immediate episodic memory	−1.50 ± 1.05	−0.74 ± 0.92	0.010**
Delay episodic memory	−1.36 ± 1.12	−0.79 ± 1.22	0.007**
Memory recognition	−0.19 ± 1.11	0.13 ± 1.18	0.293
Working memory	0.12 ± 0.65	0.15 ± 0.51	0.670
Focused attention	−0.86 ± 1.49	−0.65 ± 1.51	0.421
Divided attention	−1.51 ± 1.47	−0.50 ± 1.22	0.142
Selective attention	−2.10 ± 1.28	−0.20 ± 0.97	0.000**
Phonemic verbal fluency	−0.73 ± 1.13	−0.34 ± 1.08	0.043**
Semantic verbal fluency	−0.39 ± 1.15	−0.53 ± 1.04	0.705
Dominant hand coordination	−1.62 ± 1.27	−1.24 ± 1.57	0.258
Non dominant hand coordination	−1.58 ± 1.23	−1.18 ± 1.79	0.298

M mean, *SD* standard deviation
*z score; ** $p < 0.05$

Evaluation of depression and depressive symptoms

Twenty one patients had the three depression and depressive symptoms assessments (before, during and after HCV treatment). The baseline frequency of major depression was 9.5% (2 patients), rising to 52.4% (11 patients) during treatment ($p = 0.012$) and returning to 9.5% 6 months after the end of treatment, with no difference between patients with and without SVR ($p = 0.429$). In a similar way, depressive symptoms were observed in 19.1% before treatment, reaching 62% during ($p = 0.016$) and reducing to 28.6% after the end of treatment ($p = 0.719$). There were no differences regarding depressive symptoms according to virological response ($p = 0.597$).

Table 2 Neuropsychological domains in patients before and during antiviral treatment

Domain	Baseline (*n* = 19)	During treatment (*n* = 19)	*p*-value
	M ± SD*	M ± SD*	
Immediate episodic memory	−1.50 ± 1.05	−1.34 ± 1.01	0.758
Delay episodic memory	−1.36 ± 1.12	−1.20 ± 1.31	0.433
Memory recognition	−0.19 ± 1.11	0.61 ± 1.24	0.167
Working memory	0.12 ± 0.65	0.26 ± 0.81	0.576
Focused attention	−0.86 ± 1.49	−0.80 ± 1.35	0.850
Divided attention	−1.51 ± 1.47	−0.85 ± 1.19	0.433
Selective attention	−2.10 ± 1.28	−1.04 ± 0.93	0.004**
Phonemic verbal fluency	−0.73 ± 1.13	−0.67 ± 0.95	0.811
Semantic verbal fluency	−0.39 ± 1.15	−0.85 ± 1.09	0.136
Dominant hand coordination	−1.62 ± 1.27	−1.35 ± 1.37	0.344
Non dominant hand coordination	−1.58 ± 1.23	−1.70 ± 1.17	0.836

M mean, *SD* standard deviation
*z score; ** $p < 0.05$

Table 4 Neuropsychological domains according to the virological response to treatment

Domain	With SVR (*n* = 15)	Without SVR (*n* = 4)	*p*-value
	M ± SD*	M ± SD*	
Immediate episodic memory	−0.50 ± 0.80	−1.65 ± 0.84	0.045**
Delay episodic memory	−0.49 ± 1.12	−1.90 ± 0.99	0.040**
Memory recognition	0.38 ± 0.81	−0.80 ± 1.94	0.736
Working memory	0.17 ± 0.54	0.08 ± 0.42	0.760
Focused attention	−0.35 ± 1.39	−1.80 ± 1.58	0.064
Divided attention	−0.53 ± 1.31	−0.30 ± 0.28	1.000
Selective attention	−0.11 ± 0.68	−0.5 ± 1.80	1.000
Phonemic verbal fluency	−0.14 ± 1.05	−1.09 ± 0.93	0.160
Semantic verbal fluency	−0.40 ± 1,08	−1.02 ± 0.83	0.208
Dominant hand coordination	−1.02 ± 1.61	−2.07 ± 1.26	0.228
Non dominant hand coordination	−1.15 ± 1.92	−1.26 ± 1.44	0.920

M mean, *SD* standard deviation, *SVR* sustained virological response
*z score; ** $p < 0.05$

The covariate analysis showed the impact of higher years of schooling as a predictor of better results at neuropsychological tests ($p < 0.01$).

Discussion

In this study, the neuropsychological performance and the frequency of major depression and depressive symptoms of patients infected with HCV were compared before the beginning of treatment, right after half of the expected treatment has been reached and 6 months after the end of treatment. We observed that patients that attained viral clearance (SVR) improved significantly in the neurocognitive domains of immediate and delayed verbal episodic memory compared to patients without.

Since the seminal report by Forton et al. [32] describing an elevated choline/creatinine ratio by proton magnetic resonance spectroscopy in the frontal white matter and basal ganglia of HCV-infected patients, several studies have suggested that the brain may be affected in chronic HCV infection. Subsequent reports have documented that up to one third of HCV infected patients may have neuropsychological impairment [7, 11, 12, 33–35]. These changes are seen even in the absence of cirrhosis, decompensated liver disease, hepatic encephalopathy or previous history of abuse of psychoactive substances, suggesting an effect of the viral infection on the central nervous system. HCV locally induced inflammation and the passage of systemic pro-inflammatory cytokine through the blood-brain barrier could also impair neurologic functioning [14, 15]. The neurocognitive disturbances may be documented long before the beginning of interferon-based antiviral therapy, which is a well-known cause of neurocognitive, mood and psychiatric dysfunction.

Most studies were based on the comparison of the brain of infected versus non-infected patients by magnetic resonance imaging and functional single photon emission tomography [7, 12, 33–35]. Despite the high degree of heterogeneity of these studies, it is indisputable that chronic HCV infection is associated with impairment of attention, executive function, verbal abilities and memory. In this regard, it is noteworthy that few studies used a structured and validated neuropsychological battery of tests for diagnosing this neurocognitive dysfunction.

In contrast with a number of papers that show neuropsychological impairment in HCV infected patients, few data are available describing the potential reversibility of the cognitive disturbances after successful antiviral treatment. Byrnes et al. [36] performed ^{1}H magnetic resonance spectroscopy and a battery of neuropsychological tests before, during and after antiviral treatment with interferon and ribavirin in 15 HCV-infected patients. They concluded that HCV eradication had a beneficial effect on cerebral metabolism and improved verbal learning and visual and spatial memory. However, the sample size was limited and post-treatment assessment was carried out 12 weeks after the discontinuation of interferon, not enough to fulfill the definition of SVR. In a recent paper, Kraus et al. [37] performed a multicenter study including 168 HCV patients receiving antiviral therapy with interferon and ribavirin. Twelve months after the termination of antiviral treatment, patients with SVR had significant improvement in 3 out 5 domains (vigilance, shared attention: optical task and working memory). Our findings confirm previous few observations that HCV-associated neurocognitive impairment may be reversible after viral eradication. However, our study differs from the paper of Byrnes et al. [36] because we demonstrated that neurocognitive improvement persist long after the withdrawal of the therapy in patients with SVR, as defined by the inability to detect HCV RNA 24 weeks after completion of treatment. Despite the improvement in HVLT immediate and delay recall from baseline in those attaining SVR in our study, it is noteworthy that subjects are still performing in the impaired range. Persistent neurocognitive impairment in patients treated with interferon and ribavirin was described by Cattie et al., specifically within the domains of working memory, learning, and executive functions, even after HCV viral load undetectability [38]. Our study has also some difference with the paper of Kraus et al. [37]. We used a stringent protocol that included clinical assessment, exclusion of potential confounding variables such as unrelated conditions (severe anemia, fatigue, untreated hypothyroidism, and dementia), substance abuse and heavy alcohol intake. Cognitive function disturbances were assessed by a more comprehensive battery of neuropsychological tests, which included 11 domains of interest in HCV-infected patients. Mood was assessed with two different instruments. Furthermore, sociodemographical variables which could influence the performance of the patients were taken into account.

Our study observed that depression and depressive symptoms are common in untreated hepatitis C patients and they increase significantly during interferon based treatment. However, SVR did not lead to a significant decline in the frequency of these symptoms. It is worth restating that the majority of patients displayed a related condition. In fact, the illness, regardless of its cause, can influence the presence of mood disorders. It is possible that the frequency of major depression and related symptoms observed before antiviral treatment reflect, at least in part, the clinical background of the patients. It is well documented in the literature that the frequency of depression and depressive symptoms increases over the course of interferon based treatment [39–41], but returns to baseline levels after the cessation of treatment, indicating the reversibility of these symptoms, observations confirmed by this study. Recently Huckans et al. also reported increased symptoms of depression during interferon therapy in a cohort of 33 HCV infected patients, which decreased or remitted following treatment discontinuation [42]. Eccles et al. have demonstrated that hypothalamic-pituitary-adrenal axis hyperactivity prior to interferon based therapy evaluated through measurement of the waking salivary cortisol response was associated to depression during treatment [43]. Whale et al. showed recently that younger age, previous history of major depression disorder, higher baseline psychomotor retardation and somatic symptoms item scores using the Hamilton Depression Rating Scale and HCV genotype 2 were implicated in depression during IFN treatment [44]. In the present study we excluded patients with major depression diagnosis at baseline and we could not find predictive factors for depression during IFN treatment, maybe due to small sample evaluated. The exogenous administration of IFN in addition to the HCV chronic activation of the immune and elevated systemic cytokine levels could induce sickness behavior and depression [13]. Interestingly, depression and / or the severity of depressive symptoms related to IFN treatment seem higher in HCV mono-infected patients when compared to HIV/HCV co-infected patients and in those with chronic hepatitis B [45, 46]. It is notable that hemolytic anemia induced by ribavirin is common during antiviral treatment, contributing to the somatic effects of depression. An American study with 32 patients concluded that interferon exacerbates somatic depressive symptoms [39]. However, the major limitation of this study pertains to the fact that the data were not controlled for anemia, and only US war veterans were included in the study, which is possibly not a representative sample of the population infected with HCV. Our data were rigorously controlled for hemoglobin levels throughout the course of treatment.

The frequent impairment of attention, concentration and psychomotor skills suggests a relation with the fronto-cortical systems, which would be affected by chronic HCV infection. Chronic HCV infection, independently of viral load genotype, triggers activation of inflammatory cytokines and immune response. This response is directed towards the 5-HT receptor, which plays an important role in the pathophysiology of depression and produces changes in cognitive function and mood [4, 32, 33]. Indeed, major depression may be associated with cognitive impairments, such as executive functions and memory alterations secondary to attention deficit [47]. In our study, however, despite an increase in depression and depressive symptoms during treatment, patients experienced improvement in the domains of immediate verbal episodic memory, delayed verbal episodic memory, selective attention and phonemic verbal fluency. Besides this, depression and depressive symptoms frequencies returned to baseline while immediate verbal episodic memory and delayed verbal episodic memory improved in those attaining SVR.

HCV therapy has experienced a revolution in recent years, with interferon free regimens directed at specific steps of viral replication (direct acting antivirals, i.e., DAA), leading to highly effective, shorter and safer treatments. To date, there are limited data regarding the impact of DAA induced viral clearance on cognition and depressive symptoms. Kleefeld et al. reported in an HCV / HIV population 12 patients who achieved viral clearance with DAA [48]. Improvement in the domains visual memory, attention, processing speed and executive functioning were reported, however, the limited number of patients and practice effects may hamper firm conclusions. Another study with sofosbuvir and lepipasvir associated HCV viral suppression with normalization of cerebral N-acetyl aspartate evaluated by magnetic resonance spectroscopy [49].

A limitation of our study is the lack of an untreated HCV control group to rule out some confounders, such as practice effect on the neurocognitive domains tested. Regarding the Trail Making Test A and B, we used it exclusively to evaluate the domain of sustained and alternated attention, but additional information about processing speed components could have been obtained. Another relative weakness of our study is the small number of patients, in particular those non-responders at the end of the follow-up.

Conclusions

In summary, we demonstrated that patients which attained HCV eradication had significant improvement in immediate and delayed episodic memory. However, the frequency of depressive symptoms and depression did not decrease. The added benefit of the improvement of neurocognitive impairment after the HCV clearance with interferon-based therapy has clinical implications and the potential of making the cognitive function a valid outcome of treatment. Future studies will need to address the correlation of the performance on the battery of neurocognitive tests with depressive symptoms, quality of life or other patient reported outcomes. From the same perspective, further studies assessing the effect of the new DAA on the cognitive function are warranted.

Abbreviations

AUDIT: Alcohol Use Disorders Identification Test; BDI: Beck depression inventory; COWAT-FAS: Controlled Oral Word Association Test- Phonemic Fluency; DAA: Directing acting antivirals; HCV: Cronic hepatitis C virus; HIV: Human immunodeficiency virus; HVLT-R: Hopkins verbal learning – revised; IQ: Intelligence quotient; PRIME-MD: Primary care evaluation of mental disorders; RNA: Ribonucleic acid; SVR: Sustained virological response; TMT A and B: Trail making test A and B; WAIS III: Wechsler adult intelligent scale

Acknowledgements
Thanks to Capes (Commission for the Improvement of Higher Education Personnel) for the scholarship during the study for Barbosa ME.

Authors' contributions
MEB conceived and designed the study, collected and assembled the data, contributed to the data analysis and interpretation and wrote the manuscript. ALZ designed the study, collected and assembled the data, contributed to the data analysis and interpretation and revised the manuscript. DFM contributed to the data analysis and interpretation, wrote and revised the manuscript. MGP, CPO and FJC revised the manuscript. AFQ conceived and designed the study, contributed to the data analysis and interpretation, wrote and revised the manuscript. All authors approved the final form of the article.

Consent for publication
Not applicable.

Competing interests
The authors declare that they have no competing interest.

Author details
[1]Division of Psychology, Clinics Hospital, University of Sao Paulo School of Medicine, Avenida Dr. Eneas Carvalho de Aguiar, 255, São Paulo 05403-900, Brazil. [2]Division of Clinical Gastroenterology and Hepatology, Clinics Hospital, Department of Gastroenterology, University of São Paulo School of Medicine, Avenida Dr. Eneas Carvalho de Aguiar, 255, sala 9159, São Paulo 05403-900, Brazil. [3]Division of Gastroenterology, School of Medical Sciences, University of Campinas, Rua Carlos Chagas, 420, Campinas 13083-878, Brazil. [4]Department of Gastroenterology, University of Sao Paulo School of Medicine, Av. Dr. Enéas de Carvalho Aguiar n° 255, São Paulo 05403-000, Brazil.

References

1. Wedemeyer H, Dore GJ, Ward JW. Estimates on HCV disease burden worldwide - filling the gaps. J Viral Hepat. 2015;22(Suppl 1):1–5.
2. Ascione A, Tartaglione T, Di Costanzo GG. Natural history of chronic hepatitis C virus infection. Dig Liver Dis. 2007;39(Suppl 1):S4–7.
3. Younossi Z, Park H, Henry L, Adeyemi A, Stepanova M. Extra-hepatic manifestations of hepatitis C-a meta-analysis of prevalence, quality of life, and economic burden. Gastroenterology. 2016;150:1599–608.
4. Perry W, Hilsabeck RC, Hassanein T. Cognitive dysfunction in chronic hepatitis C: a review. Dig Dis Sci. 2008;53:307–21.
5. Forton DM, Thomas HC, Murphy CA, Allsop JM, Foster GR, Main J, et al. Hepatitis C and cognitive impairment in a cohort of patients with mild liver disease. Hepatology. 2002;35:433–9.
6. Yarlott L, Heald E, Forton D. Hepatitis C virus infection, and neurological and psychiatric disorders - a review. J Adv Res. 2017;8:139–48.
7. Thames AD, Castellon SA, Singer EJ, Nagarajan R, Sarma MK, Smith J, et al. Neuroimaging abnormalities, neurocognitive function, and fatigue in patients with hepatitis C. Neurol Neuroimmunol Neuroinflamm. 2015;2:e59.
8. Constant A, Castera L, Dantzer R, Couzigou P, de Ledinghen V, Demotes-Mainard J, et al. Mood alterations during interferon-alfa therapy in patients with chronic hepatitis C: evidence for an overlap between manic/ hypomanic and depressive symptoms. J Clin Psychiatry. 2005;66:1050–7.
9. Asnis GM, De La Garza R 2nd. Interferon-induced depression in chronic hepatitis C: a review of its prevalence, risk factors, biology, and treatment approaches. J Clin Gastroenterol. 2006;40:322–35.
10. Adinolfi LE, Nevola R, Lus G, Restivo L, Guerrera B, Romano C, et al. Chronic hepatitis C virus infection and neurological and psychiatric disorders: an overview. World J Gastroenterol. 2015;21:2269–80.
11. Hilsabeck RC, Perry W, Hassanein TI. Neuropsychological impairment in patients with chronic hepatitis C. Hepatology. 2002;35:440–6.
12. Weissenborn K, Krause J, Bokemeyer M, Hecker H, Schüler A, Ennen JC, et al. Hepatitis C virus infection affects the brain-evidence from psychometric studies and magnetic resonance spectroscopy. J Hepatol. 2004;41:845–51.
13. Dantzer R, O'Connor JC, Freund GG, Johnson RW, Kelley KW. From inflammation to sickness and depression: when the immune system subjugates the brain. Nat Rev Neurosci. 2008;9:46–56.
14. Senzolo M, Schiff S, D'Aloiso CM, Crivellin C, Cholongitas E, Burra P, et al. Neuropsychological alterations in hepatitis C infection: the role of inflammation. World J Gastroenterol. 2011;17:3369–74.
15. Iriana S, Curry MP, Afdhal NH. Neurologic manifestations of hepatitis C virus infection. Clin Liver Dis. 2017;21:535–42.
16. Brucki SM, Nitrini R, Caramelli P, Bertolucci PH, Okamoto IH. Suggestions for utilization of the mini-mental state examination in Brazil. Arq Neuropsiquiatr. 2003;61(3B):777–81.
17. Ferenci P, Lockwood A, Mullen K, Tarter R, Weissenborn K, Blei AT. Hepatic encephalopathy–definition, nomenclature, diagnosis, and quantification: final report of the working party at the 11th world congresses of gastroenterology, Vienna, 1998. Hepatology. 2002;35:716–21.
18. Bajaj JS, Saeian K, Verber MD, Hischke D, Hoffmann RG, Franco J, et al. Inhibitory control test is a simple method to diagnose minimal hepatic encephalopathy and predict development of overt hepatic encephalopathy. Am J Gastroenterol. 2007;102:754–60.
19. Babor TF Higgins-Biddle JC, Saunders JB, Monteiro MG. Audit – The alcohol use disorders identification test. Guidelines for use in primary care. [Second edition]. Switzerland: World Health Organization; 2001.
20. The French METAVIR Cooperative Study Group. Intraobserver and interobserver variations in liver biopsy interpretation in patients with chronic hepatitis C. Hepatology. 1994;20(1 Pt 1):15–20.
21. Ghany MG, Nelson DR, Strader DB, Thomas DL, Seeff LB. American Association for Study of liver diseases. An update on treatment of genotype 1 chronic hepatitis C virus infection: 2011 practice guideline by the American Association for the Study of Liver Diseases. Hepatology. 2011;54:1433–44.
22. Lezak MD, Howieson DB, Loring DW. Neuropsychological assessment. 4th ed. New York: Oxford University Press; 2004.
23. Spreen O, Strauss E. A compendium of neuropsychological tests: administration, norms, and commentary. New York: Oxford University Press; 1991.
24. Butler M, Retzlaff P, Vanderploeg R. Neuropsychological test usage. Prof Psychol Res Pract. 1991;22:510–2.
25. Crowe SF. The differential contribution of mental tracking, cognitive flexibility, visual search, and motor speed to performance on parts a and B of the trail making test. J Clin Psychol. 1998;54:585–91.
26. Benedict RH, Schretlen D, Groninger L, Brandt J, Benedict RH. Hopkings verbal learning test-revised: normative data and analysis of inter-form and test-retest reliability. Clin Neuropsychol. 1998;12:43–55.
27. Wechsler DA. Manual for the Wechsler adult intelligence scale. London: England. National Foundation for Educational Research; 1998.
28. Fraguas R Jr, Henriques SG Jr, De Lucia MS, Iosifescu DV, Schwartz FH, Menezes PR, et al. The detection of depression in medical setting: a study with PRIME-MD. J Affect Disord. 2006;91:11–7.
29. Spitzer RL, Kroenke K, Linzer M, Hahn SR, Williams JB, Degruy FV 3rd, et al. Health-related quality of life in primary care patients with mental disorders. Results from the PRIME-MD 1000 study. JAMA. 1995;274:1511–7.
30. American Psychiatric Association. DSM-IV-TR™. Manual diagnóstico e estatístico de transtornos mentais. (C. Dornelles, Trad.). 4th ed. Porto Alegre: Artmed; 2002.
31. Gorestein C, Andrade L. Inventário de depressão de Beck: propriedades psicométricas da versão em português. Rev Psiq Clin. 1998;25:245–50.
32. Forton DM, Allsop JM, Main J, Foster GR, Thomas HC, Taylor-Robinson SD. Evidence for a cerebral effect of the hepatitis C virus. Lancet. 2001; 358:38–9.
33. Forton DM, Allsop JM, Cox IJ, Hamilton G, Wesnes K, Thomas HC, et al. A review of cognitive impairment and cerebral metabolite abnormalities in patients with hepatitis C infection. AIDS. 2005;19(Suppl 3):S53–63.

34. Hilsabeck RC, Hassanein TI, Carlson MD, Ziegler EA, Perry W. Cognitive functioning and psychiatric symptomatology in patients with chronic hepatitis C. J Int Neuropsychol Soc. 2003;9:847–54.
35. Forton DM, Hamilton G, Allsop JM, Grover VP, Wesnes K, O'Sullivan C, et al. Cerebral immune activation in chronic hepatitis C infection: a magnetic resonance spectroscopy study. J Hepatol. 2008;49:316–22.
36. Byrnes V, Miller A, Lowry D, Hill E, Weinstein C, Alsop D, et al. Effects of antiviral therapy and HCV clearance on cerebral metabolism and cognition. J Hepatol. 2012;56:549–56.
37. Kraus MR, Schäfer A, Teuber G, Porst H, Sprinzl K, Wollschläger S, et al. Improvement of neurocognitive function in responders to an antiviral therapy for chronic hepatitis C. Hepatology. 2013;58:497–504.
38. Cattie JE, Letendre SL, Woods SP, Barakat F, Perry W, Cherner M, et al. Translational Methamphetamine AIDS research center (TMARC) group. Persistent neurocognitive decline in a clinic sample of hepatitis C virus-infected persons receiving interferon and ribavirin treatment. J Neuro-Oncol. 2014;20:561–70.
39. Loftis JM, Hauser P. The phenomenology and treatment of interferon-induced depression. J Affect Disord. 2004;82:175–90.
40. Leutscher PD, Lagging M, Buhl MR, Pedersen C, Norkrans G, Langeland N, et al. Evaluation of depression as a risk factor for treatment failure in chronic hepatitis C. Hepatology. 2010;52:430–5.
41. Carta MG, Angst J, Moro MF, Mura G, Hardoy MC, Balestrieri C, et al. Association of chronic hepatitis C with recurrent brief depression. J Affect Disord. 2012;141(2–3):361–6.
42. Huckans M, Fuller B, Wheaton V, Jaehnert S, Ellis C, Kolessar M, et al. A longitudinal study evaluating the effects of interferon-alpha therapy on cognitive and psychiatric function in adults with chronic hepatitis C. J Psychosom Res. 2015;78:184–92.
43. Eccles J, Lallemant C, Mushtaq F, Greenwood M, Keller M, Golding B, et al. Pre-treatment waking cortisol response and vulnerability to interferon α induced depression. Eur Neuropsychopharmacol. 2012;22:892–6.
44. Whale R, Fialho R, Rolt M, Eccles J, Pereira M, Keller M, et al. Psychomotor retardation and vulnerability to interferon alpha induced major depressive disorder: prospective study of a chronic hepatitis C cohort. J Psychosom Res. 2015;79:640–5.
45. Fialho R, Pereira M, Harrison N, Rusted J, Whale R. Co-infection with HIV associated with reduced vulnerability to symptoms of depression during antiviral treatment for hepatitis C. Psychiatry Res. 2017;253:150–7.
46. Huang YW, Hu JT, Hu FC, Chang CJ, Chang HY, Kao JH, et al. Biphasic pattern of depression and its predictors during pegylated interferon-based therapy in chronic hepatitis B and C patients. Antivir Ther. 2013;18:567–73.
47. Marazziti D, Consoli G, Picchetti M, Carlini M, Faravelli L. Cognitive impairment in major depression. Eur J Pharmacol. 2010;626:83–6.
48. Kleefeld F, Heller S, Jessen H, Ingiliz P, Kraft A, Hahn K. Effect of interferon-free therapy on cognition in HCV and HCV/HIV infection: a pilot study. Neurology. 2017;88:713–5.
49. Alsop D, Younossi Z, Stepanova M, Afdhal NH. Cerebral MR spectroscopy and patient-reported mental health outcomes in hepatitis C genotype 1 naive patients treated with ledipasvir and sofosbuvir. Hepatology. 2014;60:221A.

14

Hepatitis B reactivation among 1962 patients with hematological malignancy in Taiwan

Chien-Yuan Chen[1], Feng-Ming Tien[1], Aristine Cheng[2], Shang-Yi Huang[1], Wen-Chien Chou[1,3], Ming Yao[1], Jih-Luh Tang[1,4], Hwei-Fang Tien[1] and Wang-Huei Sheng[2*]

Abstract

Background: The risk of Hepatitis B virus (HBV) reactivation in patients with different hematological malignancy except lymphoma were rarely known before.

Methods: A total of 1962 patients with hematological malignancy were enrolled and followed-up at the National Taiwan University Hospital between 2008 and 2013. The clinical characteristics, HBV serology, and laboratory data were retrospectively reviewed and analyzed.

Results: A total of 1962 patients comprising 1048 men and 914 women were studied. The median age of the patients was 55 years (range, 15–97 years). Chronic HBV carriage was documented at diagnosis of hematological malignancy in 286 (14.6%) patients. A total of 171 (59.8%) of the 286 HBV carriers received primary prophylaxis with anti-HBV agents. Of the HBV carriers, 97 (33.9%) developed hepatitis B reactivation during or after chemotherapy, including 59 patients who had discontinued antiviral therapy. The incidence of hepatitis B reactivation among patients with hematological malignancy and HBV carriage was 10.4 per 100 person–years. A multivariate analysis revealed hepatocellular carcinoma ($p < 0.001$) and antiviral prophylaxis use ($p < 0.001$) were independent risk factors of HBV reactivation in HBV carriers. Of the 1676 patients with initial negative hepatitis B surface antigen (HBsAg) counts, 41 (2.4%) experienced hepatitis B reactivation, reverse seroconversion of HBsAg, and lost their protective hepatitis B surface antibody (anti-HBs). A multivariate analysis revealed that diabetes mellitus ($p = 0.005$, odds ratio (OR): 0.218, 95% confidence interval (CI): 0.076–0.629), allogeneic transplantation ($p = 0.013$, OR: 0.182, 95% CI: 0.047–0.701), liver cirrhosis ($p < 0.001$, OR: 0.002, 95% CI: 0–0.047), low anti-HBs titers ($p = 0.016$, OR: 0.020, 95% CI: 0.001–0.480), and positive hepatitis B core antibody ($p = 0.013$, OR: 0.070, 95% CI: 0.009–0.571) were independent risk factors of positive seroconversion of HBsAg in patients with hematological malignancy.

Conclusions: The incidence of HBV reactivation among the patients with varying subtypes of hematological malignancy is similar. Prophylaxis with anti-HBV agents critically reduced the risk of hepatitis B reactivation.

Keywords: Hepatitis B reactivation, Hematological malignancy, Antiviral prophylaxis, Chemotherapy

Background

Hepatitis B virus (HBV) is a DNA virus transmitted parenterally, sexually, and perinatally. HBV affects 350 to 400 million persons worldwide and constitutes a major global health burden [1, 2]. HBV infection can cause acute and chronic liver diseases including cirrhosis and hepatocellular carcinoma (HCC). Following immunosuppression, HBV replication along with signs of hepatocellular injury in a silent hepatitis B surface antigen (HBsAg) carrier may occur [3]. The clinical presentation of HBV reactivation ranges from asymptomatic to severe fulminant hepatitis, liver failure, and death. HBV reactivation in cancer patients undergoing cytotoxic chemotherapy has been observed in patients with lymphoma [4, 5], patients treated with corticosteroids [6, 7] and rituximab [8, 9], as well as in patients undergoing stem cell and bone marrow transplantation [10, 11]. HBV has long been endemic in Taiwan, and, previously, the seropositive rates of hepatitis B core antibody

* Correspondence: whsheng@ntu.edu.tw
[2]Division of Infectious Disease, Department of Internal Medicine, National Taiwan University Hospital, 7 Chung-Shan South Road, Taipei 10002, Taiwan

(anti-HBc) approached 80%–90% and the carrier rate of HBsAg in the population reached a level as high as 15%–20% prior to the nationwide hepatitis B vaccination program [12–14].

Hematological malignancy is a group of clonal blood disorders that affect lymphoid, myeloid, and stem cells. The clinical manifestations of hematological malignancy usually present with anemia, thrombocytopenia, leukopenia, and varying degrees of immunocompromised status. Conventional cytotoxic chemotherapy is the major treatment for hematological malignancy. Immunotherapy, graft versus host disease, immunosuppressant, and stem cell transplantation also detract from immune functions and result in HBV reactivation [4–11]. Reactivation of viral hepatitis, including hepatitis B, is a potential cause for abnormal liver function tests in leukemic patients receiving chemotherapy [15, 16]. Various chemotherapy agents and steroids are frequently used as part of a combination regimen for hematological malignancy. HBV reactivation has been highlighted as being crucial for the treatment of lymphoma [4–6]. Several comprehensive guidelines have been proposed to provide evidence-based recommendations for clinicians caring for this patient population [17–22]. However, the epidemiology and clinical risk factors among different subtypes of hematological malignancy remain unclear. We previously investigated the epidemiology and clinical manifestations of hepatitis B reactivation among 490 acute myeloid leukemia (AML) patients [23]. The incidence of hepatitis B reactivation among AML patients with HBV carriage was 9.5 per 100 person–years [23]. Hepatitis B reactivation is not uncommon in HBsAg positive AML patients. In the present study, we investigated the epidemiology of HBV reactivation for varying subtypes of hematological malignancy and analyzed the risk factors among patients with different subtypes of hematological malignancy.

Methods

Hospital setting and patients

National Taiwan University Hospital (NTUH) is a 2900-bed teaching hospital in Taipei metropolitan area. The clinical characteristics, hepatitis B serology, hepatitis B virus DNA data, and outcome results of all adult patients with hematological malignancy during the period of January 2008 to December 2013 that attended NTUH were retrospectively reviewed and analyzed. Liver function tests, hepatitis B serology titer, and HBV DNA levels were performed as clinically indicated. This study was approved by the National Taiwan University Hospital Institutional Review Board.

Definitions

The biochemistry alanine aminotransferase (ALT) was measured using the Beckman Coulter AU5800 platform (Beckman Coulter Inc., Brea, CA, USA); HBsAg, hepatitis B surface antibody (anti-HBs), anti-HBc, hepatitis B envelope antigen (HBeAg), and hepatitis C antibody (anti-HCV) were measured using the Abbott ARCHITECT i2000SR (Abbott Laboratories, Abbott Park, North Chicago, IL, USA); HBV DNA was analyzed using the COBAS® AmpliPrep /COBAS® TaqMan® HBV Test, v2.0 (Roche, Basel, Switzerland) in accordance with manufacturer instructions. The serological results were defined by the following cutoff values: HBsAg positive was ≧0.05 IU/mL; anti-HBs positive was a seroprotection threshold of 10mIU/ mL; and anti-HBc positive was ≧1.0 IU/mL. HBeAg positive was defined as ≧1.0 IU/mL. Chronic hepatitis B carrier status was defined by the detection of positive HBsAg counts for more than 6 months. Hepatitis B reactivation was defined as a greater than 10-fold increase, compared with previous nadir levels of HBV DNA, or by the reappearance of HBeAg in the serum for patients whose baseline HBeAg count was negative [5, 6]. HBV-related hepatitis was defined as a greater than 3-fold increase of the serum alanine aminotransferase (ALT) level (the upper normal limit is 41 IU/L at NTUH) accompanying or following HBV reactivation. In July 1984, the Taiwan government launched a nationwide universal HBV vaccination program [13]. The following catch-up program of the nationwide HBV vaccination had a coverage rate of 86.9% to 98.0% [14].

The diagnosis of cirrhosis was based on clinical symptoms and signs and imaging studies (ultrasound and computed tomography). The diagnostic criteria of HCC in this study were based on histologic and/or clinical findings and on the presence of the following: chronic viral hepatitis infection and liver cirrhosis, hepatic tumor with imaging (ultrasound and computed tomography) characteristics compatible with a diagnosis of HCC and without evidence of gastrointestinal or other primary tumor, and a persistent elevation of the serum level of alpha-fetoprotein to 400 ng/mL or higher.

Statistical analysis

The survival rates were estimated using the Kaplan-Meier analysis and compared using the log-rank test. Categorical variables were compared using the chi-square test. Univariate and multivariate analyses with a Cox regression analysis (log-rank test) were performed. Factors with p-values of ≤0.2 in univariate analysis were used in the multivariate model. All statistical analyses were performed using the statistical package SPSS for Windows v.18 (SPSS Inc., Chicago, IL). A p-value of ≤0.05 was considered significant and all statistical tests were two-tailed.

Results

Epidemiology

There were 2083 patients with hematological malignancy admitted to the hematological ward of the National Taiwan University Hospital between 2008 and 2013. The flow chart is illustrated in Fig. 1. A total of 1962 patients

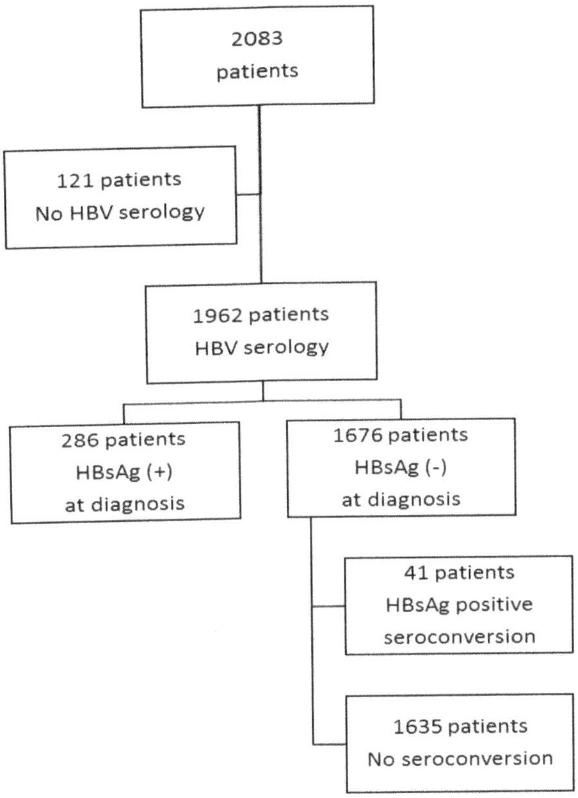

Fig. 1 Study flow and hepatitis B serological data of patients at diagnosis of hematological malignancy

with hepatitis B serological profile at diagnosis of hematological malignancy were investigated, including 1046 men and 914 women. The median age was 55 years (range 15–97 years). The detailed clinical characteristics and laboratory data are listed in Table 1. The most common diagnosis of hematological malignancy was lymphoma, with 769 people (39.2%), followed by acute myeloid leukemia (AML), with 606 people (30.9%), myeloma, with 197 people (10.0%), acute lymphoblastic leukemia (ALL), with 160 people (8.2%), myelodysplastic syndrome (MDS) or aplastic anemia (AA), with 142 people (7.2%), chronic myeloid leukemia (CML) or myeloproliferative neoplasm (MPN), with 60 people (3.1%), and chronic lymphocytic leukemia (CLL), with 27 people (1.4%). Of 1962 patients, 286 (14.6%) were diagnosed with positive HBsAg during their diagnosis of hematological malignancy. There were 174 of 286 HBsAg-positive patients had HBeAg data at diagnosis of malignancy. Positive Hbe and anti-Hbe rate were 21.3% (37 / 174) and 80.4% (107 / 133) in 286 HBV carriers. A total of 97 (33.9%) of 286 HBsAg-positive patients had HBV reactivation during follow-up. 71 (73.2%) of 97 patients with HBV reactivation developed hepatitis and the peak median alanine aminotransferase level is 613 IU/L (range 105–3506 IU/L). Ten patients died due to fulminant hepatitis and hepatic failure. For the median follow-up of 1050 days, the incidence of HBV reactivation in 286 HBV carriers was 10.4 per 100 person–years. The higher incidence value was 13.4 per 100 person–years for AML, and the lower was 7.4 per 100 person-years for CML/MPN, and there was no difference among people with varying subtypes of hematological malignancy ($p = 0.335$).

A total of 41 (2.4%) of 1676 patients whose HBsAg was negative initially displayed positive seroconversion during subsequent follow–ups and had their HBsAg become positive. Anti-HBc data existed for a total of 849 patients, and 567 (66.8%) patients showed positive anti-HBc in this cohort.

Prophylaxis of hepatitis B reactivation in patients with hematological malignancy

There were 286 patients with positive HBsAg at diagnosis of hematological malignancy. Of the 286 patients, the primary prophylaxis for 171 patients (59.8%) was antiviral agents, including 85 (49.7%) patients with entecavir, 76 (44.4%) with lamivudine, 2 (1.2%) with telbivudine, 1 (0.6%) with tenofovir, and 7 (4.1%) with adefovir. A total of 97 patients had HBV reactivation and 71 (73.2%) of the 97 patients had hepatitis. There were 59 patients who developed HBV reactivation after a discontinuance period of antiviral agent primary prophylaxis, and the median length for HBV reactivation was 210 days (range 15–2349 days) after discontinuing the antiviral drug. Even under antiviral drug use, 26 patients had HBV reactivation, including 6 who had tyrosine–methionine–aspartate– aspartate mutation. There were 12 patients who had HBV reactivation without antiviral prophylaxis. A total of 10 (10.3%) out of 97 HBV reactivation patients died of fulminant hepatitis and hepatic failure, including 5 patients who had discontinued use of the antiviral drug (median period after discontinuance was 96 days, range 44–226 days), 3 patients who did not use antiviral prophylaxis, and 2 other patients with HBV reactivation even with use of antiviral prophylaxis.

Risk of HBV reactivation in HBV carrier

We analyzed the risk factors of HBV reactivation in 286 HBsAg positive patients. The detailed results are listed in Table 2. The variables comprised hematological malignancy subtypes, age, gender, concurrent hepatitis C infection, liver cirrhosis, hepatocellular carcinoma, diabetes mellitus, allogeneic transplantation recipient, and antiviral prophylaxis use. A univariate analysis revealed that hepatocellular carcinoma ($p = 0.032$) and antiviral prophylaxis ($p < 0.001$) were risk factors of HBV reactivation in an HBV carrier, and age > 65 years was associated with a reduced rate of HBV reactivation ($p = 0.052$). A multivariate analysis revealed that both hepatocellular carcinoma ($p < 0.001$, odds ratio (OR): 0.101, 95% confidence interval (CI): 0.029–0.355), and antiviral prophylaxis ($p < 0.001$, OR: 4.631, 95% CI: 2.902–7.390) were

Table 1 Clinical and laboratory data of patients with hematological malignancy

		Total	AML	ALL	Lymphoma	CML/MPN	CLL	MM	MDS/AA	p
Number		1962	606	160	769	60	27	197	143	
Gender	Man	1048	326	83	399	36	16	108	81	0.799
	Woman	914	280	77	370	24	11	89	62	
Age, median(range), year		55(15–97)	54(17–92)	38(16–86)	57(15–97)	48(18–86)	61(37–89)	59(30–87)	55(17–94)	<0.001
HBs Ag(+) at diagnosis		286	75	13	142	6	5	31	14	0.002
HBV reactivation		97	29	3	46	1	2	10	6	0.335
HBs Ag(−) positive seroconversion		41	5	7	24	0	1	3	1	0.013
Hepatitis C		73	17	0	42	1	1	5	7	0.013
Liver cirrhosis		21	6	1	10	1	0	1	2	0.924
Hepatocellular carcinoma		9	3	0	4	2	0	0	0	0.038
Underlying diabetes		273	75	22	109	8	4	31	24	0.833
Allogeneic transplantation		439	233	81	48	18	2	3	54	<0.001

AML acute myeloid leukemia, *ALL* acute lymphoblastic leukemia, *CML/MPN* chronic myeloid leukemia/myeloproliferative neoplasm, *CLL* chronic lymphocytic leukemia, *MM* myeloma, *MDS/AA* myelodysplastic syndrome/aplastic anemia

independent risk factors of HBV reactivation in HBsAg-positive patients.

Risk factor of hepatitis B reverse seroconversion

We observed that 41 (2.4%) out of the 1676 patients who were HBsAg negative at diagnosis of hematological malignancy exhibited reverse seroconversion to HBsAg positive in the follow-up, including 7 (4.8%) out of 147 patients with ALL, 1 (4.5%) out of 22 with CLL, 24 (3.8%) out of 627 with lymphoma, 5 (0.9%) out of 531 with AML, 3 (1.8%) out of 166 with myeloma, and 1 (0.8%) out of 129 with MDS and AA, respectively. There were 54 patients with CML/MPN; however, out of them, no one acquired reverse seroconversion. The median follow–up period was 835 days (range 1–2976 days). A total of 36 (87.8%) out of 41 patients had hepatitis after reverse seroconversion, and 1 patient died of fulminant hepatitis and hepatic failure. The detailed results are provided in Table 3.

We analyzed the risk of reverse seroconversion in 1676 patients with hematological malignancy. The variables comprised hematological malignancy subtypes, age, gender, concurrent hepatitis C infection, liver cirrhosis, hepatocellular carcinoma, diabetes mellitus, allogeneic transplantation recipient, anti-HBs, and anti-HBc. A univariate analysis revealed that hematological subtypes (p = 0.038), diabetes mellitus (p = 0.04), liver cirrhosis ($p < 0.001$), low anti-HBs titer values (p = 0.002), and positive anti-HBc (p = 0.005) were risk factors of HBsAg positive seroconversion. A multivariate analysis revealed that diabetes mellitus (p = 0.005, OR: 0.218, 95% CI: 0.076–0.629), allogeneic transplantation (p = 0.013, OR: 0.182, 95% CI: 0.047–0.701), liver cirrhosis ($p < 0.001$, OR: 0.002, 95% CI: 0.000–0.047), low anti-HBs titer values (p = 0.016, OR: 0.020, 95% CI: 0.001–0.480), and positive anti-HBc (p = 0.013, OR: 0.070, 95% CI: 0.009–0.571) were independent risk factors of HBsAg positive seroconversion. Having different subtypes of hematological malignancy had no impact on HBsAg positive seroconversion in patients.

Discussion

HBV is endemic in Taiwan. Mass vaccination started in 1984 [13, 14]. However, the prevalence of HBV is still high in the general population. This is the first large cohort study to compare the incidence of HBV reactivation in different subtypes of hematological malignancy. In this retrospective cohort, 286 (14.6%) of 1962 patients were HBV carriers. HBV reactivation is critical for the clinical care of patients with hematological malignancy receiving chemotherapy. The incidence of HBV reactivation was 10.4 per 100 person–years in this study. This epidemiological result is similar to those of previous studies of lymphoma (10.4 per 100 person–years) [5] and AML (9.5 per 100 person–years) [23].

HBV reactivation in cancer patients receiving cytotoxic chemotherapy has been noted for 3 decades [3, 24, 25], especially in patients with lymphoma [4, 5], patients treated with corticosteroids [6, 7] and rituximab [8, 9], as well as in patients undergoing stem cell and bone marrow transplantation [10, 11]. There have been some reports concerning HBV reactivation in patients with AML [23, 26, 27] and myeloma [28, 29]. We observed HBV reactivation in patients with different subtypes of hematological malignancy. This study confirmed that HBV reactivation developed in patients with different subtypes of hematological malignancy. Antiviral drug prophylaxis is critical for HBV reactivation according to most guidelines and professional consensuses [17–22]. In the studied cohort, 59 (60.8%) out of 97 HBV carriers experienced HBV reactivation after discontinuing use of antiviral medication. Thus, the ideal length that HBV

Table 2 Risk factors of HBV reactivation in HBsAg-positive patients with hematological malignancy

Factors	Reactivation N = 97	No Reactivation N = 189	Univariate P value	Multivariate P Value	Odds ratio(95% CI)
Hematological malignancy			0.332	NA	
AML	29	46			
ALL	3	10			
Lymphoma	46	96			
CML/MPN	1	5			
CLL	2	3			
Myeloma	10	21			
MDS/AA	6	8			
Age > 65 year			0.052	0.198	
Yes	11	57			
No	86	132			
Gender			0.781	NA	
Man	55	106			
Woman	42	83			
Hepatitis C			0.180	0.453	
Yes	4	4			
No	93	185			
Liver cirrhosis			0.906	NA	
Yes	4	7			
No	93	182			
Hepatocellular carcinoma			0.032	<0.001	0.101(0.029–0.355)
Yes	3	1			
No	94	188			
Diabetes mellitus			0.388	NA	
Yes	10	20			
No	87	169			
Allogeneic transplantation			0.113	0.269	
Yes	28	31			
No	69	158			
Antiviral prophylaxis			<0.001	<0.001	4.631(2.902–7.390)
Yes	26	145			
No	71	44			

AML acute myeloid leukemia, *ALL* acute lymphoblastic leukemia, *CML/MPN* chronic myeloid leukemia/myeloproliferative neoplasm, *CLL* chronic lymphocytic leukemia, *MM* myeloma, *MDS/AA* myelodysplastic syndrome/aplastic anemia

patients should use antiviral medication for after chemotherapy is still a controversial topic.

Resolved hepatitis B reactivation and acquired reverse seroconversion has been investigated in recent literature [30–33]. In one such study, 33 (6.8%) out of 482 lymphoma patients acquired HBV reverse seroconversion between 2000 and 2010 [33]. HBV reverse seroconversion patients typically receive more cycles (≥6), prolonged durations of rituximab therapy, and hematopoietic stem cell transplantation than non-HBV reverse seroconversion patients do. In the present studied cohort, we observed that 41 (2.4%) of out 1676 patients acquired HBV reverse seroconversion. There were 54 patients with CML/MPN; however, out of these patients no one acquired reverse seroconversion. We also observed that HBV reverse seroconversion could be observed in patients with other subtypes of hematological malignancy other than lymphoma. Diabetes mellitus, allogeneic transplantation, liver cirrhosis, low anti-HBs titers (less than 100 mI U/mL), and positive anti-HBc were independent risk factors of HBV reverse seroconversion.

Diabetes mellitus is an immunocompromised status and may trigger spontaneous HBV reactivation [34–36]. The anti-HBc positive rate was 69% in this study. All patients with HBV reverse seroconversion displayed negative anti-HBc serology. Because the rate of HBV reverse seroconversion was 2.4% in this cohort, treating all resolved HBV patients receiving chemotherapy in Taiwan does not seem likely. The high risk factors of a stratified risk comprise diabetes mellitus, allogeneic transplantation, liver cirrhosis, low anti-HBs titers (less than 100 mIU/mL), and

Table 3 Risk factors for positive seroconversion of HBsAg in HBsAg-negative patients detected during diagnosis of hematological malignancy

	Positive Sero-conversion (*n* = 41)	No conversion (*n* = 1635)	Univariate *P* value	Multivariate *P* value	Odds ratio (95% CI)
Age			0.174	NA	
≧65 years	12	466			
< 65 years	29	1169			
Gender			0.737	NA	
Men	22	866			
Women	19	769			
Hematological malignancy			0.038	0.084	NA
AML	5	526			
ALL	7	140			
Lymphoma	24	603			
CML/MPN	0	54			
CLL	1	21			
Myeloma	3	163			
MDS / AA	1	128			
Diabetes mellitus			0.040	0.005	0.218(0.076–0.629)
Yes	10	233			
No	31	1402			
Allogeneic transplantation			0.116	0.013	0.182(0.047–0.701)
Yes	15	365			
No	26	1270			
Liver cirrhosis			<0.001	<0.001	0.002(0.000–0.047)
Yes	2	8			
No	39	1627			
Hepatocellular carcinoma			0.748	NA	
Yes	0	5			
No	41	1630			
Hepatitis C			0.216	NA	
Yes	0	65			
No	41	1570			
Negative Anti-HBs Antibody[a]			0.237	NA	
Yes	10	304			
No	24	1157			
Low Anti-HBs Antibody [a]			0.002	0.016	0.020(0.001–0.480)
Yes	30	915			
No	4	546			
Positive Anti-HBc Antibody[b]			0.005	0.013	0.070(0.009–0.571)
Yes	18	567			
No	1	263			

NA not available, [a] Anti-HBs Antibody checked, (*n* = 1495), Low Anti-HBs Antibody <100mIU/mL, [b] Anti-HBc Antibody checked (*n* = 849), *AML* acute myeloid leukemia, *ALL* acute lymphoblastic leukemia, *CML/MPN* chronic myeloid leukemia/myeloproliferative neoplasm, *CLL* chronic lymphocytic leukemia, *MM* myeloma, *MDS/AA* myelodysplastic syndrome/aplastic anemia

positive anti-HBc. Thus, predicting the risk of HBV reverse seroconversion is possible.

Conclusions

The treatment of hematological malignancy has improved during the past several decades. Conventional cytotoxic chemotherapy, rituximab-based immunotherapy, and stem cell transplantation can cause a patient to become immunocompromised and result in HBV reactivation. We observed that HBV carriers and patients with resolved HBV could experience reverse seroconversion and reactivation. The incidence of HBV reactivation did not differ significantly among various subtypes of hematological malignancy. Antiviral agent prophylaxis is the most critical method to prevent HBV reactivation. However, some patients develop HBV reactivation after discontinuing use of antiviral agents after chemotherapy. Thus, the duration of antiviral agent treatment after chemotherapy should be further investigated.

Abbreviations

AA: Aplastic anemia; ALL: Acute lymphoblastic leukemia; ALT: Alanine aminotransferase; AML: Acute myeloid leukemia; Anti-HBc: Anti-hepatitis B core antibody; Anti-HBs: Anti-hepatitis B surface antigen antibody; Anti-HCV: Anti-hepatitis C virus antibody; CI: Confidence interval; CLL: Chronic lymphocytic leukemia; CML: Chronic myeloid leukemia; HBeAg: Hepatitis B envelope antigen; HBsAg: Hepatitis B surface antigen; HBV: Hepatitis B virus; HCC: Hepatocellular cell carcinoma; MDS: Myelodysplastic syndrome; MPN: Myeloproliferative neoplasm; OR: Odds ratio

Acknowledgements

We thank the staff of the Eighth Core Lab., Department of Medical Research, National Taiwan University Hospital, for their technical support during the study. All authors disclosed no conflicts of interest or financial funding relevant to this publication.

Funding

The study received no funding.

Authors' contributions

CYC, AC, FMT, and WHS participated in the study design. SYH, WCC, MY, JLT, and HFT participated in data collection and analysis. CYC, AC, and WHS participated in editing and proofreading. All authors read and approved of the final manuscript.

Consent for publication

Not applicable.

Competing interests

The authors declare that they have no competing interests.

Author details

[1]Division of Hematology, Department of Internal Medicine, National Taiwan University Hospital, Taipei, Taiwan. [2]Division of Infectious Disease, Department of Internal Medicine, National Taiwan University Hospital, 7 Chung-Shan South Road, Taipei 10002, Taiwan. [3]Department of Laboratory Medicine, National Taiwan University Hospital, Taipei, Taiwan. [4]Tai-Cheng Stem Cell Therapy Center, National Taiwan University Hospital, Taipei, Taiwan.

References

1. Dienstag JL. Hepatitis B virus infection. N Engl J Med. 2008;359:1486–500.
2. Trépo C, Chan HL, Lok A. Hepatitis B virus infection. Lancet. 2014;384:2053–63.
3. Shouval D, Shibolet O. Immunosuppression and HBV reactivation. Semin Liver Dis. 2013;33:167–77.
4. Yeo W, Chan PK, Zhong S, Ho WM, Steinberg JL, Tam JS, et al. Frequency of hepatitis B virus reactivation in cancer patients undergoing cytotoxic chemotherapy: a prospective study of 626 patients with identification of risk factors. J Med Virol. 2000;62:299–307.
5. Hsu C, Tsou HH, Lin SJ, Wang MC, Yao M, Hwang WL, et al. Chemotherapy-induced hepatitis B reactivation in lymphoma patients with resolved HBV infection: a prospective study. Hepatology. 2014;59:2092–100.
6. Cheng AL, Hsiung CA, Su IJ, Chen PJ, Chang MC, Tsao CJ, et al. Steroid-free chemotherapy decreases risk of hepatitis B virus (HBV) reactivation in HBV-carriers with lymphoma. Hepatology. 2003;37:1320–8.
7. Yeo W, Zee B, Zhong S, Chan PK, Wong WL, Ho WM, et al. Comprehensive analysis of risk factors associating with hepatitis B virus (HBV) reactivation in cancer patients undergoing cytotoxic chemotherapy. Br J Cancer. 2004;90:1306–11.
8. Kusumoto S, Tanaka Y, Ueda R, Mizokami M. Reactivation of hepatitis B virus following rituximab-plus-steroid combination chemotherapy. J Gastroenterol. 2011;46:9–16.
9. Tsutsumi Y, Yamamoto Y, Shimono J, Ohhigashi H, Teshima T. Hepatitis B virus reactivation with rituximab-containing regimen. World J Hepatol. 2013;5:612–20.
10. Martin BA, Rowe JM, Kouides PA, DiPersio JF. Hepatitis B reactivation following allogeneic bone marrow transplantation: case report and review of the literature. Bone Marrow Transplant. 1995;15:145–8.
11. Liang R, Lau GK, Kwong YL. Chemotherapy and bone marrow transplantation for cancer patients who are also chronic hepatitis B carriers: a review of the problem. J Clin Oncol. 1999;17:394–8.
12. Hsu HM, Lu CF, Lee SC, Lin SR, Chen DS. Seroepidemiologic survey for hepatitis B virus infection in Taiwan: the effect of hepatitis B mass immunization. J Infect Dis. 1999;179:367–70.
13. Chang MH, Chen CJ, Lai MS, Hsu HM, Wu TC, Kong MS, et al. Universal hepatitis B vaccination in Taiwan and the incidence of hepatocellular carcinoma in children. Taiwan childhood Hepatoma study group. N Engl J Med. 1997;336:1855–9.
14. Ni YH, Huang LM, Chang MH, Yen CJ, Lu CY, You SL, et al. Two decades of universal hepatitis B vaccination in Taiwan: impact and implication for future strategies. Gastroenterology. 2007;132:1287–93.
15. Ishiga K, Kawatani T, Suou T, Tajima F, Omura H, Idobe Y, et al. Fulminant hepatitis type B after chemotherapy in a serologically negative hepatitis B virus carrier with acute myelogenous leukemia. Int J Hematol. 2001;73:115–8.
16. Wong GC, Tan P, Goh YT, Ng HS, Chong R, Lee LH. Exacerbation of hepatitis in hepatitis B carriers following chemotherapy for haematological malignancies. Ann Acad Med Singap. 1996;25:500–3.
17. Sandherr M, Hentrich M, von Lilienfeld-Toal M, Massenkeil G, Neumann S, Penack O, et al. Antiviral prophylaxis in patients with solid tumours and haematological malignancies-update of the guidelines of the infectious diseases working party (AGIHO) of the German Society for Hematology and Medical Oncology (DGHO). Ann Hematol. 2015;94:1441–50.
18. Artz AS, Somerfield MR, Feld JJ, Giusti AF, Kramer BS, Sabichi AL, et al. American Society of Clinical Oncology provisional clinical opinion: chronic hepatitis B virus infection screening in patients receiving cytotoxic chemotherapy for treatment of malignant diseases. J Clin Oncol. 2010;28:3199–202.
19. Manzano-Alonso ML, Castellano-Tortajada G. Reactivation of hepatitis B virus infection after cytotoxic chemotherapy or immunosuppressive therapy. World J Gastroenterol. 2011;17:1531–7.
20. Liaw YF, Kao JH, Piratvisuth T, Chan LY, Chien RN, Liu CJ, et al. Asian-Pacific consensus statement on the management of chronic hepatitis B: a 2012 update. Hepatol Int. 2012;6:531–61.
21. Koh C, Zhao X, Samala N, Sakiani S, Liang TJ, Talwalkar JA. AASLD clinical practice guidelines: a critical review of scientific evidence and evolving recommendations. Hepatology. 2013;58:2142–52.
22. Bihl F, Alaei M, Negro F. The new EASL guidelines for the management of chronic hepatitis B infection adapted for Swiss physicians. Swiss Med Wkly. 2010;140:154–9.
23. Chen CY, Huang SY, Cheng A, Chou WC, Yao M, Tang JL, et al. High risk of hepatitis B reactivation among patients with acute myeloid Leukemia. PLoS One. 2015;10:e0126037.
24. Nakamura Y, Motokura T, Fujita A, Yamashita T, Ogata E. Severe hepatitis related to chemotherapy in hepatitis B virus carriers with hematologic malignancies. Survey in Japan, 1987-1991. Cancer. 1996;78:2210–5.
25. Tassopoulos NC, Papaevangelou GJ, Roumeliotou-Karayannis A, Smedile A, Engle R, Ticehurst JR, et al. Fulminant hepatitis in asymptomatic hepatitis B surface antigen carriers in Greece. J Med Virol. 1986;20:371–9.

26. Kojima H, Abei M, Takei N, Mukai Y, Hasegawa Y, Iijima T, et al. Fatal reactivation of hepatitis B virus following cytotoxic chemotherapy for acute myelogenous leukemia: fibrosing cholestatic hepatitis. Eur J Haematol. 2002;69:101–4.
27. Yujiri T, Tanaka M, Taguchi A, Tanaka Y, Nakamura Y, Tanizawa Y. Reactivation of hepatitis B virus in a hepatitis B surface antigen-negative patient with acute promyelocytic leukemia treated with arsenic trioxide. Ann Hematol. 2014;93:351–2.
28. Mya DH, Han ST, Linn YC, Hwang WY, Goh YT, Tan DC. Risk of hepatitis B reactivation and the role of novel agents and stem-cell transplantation in multiple myeloma patients with hepatitis B virus (HBV) infection. Ann Oncol. 2012;23:421–6.
29. Lee JY, Lim SH, Lee MY, Kim H, Sinn DH, Gwak GY, et al. Hepatitis B reactivation in multiple myeloma patients with resolved hepatitis B undergoing chemotherapy. Liver Int. 2015;35:2363–9.
30. Orlando R, Tosone G, Tiseo D, Piazza M, Portella G, Ciancia R, et al. Severe reactivation of hepatitis B virus infection in a patient with hairy cell leukemia: should lamivudine prophylaxis be recommended to HBsAg-negative, anti-HBc-positive patients? Infection. 2006;34:282–4.
31. Papamichalis P, Alexiou A, Boulbou M, Dalekos GN, Rigopoulou EI. Reactivation of resolved hepatitis B virus infection after immunosuppression: is it time to adopt pre-emptive therapy? Clin Res Hepatol Gastroenterol. 2012;36:84–93.
32. Huang YH, Hsiao LT, Hong YC, Chiou TJ, Yu YB, Gau JP, et al. Randomized controlled trial of entecavir prophylaxis for rituximab-associated hepatitis B virus reactivation in patients with lymphoma and resolved hepatitis B. J Clin Oncol. 2013;31:2765–72.
33. Hsiao LT, Chiou TJ, Gau JP, Yang CF, Yu YB, Liu CY, et al. Risk of reverse Seroconversion of hepatitis B virus surface antigen in Rituximab-treated non-Hodgkin lymphoma patients: a large cohort retrospective study. Medicine (Baltimore). 2015;94:e1321.
34. Demir M, Serin E, Göktürk S, Ozturk NA, Kulaksizoglu S, Ylmaz U. The prevalence of occult hepatitis B virus infection in type 2 diabetes mellitus patients. Eur J Gastroenterol Hepatol. 2008;20:668–73.
35. Wang YY, Lin SY, Sheu WH, Liu PH, Tung KC. Obesity and diabetic hyperglycemia were associated with serum alanine aminotransferase activity in patients with hepatitis B infection. Metabolism. 2010;59:486–91.
36. Kamitsukasa H, Iri M, Tanaka A, Nagashima S, Takahashi M, Nishizawa T, et al. Spontaneous reactivation of hepatitis B virus (HBV) infection in patients with resolved or occult HBV infection. J Med Virol. 2015;87:589–600.

APOB codon 4311 polymorphism is associated with hepatitis C virus infection through altered lipid metabolism

Rie Harada[1], Masako Kimura[1], Yasushi Sato[1], Tatsuya Taniguchi[1], Tetsu Tomonari[1], Takahiro Tanaka[1], Hironori Tanaka[1], Naoki Muguruma[1], Hirohiko Shinomiya[2], Hirohito Honda[3], Issei Imoto[4], Masahiro Sogabe[5], Toshiya Okahisa[5] and Tetsuji Takayama[1*]

Abstract

Background: It has been reported that some single-nucleotide polymorphisms (SNPs) in lipid regulators such as apolipoproteins and cell surface molecules for hepatitis C virus (HCV) entry into hepatocytes are associated with HCV infection. However, it is unknown how HCV infection is affected by altered lipid metabolism resulting from the SNPs. We investigated the relationship between these SNPs and HCV infection status, and also analyzed the mechanism by which these SNPs mediate HCV infection via lipid metabolism alterations.

Methods: Serum lipid and apolipoprotein profiles were tested in 158 HCV-positive and 220 HCV-negative subjects. We selected 22 SNPs in five lipid regulator genes which were related to HCV entry into hepatocytes and to lipid metabolism (*APOA1*, *APOB*, *SR-B1*, *LDLR*, and *APOE*), and their polymorphisms were analyzed using the PCR-sequence-specific oligonucleotide probe-Luminex method.

Results: An *APOB* N4311S (g.41553a > g) SNP, rs1042034, was significantly associated with HCV positivity; the HCV positivity rate for the minor allele AA genotype was significantly higher than for genotype AG + GG ($P = 0.016$). Other SNPs except for APOB P2712L SNP rs676210, which is in linkage disequilibrium with rs1042034, showed no significant difference in genotype distribution. The serum level of low density lipoprotein-cholesterol (LDL-C) in the genotype AA group was significantly lower than in the genotype non-AA group ($P = 0.032$), whereas the triglyceride (TG) level was significantly higher ($P = 0.007$).

Conclusion: An APOB SNP, rs1042034, is closely associated with HCV infection through lipid metabolism alteration. The minor allele AA genotype might contribute to facilitating serum LDL uptake into hepatocytes via LDLR by modifying their affinity and interaction and may have an influence on HCV infection by their entry to the liver through the LDLR.

Keywords: Hepatitis C virus, Lipid metabolism, SNPs, ApoB

Background

Hepatitis C virus (HCV) infects approximately 185 million people worldwide [1]. HCV infection typically causes chronic liver disease and can lead to liver cirrhosis and hepatocellular carcinoma (HCC) [2]. Accumulating studies have revealed that the HCV life cycle is closely associated with host lipid metabolism.

It has been reported that HCV entry into hepatocytes occurs through cell surface molecules such as low density lipoprotein receptor (LDLR), scavenger receptor class B type 1 (SR-B1), claudin-1 (CLDN1), DC-SIGN, L-SIGN, and CD81. However, the details of the underlying mechanisms have not yet been clarified [3]. Among these molecules LDLR and SR-B1 also play a crucial role in lipid metabolism. Apolipoproteins are proteins on the surface of lipoprotein particles and stabilize the structure of lipoproteins. Apolipoprotein B (APOB) is one of the major apolipoproteins and it transfers lipoproteins such as chylomicron, very low density lipoprotein (VLDL),

* Correspondence: takayama@tokushima-u.ac.jp
[1]Department of Gastroenterology and Oncology, Tokushima University Graduate School of Biomedical Sciences, 3-18-15, Kuramoto-cho, Tokushima 770-8503, Japan

and low density lipoprotein (LDL) as a carrier. It is secreted from the liver as a component of the outer surface of VLDL particles, which are also produced in the liver, and circulates in blood, irreversibly associating with VLDL and LDL. APOB-100 serves as a ligand for LDLRs on the cell membrane of hepatocytes. Thus, the LDL particle enters into hepatocyte through the LDLR [4–6].

In the HCV life cycle, HCV replication begins in a membranous web on the endoplasmic reticulum membrane in hepatocytes, where VLDL assembly also occurs. Both HCV particles and VLDL particles are secreted from hepatocytes and circulate in blood as a complex referred to as a lipo-viral particle (LVP). Furthermore, APOB-100 and apolipoprotein E (APOE), which are referred to as VLDL-associated proteins, are present on the surface of the complex. They form LVP with HCV particles, indicating that they are deeply involved in the formation of infectious HCV particles [7]. After circulation in the blood, infectious HCV particles enter into hepatocytes with LDL through the LDLR [8].

It is well known that apolipoproteins and cell surface molecules such as LDLR and SR-B1 have single-nucleotide polymorphisms (SNPs), and some of the SNPs cause lipid metabolism disorders, leading to a high risk of cardiovascular events [9–11]. Regarding the association with HCV, several studies have suggested that SNPs of these lipid-metabolic regulators correlate with HCV infection; e.g., an SNP in *LDLR* exon 13 (rs5925) is associated with susceptibility to HCV infection [12]; an SNP in *LDLR* exon8 (rs11669576) is associated with severity of hepatic fibrosis; and an SNP in *LDLR* exon10 (rs5930) is associated with viral clearance and overall inflammation of the liver [13]. SNPs in *LDLR* 3'UTR region (rs1433099) and intron 14 (rs2569540) have been reported to have an association with hepatitis C viral load in the pre-treatment state [14]. Furthermore, polymorphisms of *APOE* have been reported to be associated with persistent HCV infection and the degree of liver damage [15, 16].

Thus, it is assumed that SNPs of lipid regulators have a strict association with HCV infection and lipid metabolism disorders. However, the relationship between HCV infection and lipid metabolism disorder among the SNPs of these lipid regulators have not yet been fully elucidated. Therefore, in this study, we first investigated the relationship between the SNPs of lipid regulator genes such as apolipoproteins and cell surface molecules that affect the HCV life cycle, and HCV infection status comparing HCV-positive and HCV-negative subjects. We then examined differences in lipid metabolism between each SNP genotype and analyzed the causal relationship between the SNP and HCV infection status through altered lipid metabolism.

Methods

Subjects

This study included a total of 378 subjects who visited our university hospital and affiliated hospitals from November 2010 to March 2014. All subjects were Japanese and were between 41 and 76 years old. Patients who had received prior or ongoing anti-viral therapy and treatment for lipid metabolism disorders were excluded. We also excluded patients with inherited lipid metabolism disorders such as familial hypercholesterolemia and secondary lipid metabolism disorders such as hypothyroidism and kidney diseases.

An HCV antibody test was carried out for all subjects; 158 were HCV positive and HCV RNA detectable by RT-PCR, and 220 were HCV negative. Serum HCV RNA levels were measured using COBAS TaqMan HCV Auto Assay System (Roche Diagnostics, Tokyo, Japan; lower limit of quantification, 1.2 log IU/ml). HCV genotypes were determined by direct sequence method at BML, Inc. (Saitama, Japan). Serum transaminase, total bilirubin, albumin levels, and prothrombin time were measured, and ultrasonography or contrast-enhanced computed tomography was performed to check liver function and search for HCC. Based on these results, subjects with severe liver dysfunction of Child-Pugh class B and C were excluded from the study. Patients with conditions associated with liver dysfunction such as HCC, hepatitis B virus (HBV) infection, or nonalcoholic steatohepatitis (NASH) were also excluded from the study. The study protocol was approved by the institutional review board of each hospital and all patients provided written informed consent to participate in this study.

Measurement of serum lipids and apolipoproteins

Serum lipids and apolipoproteins were tested after fasting overnight for 10 to 12 h. We measured low density lipoprotein-cholesterol (LDL-C), high density lipoprotein-cholesterol (HDL-C), and triglyceride (TG) according to standard procedures at our university hospital and affiliated hospitals. Serum levels of apolipoproteins (apolipoprotein A1 [APOA1], apolipoprotein A2 [APOA2], APOB, apolipoprotein C2 [APOC2], apolipoprotein C3 [APOC3], and APOE) were measured by immune nephelometry at SRL, Inc. (Tokyo, Japan).

SNP selection

We selected 22 SNPs in five genes (*APOA1*, *APOB*, *SR-B1*, *LDLR*, and *APOE*) which are related to HCV entry into hepatocytes and are associated with lipid metabolism disorders according to previous studies; three SNPs (rs613808, rs2727784, and rs11216158) in *APOA1* [17], five SNPs (rs676210, rs1042031, rs693, rs1801701, and rs1042034) in *APOB* [9], three SNPs (rs4238001, rs61932577, and rs5888) in *SR-B1* [10], nine SNPs (rs17249134, rs17249141, rs2228671, rs11669576, rs5930, rs688, rs5925, rs2569542, and rs14158) in *LDLR* [13], and two SNPs (rs429358 and rs7412) in *APOE* [18].

Genotyping

Genomic DNA was extracted from peripheral blood using the phenol-chloroform method and stored at −4 °C. Genotypes of all SNPs selected in this study were analyzed at G&G Science Co., Ltd. (Fukushima, Japan) using the PCR-sequence-specific oligonucleotide probe-Luminex method, as described previously [19].

Statistical analysis

Student's *t*-test was used to compare serum lipid and apolipoprotein levels between the two subject groups (HCV-positive and HCV-negative) as well as the genotype groups for each SNP. The genotype distributions for each SNP were analyzed using χ^2 test. A *P* value of less than 0.05 was considered statistically significant. The statistical analyses were performed using Statcel 4 (OMS Ltd., Saitama, Japan). Linkage disequilibrium was analyzed using the program Haploview from the Broad Institute website (https://www.broadinstitute.org/haploview/haploview).

Results

Characteristics of the subjects

The study included 158 patients with HCV infection and 220 subjects without HCV infection. The age and sex ratio were well balanced between the groups. There was no significant difference in serum total bilirubin, AST, ALT and albumin levels, and prothrombin values (%), which are indicative of hepatic functional reserve, and were also well balanced between groups. HCV infected patients were genotype 1b ($n = 128$), 2a ($n = 5$), 2b ($n = 9$), 3a ($n = 1$), and undetermined ($n = 6$). The remaining nine patients received only serotype analysis: serotype I ($n = 7$) and serotype II ($n = 2$).

Among 158 subjects with HCV infection, the estimated median duration of HCV infection was 51 (IQR 44.3–55.0) years, and the median HCV RNA concentration in HCV-infected patients was 6.5 (IQR 6.0–6.9) log IU/ml.

Profile of serum lipids and apolipoproteins in HCV-positive and HCV-negative subjects

Since HCV infection reportedly causes a change in serum lipid levels, we first compared the serum lipid levels between 158 HCV-positive subjects and 220 HCV-negative subjects (Table 1). The serum levels of total cholesterol (TC), LDL-C, and HDL-C in HCV-positive subjects were significantly lower than in HCV-negative subjects, whereas the serum TG level in HCV-positive subjects was higher than in HCV-negative subjects, although the difference was not statistically significant. Moreover, serum levels of all six apolipoproteins (APOA1, APOA2, APOB, APOC2, APOC3, and APOE) in HCV-positive subjects were significantly lower than in HCV-negative subjects. These results were fairly consistent with previous reports [6, 20, 21].

Table 1 Profile of serum lipids and apolipoproteins in HCV-positive and HCV-negative subjects

		Normal range	HCV+	HCV-	*P*-value
TC	(mg/dl)	120.0–219.0	169.4 ± 31.3	207.2 ± 32.0	< 0.001
LDL-C	(mg/dl)	65.0–139.0	96.8 ± 24.3	124.8 ± 29.5	< 0.001
HDL-C	(mg/dl)	40.0–90.0	53.1 ± 18.5	62.9 ± 17.6	< 0.001
TG	(mg/dl)	30.0–149.0	106.6 ± 52.2	98.3 ± 56.6	0.173
APOA1	(mg/dl)	120.0–160.0	139.6 ± 31.3	155.2 ± 29.2	< 0.001
APOA2	(mg/dl)	25.0–34.6	29.6 ± 5.5	30.8 ± 4.9	0.022
APOB	(mg/dl)	70.0–106.0	77.2 ± 17.9	96.7 ± 22.8	< 0.001
APOC2	(mg/dl)	1.6–4.2	2.1 ± 1.0	4.0 ± 1.7	< 0.001
APOC3	(mg/dl)	5.6–9.5	6.0 ± 2.3	9.2 ± 3.1	< 0.001
APOE	(mg/dl)	2.7–4.5	4.4 ± 1.1	4.7 ± 1.2	0.011

Data represent mean and standard deviation values and *P*-values were calculated using Student's t-test

Association of SNP genotype with HCV infection

To examine the relationship between SNP genotype in lipid regulator genes and HCV infection status, we analyzed the genotype distribution of the selected 22 SNPs in *APOA1*, *APOB*, *SR-B1*, *LDLR*, and *APOE*, and compared them between HCV-positive and HCV-negative groups (Table 2). Of the 22 SNPs examined, five were monomorphic in our study population; rs1801701 in *APOB*; rs61932577 in *SR-B1*; rs17249134, rs17249141, and rs11669576 in *LDLR*.

In the comparison of overall genotype distributions for each SNP, an *APOB* N4311S (g.41553a > g) SNP, rs1042034, showed a marginally non-significant trend with respect to HCV positivity ($P = 0.051$, $\chi^2 = 5.963$); the frequency of the A allele in HCV-positive subjects was higher than in HCV-negative subjects. In the comparison of specific genotypes (GG + AG vs. AA), the HCV positivity rate in the genotype AA group was significantly higher than in the genotype GG + AG group ($P = 0.016$, $\chi^2 = 5.828$). These results suggest that minor allele homozygosity (genotype AA) in rs1042034 might be associated with HCV infection. Moreover, an *APOB* P2712L (g.35310c > t) SNP, rs676210, showed a similar tendency to that of rs1042034; i.e., the frequency of the genotype CC allele in rs676210 was significantly higher than that of genotype TT + CT in HCV-positive subjects ($P = 0.031$, $\chi^2 = 4.673$). Other SNPs aside from these two showed no significant difference in genotype distribution between HCV-positive and HCV-negative subjects.

Table 2 Association of SNP genotype with HCV infection

		Alleles	HCV	Overall genotype distribution(n)			P-value (χ2 value)	Comparison of specific genotypes	P-value (χ2 value)
APOA1	rs613808	G/A		AA	GA	GG			
			+	72	74	12	0.192		
			−	120	83	17	(3.297)		
	rs2727784	G/A		GG	GA	AA			
			+	75	71	12	0.290		
			−	122	82	16	(2.473)		
	rs11216158	A/G		GG	AG	AA			
			+	99	56	3	0.231		
			−	150	62	8	(2.933)		
APOB	rs676210	C/T		TT	CT	CC			
			+	88	57	13	0.091	TT + CT vs CC	0.031
			−	133	80	7	(4.784)		(4.673)
	rs1042031	G/A		GG	GA	AA			
			+	150	8	0			
			−	205	15	0			
	rs693	C/T		CC	CT	TT			
			+	147	11	0			
			−	199	21	0			
	rs1801701	G/A		GG	GA	AA			
			+	158	0	0			
			−	220	0	0			
	rs1042034	A/G		GG	AG	AA			
			+	88	57	13	0.051	GG + AG vs AA	0.016
			−	134	80	6	(5.963)		(5.828)
SR-B1	rs4238001	G/A		GG	GA	AA			
			+	157	1	0			
			−	220	0	0			
	rs61932577	C/T		CC	CT	TT			
			+	158	0	0			
			−	220	0	0			
	rs5888	C/T		CC	CT	TT			
			+	96	54	10	0.761		
			−	128	82	10	(0.546)		
LDLR	rs17249134	T/G		GG	TG	TT			
			+	158	0	0			
			−	220	0	0			
	rs17249141	T/C		CC	TC	TT			
			+	158	0	0			
			−	220	0	0			
	rs2228671	C/T		CC	CT	TT			
			+	156	2	0			
			−	219	1	0			

Table 2 Association of SNP genotype with HCV infection *(Continued)*

		Alleles	HCV	Overall genotype distribution(n)			*P*-value (χ2 value)	Comparison of specific genotypes	*P*-value (χ2 value)
	rs11669576	A/G		GG	AG	AA			
			+	158	0	0			
			−	220	0	0			
	rs5930	G/A		GG	GA	AA			
			+	66	73	19	0.957		
			−	89	105	26	(0.088)		
	rs688	T/C		CC	TC	TT			
			+	120	36	2	0.664		
			−	160	55	5	(0.820)		
	rs5925	C/T		TT	CT	CC			
			+	114	42	2	0.479		
			−	149	65	6	(1.472)		
	rs2569542	A/G		GG	AG	AA			
			+	138	19	1	0.935		
			−	190	28	2	(0.135)		
	rs14158	G/A		GG	GA	AA			
			+	58	75	25	0.928		
			−	84	100	36	(0.150)		
APOE	rs429358	T/C		TT	TC	CC			
			+	131	27	0	0.564		
			−	177	41	2	(0.333)		
	rs7412	C/T		CC	CT	TT			
			+	142	16	0			
			−	196	24	0			

The rs1042034 SNP is located at the *APOB* carboxyl-terminal site, 6243 nucleotides away from rs676210, and this is reportedly in strong linkage disequilibrium [9]. The degree of linkage disequilibrium between these SNPs in our study population was also strong (D' = 1, $r^2 = 0.98$). Therefore, we confined the following association analysis of these SNPs with serum lipids only to rs1042034.

Association of serum lipid and apolipoprotein levels with the rs1042034 genotype

Since APOB is reported to be associated with serum lipid levels [9], we compared the serum lipid levels between genotypes AA and non-AA (GG + AG) in rs1042034 (Table 3). The serum LDL-C level in the genotype AA group was significantly lower than that in the genotype non-AA group (98.7 ± 39.4 vs. 115.1 ± 30.1, $P = 0.032$), whereas the TG level was significantly higher in the genotype AA group than in the genotype non-AA group (137.7 ± 67.7 vs. 100.7 ± 55.3, $P = 0.007$). There were no significant differences in serum levels of APOA1, APOA2, APOB, APOC2, APOC3, and APOE.

Table 3 Association of serum lipid and apolipoprotein levels with the rs1042034 genotype

		Genotype of rs1042034		*P*-value
		AA (n)	GG + AG (n)	
TC	(mg/dl)	176.7 ± 46.5 (17)	191.8 ± 36.2 (332)	0.100
LDL-C	(mg/dl)	98.7 ± 39.4 (17)	115.1 ± 30.1 (316)	0.032
HDL-C	(mg/dl)	50.8 ± 19.4 (15)	59.6 ± 18.4 (302)	0.074
TG	(mg/dl)	137.7 ± 67.7 (18)	100.7 ± 55.3 (321)	0.007
APOA1	(mg/dl)	137.5 ± 34.1 (19)	149.3 ± 30.9 (355)	0.105
APOA2	(mg/dl)	29.6 ± 4.9 (19)	30.4 ± 5.2 (355)	0.547
APOB	(mg/dl)	83.6 ± 29.5 (19)	88.9 ± 22.6 (355)	0.335
APOC2	(mg/dl)	3.2 ± 1.9 (19)	3.2 ± 1.7 (355)	0.945
APOC3	(mg/dl)	7.9 ± 3.6 (19)	7.9 ± 3.2 (355)	0.975
APOE	(mg/dl)	4.8 ± 1.9 (19)	4.5 ± 1.1 (355)	0.390

Values are expressed as mean ± standard deviation. The number of subjects available for the analysis is shown in parentheses. *P*-values were calculated using Student's t-test

To assess the effect of HCV status on lipid levels, we compared serum lipid and apolipoprotein levels between AA and non-AA genotypes of rs1042034 in HCV-positive and HCV-negative subjects (Table 4). No significant differences were observed in the levels of apolipoproteins between the AA and non-AA groups regardless of HCV status.

Discussion

In this study, we demonstrated that the AA genotype of rs1042034 in the APOB gene is significantly related to HCV infection status and might be associated with the regulation of serum LDL-C and TG levels. These results could suggest a close association between HCV infection status and lipid metabolism alterations due to the APOB SNP.

HCV exists in blood as an LVP, with which APOB and APOE are also combined [22]. HCV in LVPs can enter into hepatocytes through LDLRs on the cell membrane [23]. APOB-100 is deeply involved in these steps as a ligand for the LDLR; however, the underlying mechanisms have not yet been clarified in detail [24].

Table 4 Associations of serum lipid and apolipoprotein levels with rs1042034 genotype in HCV-positive and HCV-negative subjects

		HCV	Genotype of rs1042034		*P*-value
			AA (n)	GG + AG (n)	
TC	(mg/dl)	+	160.9 ± 43.5 (11)	170.3 ± 30.1 (138)	0.342
		–	205.7 ± 39.7 (6)	207.1 ± 32.0 (194)	0.917
LDL-C	(mg/dl)	+	86.2 ± 31.9 (11)	97.7 ± 23.2 (114)	0.134
		–	121.5 ± 44.4 (6)	124.9 ± 29.1 (202)	0.779
HDL-C	(mg/dl)	+	47.1 ± 22.6 (9)	53.6 ± 18.2 (110)	0.313
		–	56.5 ± 13.1 (6)	63.1 ± 17.7 (192)	0.370
TG	(mg/dl)	+	135.3 ± 66.1 (12)	106.3 ± 54.8 (127)	0.088
		–	142.5 ± 31.5 (6)	97.0 ± 55.4 (194)	0.052
APOA1	(mg/dl)	+	130.6 ± 35.8 (13)	140.5 ± 31.1 (144)	0.278
		–	152.3 ± 27.0 (6)	155.3 ± 29.3 (211)	0.805
APOA2	(mg/dl)	+	29.9 ± 5.6 (13)	29.6 ± 5.5 (144)	0.868
		–	29.1 ± 3.5 (6)	30.9 ± 4.9 (211)	0.374
APOB	(mg/dl)	+	74.1 ± 21.8 (13)	77.7 ± 17.6 (144)	0.490
		–	104.3 ± 35.3 (6)	96.5 ± 22.4 (211)	0.407
APOC2	(mg/dl)	+	2.6 ± 1.3 (13)	2.1 ± 1.0 (144)	0.056
		–	4.5 ± 2.6 (6)	4.0 ± 1.6 (211)	0.505
APOC3	(mg/dl)	+	6.6 ± 2.7 (13)	6.0 ± 2.3 (144)	0.394
		–	10.7 ± 3.9 (6)	9.1 ± 3.0 (211)	0.210
APOE	(mg/dl)	+	4.8 ± 2.0 (13)	4.3 ± 1.0 (144)	0.114
		–	4.7 ± 1.7 (6)	4.7 ± 1.2 (211)	0.979

Values are presented as mean ± standard deviation. The number of subjects available for the analysis is shown in parentheses. *P*-values were calculated using Student's t-test

Previously, Li and colleagues reported that an SNP in *LDLR* exon 13 (rs5925) was associated with susceptibility to HCV infection [12], but we did not detect a significant difference in the SNP in our cohort. This difference may be due to the fact that the previous study involved a smaller subject cohort (a total of 156 subjects) as compared with our study (378 subjects). Zhu and associates reported that an SNP in the *APOB* promoter region (rs934197) was associated with susceptibility to HCV infection, and showed that HCV-infected patients had significantly lower levels of LDL-C as compared with healthy individuals [25]. Although we did not analyze SNPs in the promoter region, a similar tendency of lower LDL-C levels was observed; HCV-positive subjects with AA genotype of *APOB* exhibited lower LDL-C levels than the other genotypes. Moreover, rs1042034 in *APOB* is known to regulate biding to the LDLR and is therefore assumed to cause a change in the binding affinity of APOB to LDLRs [26]. These findings are further supportive of a close relationship between the life cycle of HCV and host *APOB* polymorphism.

Since serum lipid levels are very important risk factors for cardiovascular disease, several large-scale screenings for SNPs concerning serum lipid-regulator genes have been reported. Regarding studies of the *APOB* SNP rs1042034, the genome-wide association study (GWAS), which included more than 100,000 individuals of European ancestry, reported that polymorphism of rs1042034 was significantly associated with decreased TG and increased HDL-C levels [27]. In a study involving several ethnic groups, rs1042034 was significantly associated with lower TC and LDL-C levels only in Hispanics [28]. As for Asians, rs1042034 was significantly associated with lower TG and higher HDL-C levels in South Asians, compatible with the European GWAS, but there was no significant association in East Asians [27]. Although the underlying mechanism of the changes in serum lipid levels caused by this SNP have still not been elucidated, it appears *APOB-100* mutations and polymorphisms may change the conformation of APOB-100, thereby leading to a change in LDL metabolism through the interaction of APOB-100 with the LDLR.

Based on the findings mentioned above, we can speculate that a relationship exists between HCV infection and lipid metabolism disorders through SNPs of APOB-100, whereby the AA genotype (minor allele homozygote) of rs1042034 could facilitate serum LDL uptake via LDLR on hepatocytes by modifying their mutual affinity and interaction, and consequently, the serum LDL-C level could be decreased. As a result, the susceptibility to HCV infection could be increased because HCV particles exist as LVPs and enter into the liver with LDL. However, it is not clear why genotype AA was associated with higher serum TG levels as compared with genotype non-AA, and further studies are needed to investigate this relationship in greater detail.

In the comparison of lipid levels by genotype, serum levels of LDL-C and TG showed significant differences between AA and non-AA genotype (Table 3), whereas these differences disappeared when comparing by HCV status (Table 4), indicating that HCV infection itself did not have much influence on lipid metabolism, which supports our hypothesis.

Interestingly, a large Japanese cohort study revealed that HCV infection causes not only lower TC and LDL-C levels but also significant lower serum HDL-C and TG levels [21] and they suggest that the HCV infection itself might directly cause hypolipidemia, irrespective of host factors including age, hepatic damage, and nutritional state. Furthermore, it has been reported that HCV genotype 3a and 4 are associated with hypocholesterolemia in western patients [29, 30]. However, there was no association between HCV genotypes and lipid profile or SNP pattern in our cohort (data not shown). This may be partly explained by the fact that the most frequent genotype was 1b (81%), which is the most common genotype in the Japanese population, while genotypes 3a and 4 are very rare.

Therefore, the possibility of a direct interaction of HCV with lipid metabolism could not be completely ruled out in our study and need to be confirmed in a more detailed investigation.

There are some potential limitations of our study. First, regarding the HCV negative cohort, we could not completely rule out the possibility of including individuals in whom HCV had been eradicated naturally because we enrolled subjects who were negative for serum anti-HCV antibody. Second, the lipid metabolism profiles could have been altered by differences in liver function, which can be affected by various hepatic disorders. However, in the present study, we carefully limited the participants to Child-Pugh A, and excluded subjects with NASH, HBV infection, or HCC, and therefore the baseline characteristics and liver function levels of the participants were well balanced between the two groups. Although our study had a limitation in terms of not covering all SNPs in lipid regulators, our results suggested the possibility that an *APOB-100* SNP, rs1042034, influences the susceptibility to HCV infection by their entry into the liver through the LDLR. Our data may have important implications for identifying individuals with higher susceptibility to HCV infection via SNP of lipid regulators. Exploring the molecular mechanism underlying these results could provide important information for controlling the process of HCV infection and limiting the expansion of HCV infection.

In addition, in the treatment of chronic HCV infection, the rate of sustained virological response (SVR) subsequent to the approval of direct-acting antiviral agents has been dramatically increasing and the change in serum lipid levels after SVR is gaining attention [31]. Therefore, focusing on the influence of SNPs concerning lipid metabolism in HCV patients should have important implications for antivirus therapy in the future.

Conclusions

In conclusion, this study demonstrated that an APOB SNP, rs1042034, is closely associated with HCV infection through lipid metabolism alteration. The minor allele AA genotype may facilitate serum LDL uptake into hepatocytes via LDLR by modifying their affinity and interaction and may have an influence on HCV infection by their entry into the liver through the LDLR. Further studies are needed to explore the mechanism underlying these results, which could provide important information for controlling the process of HCV infection.

Abbreviations

APOA1: Apolipoprotein A1; APOA2: Apolipoprotein A2; APOB: Apolipoprotein B; APOC2: Apolipoprotein C2; APOC3: Apolipoprotein C3; APOE: Apolipoprotein E; HCV: Hepatitis virus C; HDL-C: High density lipoprotein cholesterol; LDL-C: Low density lipoprotein cholesterol; TC: Total cholesterol; TG: Total triglycerides

Acknowledgments

The authors wish to acknowledge Mitsuyasu Yano, Hiroshi Shibata, Toshihiro Omoya, Mari Urata, Kanako Otsuka (Tokushima Prefectural Central Hospital), Masako Sei (Tokushima Health Screening Center), Akemi Tsutsui, Hiroshi Fukuno, Fumiko Kishi (Tokushima Municipal Hospital), Masahiko Nakasono (Handa Hospital), Tatsuhiko Shiraishi (Tokushima Prefectural Miyoshi Hospital), Katsuyoshi Tamaki (Ohkubo Hospital), Yoshitaka Imoto, Sayo Takahashi and Tatsunao Sueuti, (Yoshinogawa Medical Center), who provided coordination in enrolling the subjects, and Yoshihiro Okayama (Clinical Trial Center for Developmental Therapeutics, Tokushima University Hospital) who provided advice to statistical analyses.

Funding

None

Authors' contributions

Designed and coordinated the study: RH, MK, YS, TT and TT. Performed the statistical analyses: RH, MK and II. Collected the data and critically reviewed the manuscript: RH, MK, YS, TT, TT, TT, HT, NM, HS, HH, II, MS, TO and TT. Wrote the manuscript: RH, MK, YS and TT. All authors approved the final version of the manuscript.

Consent for publication

Not applicable.

Competing interests

The authors declare that they have no competing interests.

Author details

[1]Department of Gastroenterology and Oncology, Tokushima University Graduate School of Biomedical Sciences, 3-18-15, Kuramoto-cho, Tokushima 770-8503, Japan. [2]Department of Gastroenterology, Yoshinogawa Medical Center, Yoshinogawa, Tokushima 776-8511, Japan. [3]Department of Internal Medicine, Tokushima Health Screening Center, 1-10-3, Kuramoto-cho, Tokushima 770-0042, Japan. [4]Department of Human Genetics, Tokushima University Graduate School of Biomedical Sciences, 3-18-15, Kuramoto-cho, Tokushima 770-8503, Japan. [5]Department of General Medicine and Community Health Science, Tokushima University Graduate School of Biomedical Sciences, 3-18-15, Kuramoto-cho, Tokushima 770-8503, Japan.

References

1. Mohd Hanafiah K, Groeger J, Flaxman AD, Wiersma ST. Global epidemiology of hepatitis C virus infection: new estimates of age-specific antibody to HCV seroprevalence. Hepatology. 2013;57(4):1333–42.
2. Webster DP, Klenerman P, Dusheiko GM. Hepatitis C. Lancet. 2015;385:1124–35.
3. Zeisel MB, Fofana I, Fafi-Kremer S, Baumert TF. Hepatitis C virus entry into hepatocytes: molecular mechanisms and targets for antiviral therapies. J Hepatol. 2011;54(3):566–76.
4. Kim DS, Burt AA, Ranchalis JE, Jarvik ER, Rosenthal EA, Hatsukami TS, et al. Novel gene-by-environment interactions: APOB and NPC1L1 variants affect the relationship between dietary and total plasma cholesterol. J Lipid Res. 2013;54(5):1512–20.
5. Powell LM, Wallis SC, Pease RJ, Edwards YH, Knott TJ, Scott J. A novel form of tissue-specific RNA processing produces apolipoprotein-B48 in intestine. Cell. 1987;50(6):831–40.
6. Aizawa Y, Seki N, Nagano T, Abe H. Chronic hepatitis C virus infection and lipoprotein metabolism. World J Gastroenterol. 2015;21(36):10299–313.
7. Fukuhara T, Ono C, Puig-Basagoiti F, Matsuura Y. Role of lipoproteins and apolipoproteins in particle formation of hepatitis C virus. Trends Microbiol. 2015;23(10):618–29.
8. Agnello V, Abel G, Elfahal M, Knight GB, Zhang QX. Hepatitis C virus and other Flaviviridae viruses enter cells via low density lipoprotein receptor. Proc Natl Acad Sci U S A. 1999;96(22):12766–71.
9. Benn M. Apolipoprotein B levels, APOB alleles, and risk of ischemic cardiovascular disease in the general population, a review. Atherosclerosis. 2009;206(1):17–30.
10. Cerda A, Genvigir FD, Arazi SS, Hirata MH, Dorea EL, Bernik MM, et al. Influence of SCARB1 polymorphisms on serum lipids of hypercholesterolemic individuals treated with atorvastatin. Clin Chim Acta. 2010;411(9–10):631–7.
11. Yang KC, Su YN, Shew JY, Yang KY, Tseng WK, Wu CC, et al. LDLR and ApoB are major genetic causes of autosomal dominant hypercholesterolemia in a Taiwanese population. J Formos Med Assoc. 2007;106(10):799–807.
12. Li H, Liu Z, Han Q, Li Y, Chen J. Association of genetic polymorphism of low-density lipoprotein receptor with chronic viral hepatitis C infection in Han Chinese. J Med Virol. 2006;78(10):1289–95.
13. Hennig BJ, Hellier S, Frodsham AJ, Zhang L, Klenerman P, Knapp S, et al. Association of low-density lipoprotein receptor polymorphisms and outcome of hepatitis C infection. Genes Immun. 2002;3(6):359–67.
14. Caruz A, Neukam K, Rivero-Juárez A, Herrero R, Real LM, Camacho A, et al. Association of low-density lipoprotein receptor genotypes with hepatitis C viral load. Genes Immun. 2014;15(1):16–24.
15. Price DA, Bassendine MF, Norris SM, Golding C, Toms GL, Schmid ML, et al. Apolipoprotein epsilon3 allele is associated with persistent hepatitis C virus infection. Gut. 2006;55(5):715–8.
16. Wozniak MA, Itzhaki RF, Faragher EB, James MW, Ryder SD, Irving WL. Apolipoprotein E-epsilon 4 protects against severe liver disease caused by hepatitis C virus. Hepatology. 2002;36(2):456–63.
17. Delgado-Lista J, Perez-Jimenez F, Ruano J, Perez-Martinez P, Fuentes F, Criado-Garcia J, et al. Effects of variations in the APOA1/C3/A4/A5 gene cluster on different parameters of postprandial lipid metabolism in healthy young men. J Lipid Res. 2010;51(1):63–73.
18. Kuhlmann I, Minihane AM, Huebbe P, Nebel A, Rimbach G. Apolipoprotein E genotype and hepatitis C, HIV and herpes simplex disease risk: a literature review. Lipids Health Dis. 2010;9:8.
19. Itoh Y, Mizuki N, Shimada T, Azuma F, Itakura M, Kashiwase K, et al. High-throughput DNA typing of HLA-A, -B, -C, and -DRB1 loci by a PCR-SSOP-Luminex method in the Japanese population. Immunogenetics. 2005;57(10):717–29.
20. Butt AA, Xiaoqiang W, Budoff M, Leaf D, Kuller LH, Justice AC. Hepatitis C virus infection and the risk of coronary disease. Clin Infect Dis. 2009;49(2):225–32.
21. Miyazaki T, Honda A, Ikegami T, Saitoh Y, Hirayama T, Hara T, et al. Hepatitis C virus infection causes hypolipidemia regardless of hepatic damage or nutritional state: an epidemiological survey of a large Japanese cohort. Hepatol Res. 2011;41(6):530–41.
22. Gastaminza P, Cheng G, Wieland S, Zhong J, Liao W, Chisari FV. Cellular determinants of hepatitis C virus assembly, maturation, degradation, and secretion. J Virol. 2008;82(5):2120–9.
23. André P, Komurian-Pradel F, Deforges S, Perret M, Berland JL, Sodoyer M, et al. Characterization of low- and very-low-density hepatitis C virus RNA-containing particles. J Virol. 2002;76(14):6919–28.
24. Huang H, Sun F, Owen DM, Li W, Chen Y, Gale M, et al. Hepatitis C virus production by human hepatocytes dependent on assembly and secretion of very low-density lipoproteins. Proc Natl Acad Sci U S A. 2007;104(14):5848–53.
25. Zhu C, Zhang R, Liu D, Mukhtar MM, Liu W, Peng G, et al. Association of functional polymorphism of ApoB promoter with hepatitis C virus infection. Clin Chim Acta. 2009;401(1–2):124–7.
26. Boren J, Lee I, Zhu W, Arnold K, Taylor S, Innerarity TL. Identification of the low density lipoprotein receptor-binding site in apolipoprotein B100 and the modulation of its binding activity by the carboxyl terminus in familial defective apo-B100. J Clin Invest. 1998;101(5):1084–93.
27. Teslovich TM, Musunuru K, Smith AV, Edmondson AC, Stylianou IM, Koseki M, et al. Biological, clinical and population relevance of 95 loci for blood lipids. Nature. 2010;466(7303):707–13.
28. Bryant EK, Dressen AS, Bunker CH, Hokanson JE, Hamman RF, Kamboh MI, et al. A multiple replication study of plasma lipoprotein levels-associated SNPs identified in recent GWAS. PLoS One. 2013;8(5):e63469.
29. Hofer H, Bankl HC, Wrba F, Steindl-Munda P, Peck-Radosavljevic M, Osterreicher C, et al. Hepatocellular fat accumulation and low serum cholesterol in patients infected with HCV-3a. Am J Gastroenterol. 2002;97(11):2880–5.
30. Marzouk D, Sass J, Bakr I, El Hosseiny M, Abdel-Hamid M, Rekacewicz C, et al. Metabolic and cardiovascular risk profiles and hepatitis C virus infection in rural Egypt. Gut. 2007;56(8):1105–10.
31. Meissner EG, Lee YJ, Osinusi A, Sims Z, Qin J, Sturdevant D, et al. Effect of sofosbuvir and ribavirin treatment on peripheral and hepatic lipid metabolism in chronic hepatitis C virus, genotype 1-infected patients. Hepatology. 2015;61(3):790–801.

16

Hepatitis C-related cryoglobulinemic neuropathy: potential role of oxcarbazepine for pain control

Rita Moretti[1], Paola Caruso[1], Matteo Dal Ben[1,2], Silvia Gazzin[2*] and Claudio Tiribelli[2]

Abstract

Background: Peripheral neuropathy is one most common, limiting and invalidating neurological symptom in subjects with hepatitis C virus and mixed cryoglobulinemia. Notably, the medical therapy proposed to eradicate HCV, can frequently exacerbate the painful neuropathy. Therefore, neuropathy therapies are insufficient and inadequate, and comprise immunosuppressive drugs, such as steroid or cyclosporine, intravenous immunoglobulin or plasma exchange. These have shown variable success in case reports, with a presumably temporary effect, but with major side effects.

Methods: We assessed the effects of oxcarbazepine treatment in 67 cases of cryoglobulinemia related neuropathy, who did not respond to either steroid or Gabapentin, or Pregabalin. Oxcarbazepine was chosen based on the promising preliminary results.

Results: Patients treated with Oxcarbazepine showed a rapid, discrete and persistent relief of polyneuropathic signs, without consistent side effects, and with a limited interaction with concomitant drugs.

Conclusions: These data favor the use of oxcarbazepine as a useful tool in the management of neuropathic pain associated with Hepatitis–C cryoglobulin neuropathy.

Keywords: HCV, Oxcarbazepine, Neuropathy, Pain

Background

Cryoglobulins are cold-precipitating immunoglobulins [1], which form aggregates and immune complexes, outstripping the reticuloendothelial-clearing activity, depositing in the human tissues, activating the complement, and finally leading to tissue damage, promoting systemic inflammation (usually occurring at the level of skin or kidneys). Otherwise healthy individuals could present cryoglobulins, making difficult to estimate their real prevalence in medical sets, finally considered rare. Nevertheless, the variable clinical manifestations reported in literature, might leads to underestimation of cryoglobulinemia diffusion.

Cryoglobulins can be divided into three types, following the Brouet classification [2], essential, or secondary to autoimmune pathologies and chronic medical conditions (primarily chronic infections) and related to lymphoproliferative diseases [2]. The second and third types, also defined as mixed cryoglobulins [2, 3], composed by monoclonal Ig rheumatoid factor and polyclonal IgG and IgM rheumatoid factor, are seen very frequently in HCV infections [3–7].

Despite varying from country to country, the prevalence of peripheral neuropathies in HCV-associated cryoglobulinemia substantially varies in the Mediterranean [1, 3, 8]. Of note, HCV-related proteins are present in damaged skin, blood vessels, and kidneys and seem to play a direct role in the pathogenesis of the damages seen in the peripheral nerve [1, 9, 10].

Pathological findings suggest a direct damage of the small vessels around nerve, the so-called *vasa nervorum* [3, 11, 12], due to a vasculitis or to necrotizing arteritis. Both these conditions cause an ischemic damage of nerve [3, 10, 13, 14]. HCV is directly responsive for inducing the

* Correspondence: silvia.gazzin@fegato.it
[2]Italian Liver Foundation, Centro Studi Fegato, AREA Science Park, Bldg. Q, Ss 14, km 163.5, 34149 Trieste, Italy

inflammation cascade of events in the vessels, since it has been demonstrated HCV-RNA in epineurial cells [15–17].

Peripheral neuropathy is the most common reported symptom in patients with HCV-associated mixed cryoglobulinemia [18–20], where it may be the first clinical manifestation, despite its prevalence is still unknown. There is only a report [14] assessing the prevalence of peripheral neuropathy in HCV; neuropathy was found in 33% of patients without other cryoglobulinemia-related symptoms and clinically, most frequently, patients present a symmetrical sensory or motor-sensory polyneuropathy, or less frequently as a mono-neuropathy, or as a multiple mononeuropathy [3, 15].

At biopsy, axonal degeneration is shown, possibly triggered by the deposit of cryoglobulins at the level of *vasa nervosum* microcirculation and vasculitis-induced ischemia, as well, despite seldom reported, by an immunological mediated demyelination. Electrophysiological studies and teased nerve fiber studies allowed neuropathies to be classified as predominantly sensory axonopathies [21, 22], even if there are some descriptions of demyelinating peripheral neuropathies [3, 21–24].

There is no conventional treatment for HCV cryoglobulin neuropathy. It is accepted nowadays that prolonged antiviral therapy led to a reduction of HCV-RNA levels, associated with a reduction of cryoglobulinemia [25]. The reduction of cryoglobulins under the detectable levels has been obtained by treating patients with interferon-alpha (IFN alpha) plus ribavirin, obtaining an amelioration of painful polyneuropathy. On the other hand, the side effects of IFN alpha therapy are known, with the exacerbation of the symptoms of mixed cryoglobulinemia, with an exacerbation of the neuropathy, whit severe myalgia, arthralgia [26, 27]. Moreover, there are different cases of described side effects of IFN alpha, such as demyelinating sensory neuropathy, neuropsychiatric symptoms, a possible bone marrow dyscrasia, a transient or definite worsening of hepatitis [22, 28, 29]. For cryoglobulin-related neuropathy, other options have been proposed, including alternative immunosuppressive agents, such as steroid or cyclosporine [30], and plasma exchange [31]. They showed variable success and the effect is presumably temporary. There are some works which stressed the importance of steroids and cyclophosphamide [12]. Considering that peripheral cryoglobulin-related neuropathy in HCV patients give, as the most frequent symptom, the neuropathic pain, the principle target should be its earliest relief and without (or with the most limited) side effects.

After the promising results of a previous work [11], we present a series of many patient, with HCV cryoglobulinemia related polineuropathy, who did not respond to steroid and Gabapentin treatment, but have been successfully managed with Oxcarbazepine.

Methods

Patients

Sixty-seven HCV-positive patients (details in Tables 1 and 2) followed by the Liver Center of the University of Trieste from 1st January 2000-to 1st January 2015, have been studied in the Neurology Unit due to the detection of peripheral neuropathic signs. All the patients were treated with IFN-αlpha and ribavirin therapy, three times a week; a progressive decrease of their viral load was observed in all of them. Neurological signs of peripheral neuropathic signs appeared for 11 patients 9.7 ± 2.1 months after the cessation of antiviral therapy even with a sustained viral response, and increase in the cryoglobulins serum level. Forty-four patients interrupted antiviral therapy (mean period of treatment of 7.6 9.7 ± 2.1) due to neurological symptoms such as anxiety and depression (18 patients), suicidal thoughts (6 patients), major sleeping disturbances, concentration difficulties and daily living executive complications (8 patients), apathy, chronic fatigue, loss of weight (12 patients). Drop out are in line with some data presented in Literature, i.e. by Manns et al. [32, 33] All the 44 patients showed cryoglobulin neuropathic polyneuropathy 3.4 ± 1.2 months after stopping antiviral therapy. Twelve patients were strained to interrupt the IFN and ribavirin therapy (after mean time of therapy duration of 6.2 ± 3.9 months) due to the appearance of painful peripheral

Table 1 Epidemiological and biological features in 67 patients with HCV and cryoglobulinemia

Patients (total 67)	Features
Age (years)	50.4 ± 2.7
Sex ratio (M/F)	31/36
Apparent duration of disease (years)	4.1 ± 1.3
Albumin level (g/L)	39.7 ± 8.5
ALT (IU/L)	131.4 ± 16.7
Prothrombin time (%)	84.1 ± 12.2
Rheumatoid factors (n of pts. and %)	41/67 (61%)
Mean Cryoglobulinemia(g/L)	0.27 ± 0.8
Cryoglobulinemia type	
CGS TYPE II (n of pts. and %)	42/67 (64%)
CGS TYPE III (n of pts. and %)	25/67 (36%)
ANTI HCV Antibodies (n of pts. and %)	67/67 (100%)
ANTI HBV Antibodies (n of pts. and %)	35/67 (52%)
Anti HBC	30 (86%)
HBsAg	5 (14.2)
Anti HBS	30 (86%)
HBeAG	0
AntiHBe	0
HCV RNA sequences in sera (n of pts. and %)	49/67 (73%)

Table 2 HCV status of the 67 patients

Patients (total 67) (number and %)	Features
Anti HCV antibodies	67/67 (100%)
Chronic Hepatitis	67/67 (100%)
Cirrhosis	6/67 (8.9%)
Presumed disease duration (years)	6.1 ± 2.7
Fibrosis score	1.9 ± 0.7
HAI score [47]	6.5 ± 1.2
HCV genotype (number and %)	
1	43 (64.1%)
2	1 (1.5%)
3	21 (31.3%)
4	2 (3%)

neuropathy, associated with an elevation of cryoglobulinemia, and therefore excluding the IFN-related neuropathy.

The new antiviral drugs (sofusbuvir, simeprevir, daclatasvir, etc.) were not used, since at the time of the recruitment they were not available. All of the 67 patients reported progressive painful paresthesias, shock pain episodes, boot-glove dysesthesia sensations. All the patients showed signs of cryoglobulinemia (mean 0.27 +/− 0.8 g/L; range 0.05–1.6 g/L). Cryocrit levels were measured as the percentage of packed cryoglobulins after cold centrifugation of the serum, and cryoglobulin composition was determined by immunodiffusion on Ouchterlony plates against specific antisera. Fifty-eight had polyneuropathy and 9 had mononeuropathy multiplex. All subjects had an electroneurographic confirmation of peripheral neuropathy, 57 presented the axonal profile and 10 showed the axonal-demyelinating signs of damage (Table 3). Thirty-six patients referred a relatively acute onset of pain and numbness in feet and legs together with a rash on the dorsal surface of low limbs, in particular, starting from the feet, extending midway up to the legs. Seventeen patients presented with the acute onset of pain, described as "electric shocks" which is followed by numbness in legs. These symptoms started approximately two years prior presentation of overt liver disease, and gradually worsened. Fourteen patients (all women) presented a mainly sensory neuropathy, asymmetrical, with dysesthesia symptoms and

Table 3 Electrophysiological and clinical features of the examined patients

Symptoms	Patients
Neuropathy type	
Polyneuropathy	58
Mononeuropathy	9
Electrophisiological features	
Demyelination	10
Axonal	57

were committed due to a presumptive restless leg syndrome, which was not confirmed by the neurologist. All the patients denied any other symptom such as fever, chills, arthralgias or skin alterations, apart from those described above, or other general hepatic-referable symptoms; 24 patients admitted alcohol consumption before the beginning of IFN-alpha and ribavirin therapy.

Reduced complement C4 activity has been found in 39 patients; positive search for antinuclear antibodies has been found in 13 patients, anti-mitochondrial in 19 patients and C-reactive protein has been found in 32 patients.

Pharmacological treatment

As shown in Fig. 1, after the electroneurographic confirmation of the clinical diagnosis of cryoglobulinemia related polineuropathy, patient started a cycle of steroids for 14 days, followed by Gabapentin if steroids failed to improve the simptoms. If Gabapentin treatement was not successful or accompained by side effects, it was substituted with Pregabalin, witch was soon interrupted for severe side effects. After one month of wash-out, all the 67 patients, who still complained for the neurological sympotms began

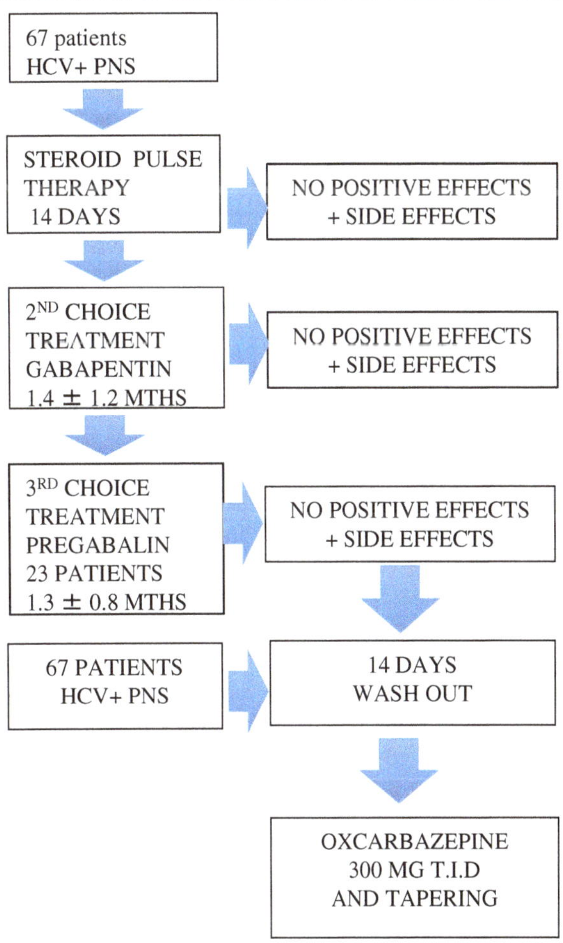

Fig. 1 Patients flowchart

Oxcarbazepine. A neuriological assesemsnt was performed every month for 12 months after the start of Oxcarbazepine treatement.

Statistical analyses

Statistical analyses were performed using SAS® software (version 16.0 SAS® Software Inc., Cary, NC, USA). Within-group changes from baseline were tested using the Wilcoxon Signed Ranks test. Between-group comparisons of changes from baseline were tested using the Marginal Homogeneity Test. Spearman correlation test has been employed for each significant variable. This was done for each efficacy variable. Results are presented as mean changes from baseline with standard deviations, and p-values are provided where appropriate.

Results

As in Fig. 1, after the clinical diagnosis all patients were treated with steroids (up to 100 mg/daily of prednisone); 10 patients partially responded, 40 experienced steroidal side effects, which causes interruption, and 17 did not show any benefit.

One month after the steroid washout, gabapentin. It was prescribed (1887 ± 205 mg/day) followed by a moderate improvement in the painful sensation (average visual analog scale from 8 to 9 to 6–7). After one month of follow-up, due to daytime sleepiness, nausea, dizziness and gait alteration the drug was stopped. The average duration of the treatment was 1.4 ± 1.2 months.

In 23 strongly motivated patients, pregabalin (50 mg, t.i.d) was prescribed; 14 patients showed cholestatic and liver damage, 2 presented overt jaundice and 7 patients a prolongation of the prothrombin time. All side effects subsided after the medication was stopped. No amelioration of pain symptoms was observed.

At the end of this period of treatment (average time of 5.6 months), all the 67 patients reported side effects and persistence of pain. After two weeks of washout of any other pain-relief drug(s), oxcarbazepine was given at a dose of 300 mg/day for a week, increased to 600 mg/day the following week, and then further increased to 900 mg/day. The dosage was increased to 1200 mg/day in 11 patients for 10.2 ± 2.3 days, due to persistence of pain, to be then readjusted to 900 mg/day. Each patients was follow-up monthly for 12 months, and each check-up, the Short form McGill Pain Assessment Questionnaire (SF-MPQ) [34] was administered. The average SF-MPQ was 32.1 ± 5.7 at baseline (average scores 24–36), and decreased to 21.3 ± 2.3 (average scores 17–25, $p < 0.001$) after one month. The average SF-MPQ at 6-month was 12.5 ± 3.7 (average scores 9–14; $p < 0.001$ over baseline). At the 6th month of follow-up, the dose of Oxcarbazepine was reduced to 600 mg/day; 33 patients were pain free and maintained the dose for two additional months while 34 increased to 900 mg/day. All the 67 patients, who have been prescribed Oxcarbazepine, completed the 12 months follow-up: 46 patient arte asymptomatic and do not take any anti-epileptic drug. All patients referred sleepiness and drowsiness at the beginning of the therapy that rapidly disappeared; no other side effects were observed.

Discussion

Hepatitis C is a serious health concern, affecting millions of people worldwide. The majority of the subject positive for HCV antibody are asymptomatic. More recently, central (CNS) and peripheral nervous system (PNS) have been studied as focal collateral damage regions, tightly involved in HCV.

The treatment of HCV-cryoglobulins -associated PNS is actually based IFN plus ribavirin therapy, eventually associated with steroids [4, 35–37]. Studies have showed that patients with HCV-associated cryoglobulinemia and extra-hepatic manifestations treated with IFN-alpha alone were reported to be responders (resolution of symptoms, disappearance of cryoprecipitates and HCV RNA), with only one tapering off of IFN-alpha after 3 years of treatment with sustained resolution of HCV and cryoglobulinemia [34]. However, long-term studies were not performed and the results of long term follow-up are not available [38–40]. The few data available seems to indicate favorable outcomes in cryoglobulinemia HCV subjects treated with corticosteroids [10, 39, 40]. Since chronic steroid administration also increases the level of HCV RNA, this treatment should be limited. Therefore, intravenous immunoglobulin or plasmapheresis should be considered as a therapeutic option [24]. In addition, in patients with severe cryoglobulinemia-associated vasculitis as those with rapidly progressive renal failure or neurological involvement, the antiviral therapy should be delayed for 2–4 months while they are treated with aggressive scheme with plasmapheresis, high doses of corticosteroids and either cyclophosphamide or rituximab [41]. Rituximab therapy has been used predominantly in HCV-related mixed cryoglobulinemia refractory to or unsuitable for corticosteroids and antiviral (IFN-α) therapy [41]. The role of interferon to exacerbate cryoglobulinemia related neuropathy is still under evaluation, although recent data obtained in 24 patients showed that interferon-free regimen with new drugs as sofosbuvir resulted in an almost complete clinical response of the vasculitis but still undefined effect on pain relief [42].

Painful neuropathy is a dramatic and persistent condition, which affects many patients, and is an invalidating condition. The several options available for pain control are confusing and daunting. The best solution seems to be an escalating regime matching the intensity and nature of the sensory components of the pain state. Moreover, in chronic conditions, such as HCV- related hepatitis, where many different clinical details should be considered, pain relief therapies should not interfere with the underline disease and the concomitant antiviral treatment. Therefore, pain-treatment should be efficacious, should not interfere with their general and hepatic condition, should not create side effects as, in particular, disequilibrium, gait imbalance, drowsiness and reduced vigilance.

Oxcarbazepine is a safe drug, without significant side effects, and the rarely described hepato-toxicity seems to be related to a hypersensitivity or to a immune –mediated response to some metabolites of the drug, rapidly and totally reversible [43]. Oxcarbazepine should be careful monitored by specialists, with reported side effects, which can be distinguished in: *more common, but rapidly and spontaneously solving side effects (1:100):* Blurred vision, disequilibirum, mental depression, emotional incontinence, cough and sore throat sensation. *Less common (less than 1:1000):* Agitation, awkwardness, mental confusion, persistent disequilibrium associated with orthostatic hypotension, fast or irregular heartbeat, thirst, muscle cramps, headache, skin rash, weakness. Usually they spontaneously disappeared, and they do not need a suspension of therapy. *Rare (less than 1: 3500)*: Anxiety, burning feeling in the chest or stomach, hives or itching, irritability, restlessness, muscle pain or weakness, purple spots on the skin and rectal bleeding; these needs a careful medical examination, and the consequent decision to stop it.

Oxcarbazapine possess intrinsic pain-relief properties [44], either considering acute or chronic pain [44, 45] and neuropathic pain [46]. The efficacy of previous studies, its safety, the good tolerance and the limited side effects leads to this study, which confirmed the previously reported data [10]. Results are stable, we have not reported serious adverse side effects and pain relief is stable. Our study demonstrated that treatment of HCV-cryoglobulins related neuropathy with oxcarbazapine is effective in the large majority of patients at a dosage which is rather well tolerated and is not associated with any relevant side effect. The particular condition of these patients (particularly vulnerable to hepatotoxicity), the conspicuous potential interactions with concomitant drugs taken by the patients (antiviral, etc), the rapid beneficial effect (demonstrated by the decrease of the average SF-MPQ), and the absence of consistent side effects (demonstrated by a good pattern of labs values) favour to the useof oxcarbazepine in the management of neuropathic pain.

Conclusions

In this work, patients not responsive to steroids, gabapentin at high dosage and to pregabalin, benefit from oxcarbazepine. The limited side effects, associated to the favourable and rapid response, the reduced interaction with concomitant drugs support the use of oxcarbazepine as an effective and safe treatment of the of HCV-cryoglobulins related neuropathy.

Abbreviations

CNS: Central nervous system; GGT: Gamma-glutamyltranspeptidase; HAV: Hepatitis A virus; HBV: Hepatitis B virus; HCV: Hepatitis C virus; IFN: Interferon; IFN-alpha: Interferon-alpha; MHD: 10-hydroxcarbazepine; PNS: Peripheral nervous system; SF-MPQ: Short form McGill Pain Assessment Questionnaire; VAS: Visual analogue scale

Acknowledgments

Not applicable.

Funding

MDB was partially supported by the fellowship U12GPFIRB11. This study was supported in part by ad in house grant of Fondazione Italiana Fegato (Italian Liver Foundation).

Authors' contributions

RM designed the experimental plan, evaluated the patients, collected and analyzed data. RM, PC, MDB, CT, SG critical revised the work and prepared the manuscript. All authors have read and approved the final version of the submitted manuscript.

Consent for publication

The patients gave their written informed consent to publish the study.

Competing interests

The authors declare that they have no competing interests.

Author details

[1]Neurology Clinic, Department of Medical, Surgical, and Health Sciences, University of Trieste, 34100 Trieste, Italy. [2]Italian Liver Foundation, Centro Studi Fegato, AREA Science Park, Bldg. Q, Ss 14, km 163.5, 34149 Trieste, Italy.

References

1. Ramos-Casals M, Stone JH, Cid MC, Bosch X. The cryoglobulinaemias. Lancet Lond Engl. 2012;379:348–60.
2. Brouet JC, Clauvel JP, Danon F, Klein M, Seligmann M. Biologic and clinical significance of cryoglobulins. A report of 86 cases. Am J Med. 1974;57:775–88.
3. Lidove O, Cacoub P, Maisonobe T, Servan J, Thibault V, Piette JC, et al. Hepatitis C virus infection with peripheral neuropathy is not always associated with cryoglobulinaemia. Ann Rheum Dis. 2001;60:290–2.
4. Trejo O, Ramos-Casals M, García-Carrasco M, Yagüe J, Jiménez S, de la Red G, et al. Cryoglobulinemia: study of etiologic factors and clinical and immunologic features in 443 patients from a single center. Medicine (Baltimore). 2001;80:252–62.
5. Nemni R, Sanvito L, Quattrini A, Santuccio G, Camerlingo M, Canal N. Peripheral neuropathy in hepatitis C virus infection with and without cryoglobulinaemia. J Neurol Neurosurg Psychiatry. 2003;74:1267–71.
6. Trendelenburg M, Schifferli JA. Cryoglobulins are not essential. Ann Rheum Dis. 1998;57:3–5.
7. Gorevic PD, Kassab HJ, Levo Y, Kohn R, Meltzer M, Prose P, et al. Mixed cryoglobulinemia: clinical aspects and long-term follow-up of 40 patients. Am J Med. 1980;69:287–308.
8. Bonetti B, Monaco S, Giannini C, Ferrari S, Zanusso GL, Rizzuto N. Human peripheral nerve macrophages in normal and pathological conditions. J Neurol Sci. 1993;118(2):158–68.
9. Sansonno D, Cornacchiulo V, Iacobelli AR, Di Stefano R, Lospalluti M, Dammacco F. Localization of hepatitis C virus antigens in liver and skin tissues of chronic hepatitis C virus-infected patients with mixed cryoglobulinemia. Hepatol Baltim Md. 1995;21:305–12.
10. Moretti R, Torre P, Antonello RM, Cattaruzza T, Pizzolato G. Peripheral neuropathy in hepatitis C virus-related mixed cryoglobulinaemia: existing treatments and a positive symptomatic response to oxcarbazepine. Funct Neurol. 2006;21:137–40.

11. Tembl JI, Ferrer JM, Sevilla MT, Lago A, Mayordomo F, Vilchez JJ. Neurologic complications associated with hepatitis C virus infection. Neurology. 1999;53:861–4.
12. Heckmann JG, Kayser C, Heuss D, Manger B, Blum HE, Neundörfer B. Neurological manifestations of chronic hepatitis C. J Neurol. 1999;246:486–91.
13. Monaco S, Ferrari S, Gajofatto A, Zanusso G, Mariotto S. HCV-related nervous system disorders. Clin Dev Immunol. 2012;2012:236148.
14. Carvalho-Filho RJ, Narciso-Schiavon JL, Tolentino LHL, Schiavon LL, Ferraz MLG, AEB S. Central nervous system vasculitis and polyneuropathy as first manifestations of hepatitis C. World J Gastroenterol. 2012;18:188–91.
15. Zaltron S, Puoti M, Liberini P, Antonini L, Quinzanini M, Manni M, et al. High prevalence of peripheral neuropathy in hepatitis C virus infected patients with symptomatic and asymptomatic cryoglobulinaemia. Ital J Gastroenterol Hepatol. 1998;30:391–5.
16. De Martino L, Sampaolo S, Tucci C, et al. Viral RNA in nerve tissue of patients with hepatitis C infection and peripheral neuropathy. Muscle Nerve. 2003;27(1):102–4.
17. Younis LK, Talaat FM, Deif AH, Borei MF, Abdel Reheim SM, El Salmawy DH. Immunohistochemical detection of HCV in nerves and muscles of patients with HCV associated peripheral neuropathy and Myositis. Int J Health Sci (Qassim). 2007;1(2):195–202.
18. Mehta S, Levey JM, Bonkovsky HL. Extrahepatic manifestations of infection with hepatitis C virus. Clin Liver Dis. 2001;5:979–1008.
19. Lidove O, Maisonobe T, Servan J, Thibault V, Léger JM, Piette JC, et al. Peripheral neuropathy and hepatitis C virus infection: more than cryoglobulinemia. Rev Méd Interne. 2001;22:939–47.
20. Bonetti B, Scardoni M, Monaco S, Rizzuto N, Scarpa A. Hepatitis C virus infection of peripheral nerves in type II cryoglobulinaemia. Virchows Arch Int J Pathol. 1999;434:533–5.
21. Apartis E, Léger JM, Musset L, Gugenheim M, Cacoub P, Lyon-Caen O, et al. Peripheral neuropathy associated with essential mixed cryoglobulinaemia: a role for hepatitis C virus infection? J Neurol Neurosurg Psychiatry. 1996;60:661–6.
22. Gemignani F, Melli G, Inglese C, Marbini A. Cryoglobulinemia is a frequent cause of peripheral neuropathy in undiagnosed referral patients. J Peripher Nerv Syst JPNS. 2002;7:59–64.
23. Chin RL, Sander HW, Brannagna TH, De Sousa E, Latov N. Demyelinating neuropathy in patients with hepatitis C virus infection. J Clin Neuromuscular Disease. 2010;11(4):209–12.
24. Vishal S, Yoihenba K, Biplab Singh N, Ningshen R, Bhimo Singh T. Demyelinating neuropathy- a rare presentation of HCV infection without mixed cryoglobulinaemia. JIACM. 2016;17(1):50–3.
25. Conca P, Caffaro G, de Renzo A, Coppola A, Cimino E, Tarantino G. Successful and safe long-term standard anti-viral therapy in a patient with explosive immune response in course of HCV-related liver cirrhosis. Int J Mol Sci. 2015;16:14075–85. https://doi.org/10.3300/ijms160614075.
26. Carvalho A, Santos Garcia JB, de Sousa Furtado I. Peripheral neuropathy associated to cryoglobulinemia in patients with hepatitis C. Case report and literature review. Rev. Dor Sao Paulo. 2013;14(1):71–5.
27. Levine JW, Gota C, Fesslerb J, Calabrese LH. Peristent cryoglobulinemic vasculitis following successful treatment of hepatitis virus. The J Rheumatol. 2005;32(6):1164–7.
28. La Civita L, Zignego AL, Lombardini F, Monti M, Longombardo G, Pasero G, et al. Exacerbation of peripheral neuropathy during alpha-interferon therapy in a patient with mixed cryoglobulinemia and hepatitis B virus infection. J Rheumatol. 1996;23:1641–3.
29. Boonyapisit K, Katirji B. Severe exacerbation of hepatits C-associated vasculitic neuropathy following treatment with interferon alpha: a case report and literature review. Muscle Nerve. 2022;25.909–13.
30. Ballarè M, Bobbio F, Poggi S, Bordin G, Bertoncelli MC, Catania E, et al. A pilot study on the effectiveness of cyclosporine in type II mixed cryoglobulinemia. Clin Exp Rheumatol. 1995;13(Suppl 13):S201–3.
31. Murai H, Inaba S, Kira J, Yamamoto A, Ohno M, Goto I. Hepatitis C virus associated cryoglobulinemic neuropathy successfully treated with plasma exchange. Artif Organs. 1995;19:334–8.
32 Manns MP, Wedemeyer H, Cornberg M. Treating viral hepatitis C: efficacy, side effects, and complications. Gut. 2006;55(9):1350–9.
33 Schaefer M, Schmidt F, Folwaczny C, Lorenz R, Martin G, et al. Adherence and mental side effects during hepatitis C treatment with Interferon alfa and ribavirin in psychiatric risk groups. Hepatology. 2003;37:443 51.
34 Melzack R. The short form McGill pain questionnaire. Pain. 1987;30:191–7.
35 Naarendorp M, Kallemuchikkal U, Nuovo GJ, Gorevic PD. Longterm efficacy of interferon-alpha for extrahepatic disease associated with hepatitis C virus infection. J Rheumatol. 2001;28:2466–73.
36 Cacoub P, Lidove O, Maisonobe T, Duhaut P, Thibault V, Ghillani P, et al. Interferon-alpha and ribavirin treatment in patients with hepatitis C virus-related systemic vasculitis. Arthritis Rheum. 2002;46:3317–26.
37 Cacoub P, Saadoun D, Limal N, Sene D, Lidove O, Piette J-C. PEGylated interferon alfa-2b and ribavirin treatment in patients with hepatitis C virus-related systemic vasculitis. Arthritis Rheum. 2005;52:911–5.
38 Toyooka K, Fujimura H. Iatrogenic neuropathies. Curr Opin Neurol. 2009;22:475–9.
39 Cacoub P, Sbaï A, Hausfater P, Papo T, Gatel A, Piette JC. Central nervous system involvement in hepatitis C virus infection. Gastroentérol Clin Biol. 1998;22:631–3.
40 Dawson TM, Starkebaum G. Isolated central nervous system vasculitis associated with hepatitis C infection. J Rheumatol. 1999;26:2273–6.
41 Kamar N, Rostaing L, Alric L. Treatment of hepatitis C-virus-related glomerulonephritis. Kidney Int. 2006;69:436–9.
42 Saadoun D, Thibault V, Si Ahmed SN, Alric L, Mallet M, Guillaud C, Izzedine H, Plaisier A, Fontaine H, Costopoulos M, Le Garff-Tavernier M, Hezode C, Pol S, Musset L, Poynard T, Cacoub P. Sofosbuvir plus ribavirin for hepatitis C virus-associated cryoglobulinaemia vasculitis: VASCUVALDIC study. Ann Rheum Dis. 2016;75(10):1777–82. https://doi.org/10.1136/annrheumdis-2015-208339.
43 Shannon HE, Eberle EL, Peters SC. Comparison of the effects of anticonvulsant drugs with diverse mechanisms of action in the formalin test in rats. Neuropharmacology. 2005;48:1012–20.
44 Criscuolo S, Auletta C, Lippi S, Brogi F, Brogi A. Oxcarbazepine (Trileptal) monotherapy dramatically improves quality of life in two patients with postherpetic neuralgia refractory to carbamazepine and gabapentin. J Pain Symptom Manag. 2004;28:535–6.
45 Criscuolo S, Auletta C, Lippi S, Brogi F, Brogi A. Oxcarbazepine monotherapy in postherpetic neuralgia unresponsive to carbamazepine and gabapentin. Acta Neurol Scand. 2005;111:229–32.
46 Luef G, Poewe W. Oxcarbazepine in glossopharyngeal neuralgia: clinical response and effect on serum lipids. Neurology. 2004;63:2447–8.
47 Knodell RG, et al. Formulation and application of a numerical scoring system for assessing histological activity in asymptomatic chronic active hepatits. Hepatology. 1981;1(5):431–5.

Characterization of the hepatitis B virus DNA detected in urine of chronic hepatitis B patients

Surbhi Jain[1†], Ying-Hsiu Su[2†], Yih-Ping Su[2], Sierra McCloud[1], Ruixia Xue[3], Tai-Jung Lee[2], Shu-Chuan Lin[4], Selena Y. Lin[5], Wei Song[1,5], Jamin D. Steffen[1,6] and Chi-Tan Hu[4*]

Abstract

Background: Detection of human hepatitis B virus (HBV) DNA in the urine of patients with chronic hepatitis B infection (CHB) has been reported previously, suggesting urine could provide a potential route of horizontal HBV transmission. However, it is not clear whether the HBV DNA detected in urine is indeed full-length, infectious viral DNA. The aim of this study is to assess the potential infectivity of urine from patients with CHB and to correlate HBV DNA detection in urine with clinical parameters, such as serum viral load and HBeAg status.

Methods: Urine from 60 CHB patients with serum viral loads ranging from undetectable to 10^8 IU/mL were analyzed for HBV DNA and serum immune markers. HBV DNA was detected from total urine DNA and size-fractionated urine DNA (separated into ≤1 kb and > 1 kb fractions) by PCR analysis of six regions of the HBV genome.

Results: Twenty-seven of 59 (45.7%) patients with HBV serum viral load (≥20 IU/mL) contained at least 20 copies per mL of fragmented HBV DNA in urine detected in at least 1 of the 6 PCR assay regions. Only one patient contained HBV DNA detected by all six regions, and was found to have evidence of blood in the urine. Sixteen of 25 urine samples with high viral load (> 10^5 IU/mL) and 11 of 34 urine samples with low viral load (< 10^5 IU/mL) contained detectable HBV DNA. Twelve of 27 (44.44%) patients with detectable HBV DNA in urine were HBeAg positive, and only 5 of these HBeAg positive patients were in the group of 33 (15.15%) patients with no detectable HBV DNA in urine. By Fishers' exact test, HBV DNA in urine is significantly associated with high serum viral load ($P = 0.0197$) and HBeAg ($P = 0.0203$).

Conclusions: We conclude that urine from CHB patients with healthy kidney function should not contain full-length HBV DNA, and therefore should not be infectious.

Keywords: Hepatitis B virus, Hepatitis B virus DNA, Urine, Infection, HBV DNA PCR assays

Background

Human hepatitis B virus (HBV) infection affects primarily the liver, which can result in chronic HBV infection (CHB) and a heightened risk for cirrhosis and liver cancer. Despite the availability of a vaccine, HBV infection remains a major global health problem affecting about 240 million people worldwide [1–7]. In highly endemic areas, HBV is commonly transmitted perinatally or through horizontal transmission via exposure to infected blood. HBV can also spread by percutaneous or mucosal exposure to infected body fluids [2–8].

We have previously reported the detection of HBV DNA in the urine of patients with CHB [9] along with others [8, 10–14], suggesting urine from CHB patients could be a potential route of horizontal and nosocomial transmission. We and others have shown that urine contains fragmented DNA from circulation [9, 15–18]. Circulating cell-free DNA is known to derive from apoptosis or necrosis of host cells [17, 19–21]. It is not clear whether

* Correspondence: chitan.hu@msa.hinet.net
†Equal contributors
[4]Buddhist Tzu Chi General Hospital and Tzu Chi University, 707, Sec. 3, Chung-Yang Rd, Hualien 970, Taiwan, R.O.C.

HBV DNA detected in urine consists of the full-length 3.2 kb viral DNA (a potential indicator of infectious virus), or is merely fragmented HBV DNA derived from the infected liver. Detection of short regions of HBV DNA by PCR cannot discriminate between fragmented and full-length DNA. Therefore, a more thorough understanding of the HBV DNA detected in urine is important to better provide proper handling guidelines of urine samples from HBV infected patients.

In this study, we evaluate the nature of the DNA detected in urine from patients with CHB to assess the potential infectivity and to correlate HBV DNA detection in urine with clinical parameters, such as serum viral load and HBeAg status.

Methods

Study subjects

Urine and blood samples were obtained with written informed consents from 60 patients with CHB and were acquired under institutional review board approvals from the Buddhist Tzu Chi Medical Center in Hualien, Taiwan. Detailed patient information is provided in Table 1 and summarized in Table 2. We excluded patients with autoimmune diseases, which might have caused immune complex deposition to compromise renal filtration function.

Blood and urine analyses

Blood samples were collected immediately following urine sample collection. Sera were examined for alanine transaminase (ALT), aspartate (AST) transaminase, HBV viral load (Roche Molecular Diagnostics, USA), Hepatitis B envelope antigen (HBeAg), and Hepatitis B surface antigen (HBsAg). Alpha-fetoprotein and C-reactive protein (CRP) in blood were also determined by high sensitivity CRP (Dade Behring Inc., Marburg, Germany). The presence of antibodies directed against nuclear antigens in urine was examined using the ANA kit (Antibodies Incorporated, Davis, California). The levels of rheumatic factor were examined using the Rheumatoid Factor ELISA Kit, (Hycor Biomedical, California, United States). The levels of cryoglobulin were examined using the Cryoglobulin ELISA Kit (Cryoglobulin ELISA Kit, MyBioSource, California, United States). The levels of serum immunoglobulins were examined using the Immunoglobulin kit (Dade Behring Inc., Marburg, Germany). The levels of viral markers, including CMV IgM and IgG, EB-VCA IgM and IgG, EBEA and EBNA, and HSV IgM were examined using the Euroimmun ELISA kit (Euroimmun, Luebeck, Germany). The presence of red blood cells in urine was confirmed by examination under the microscope.

Urine collection, DNA isolation, and low molecular weight urine DNA fractionation

Freshly collected urine was immediately mixed with 0.5 mol/L EDTA, pH 8.0, to a final concentration of 10 mmol/L EDTA and stored at − 20 °C. Total urine DNA was isolated by adding an equal volume of 6 mol/L guanidine thiocyanate (Sigma, St. Louis, MO) to thawed urine as described previously [17]. The fractionated high molecular weight (HMW) urine DNA (> 1 kb) and low molecular weight (LMW) urine DNA (≤1 kb) was obtained from total urine DNA using carboxylated magnetic beads (Agentcourt Bioscience Corporation, Beverly, MA), as previously described [22].

Quantification of DNA

HBV DNA was quantified using the HBV DNA quantification kit (JBS Science, Inc. Doylestown, PA) according to the manufacturer's specifications. The schematic diagram of the region of each PCR assay used in this study in the HBV genome is illustrated in Fig. 1. The HBV DNA quantification kit (JBS Science Inc., Doylestown, PA) consists of five quantitative PCR assays that provide quantification of four different regions of the HBV genome (NC_003977·1): The HBV polymerase /Surface antigen (pol/S, nt. 246–309 and nt. 49–265), HBV DR2/X (nt. 1633–1680), HBV DR1/X (nt. 1741–1791), and HBV core (nt. 2294–2347). Note the limit of detection (LOD) is 10 copies per reaction for HBV pol/S (nt. 246–309), DR2/X, DR1/X, and HBV core assays, and 50 copies per reaction for the HBV pol/S (nt. 49–265) assay, as determined by the standards per manufacturer's specification. The existence of DNA containing 709 bp of the HBV pol/X region (nt. 1108–1816) was determined by an end-point PCR assay. The end-point PCR reactions were set up with 1 × Qiagen PCR buffer, 250 μM deoxyribonucleotide triphosphate mix, 1.0 μmol/L primers (F:TTCTCGCCAACTTACAAGGC, R:AAAAAGTTG-CATGGTGCTG), Hotstart Taq Polymerase Plus (Qiagen, Valencia, CA), at 95 °C for 5 min, then (95 °C for 30 s, 56 °C for 30 s, 72 °C for 30 s) for 40 cycles. The input of isolated DNA for each assay was from 0.5 mL urine and was performed in duplicate. Quantification of human genomic DNA was carried out using the *TP53* DNA quantification assay as described previously [18].

Statistical analysis

The association of HBV DNA in urine with serum viral load and HBeAg were analyzed by Fisher's exact test. Kruskal-Wallis test was performed to determine the correlation between urinary HBV DNA and age, gender, and AST or ALT levels. All statistical tests were performed using SPSS Statistics 20 (IBM, Armonk, NY) and QuickCals (GraphPad Software, La Jolla, CA).

Table 1 Detailed clinicopathological characteristics of the patient population

Sample ID	Age	Gender	Liver Disease	Serum Analysis							Urine analysis		Any known kidney disease	Anti-viral therapy
				HBV viral load category	HBV viral Load (IU/mL)	HBeAg (+/–)	HBsAg (+/–)	AST (IU/L)	ALT (IU/L)	AFP (ng/ml)	RBC/ High power field	Urine albumin (mg/dL)		
1	29	F	Cirrhosis	High	1.70E + 08	+	+	44	36	< 1.3	2~ 5	30	–	No
2	36	F	CHB	High	1.70E + 08	+	+	20	17	1.7	0	–	CKD	No
3	32	M	CHB	High	1.70E + 08	+	+	33	64	1.3	0~ 2	–	–	No
4	41	F	Cirrhosis	High	1.34E + 08	–	+	191	126	5.8	2~ 5	–	–	Yes
5	52	F	CHB	High	6.07E + 07	+	+	23	21	4	0~ 2	10	FSGS,CGN	No
6	52	M	Cirrhosis	High	5.81E + 07	+	+	109	48	81	0~ 2	–	–	Yes
7	68	F	Cirrhosis	High	4.57E + 07	+	+	73	38	3.6	2~ 5	200	–	Yes
8	29	F	CHB	High	4.53E + 07	+	+	48	60	1.8	0~ 2	–	–	No
9	32	M	CHB	High	4.13E + 07	+	+	394	921	16.4	0~ 2	–	–	Yes
10	22	M	CHB	High	3.04E + 07	+	+	160	556	5.2	0	–	–	No
11	54	M	CHB	High	1.44E + 07	–	+	24	25	2.8	0	–	–	No
12	72	F	CHB	High	3.89E + 06	–	+	58	62	35.1	0~ 2	–	–	No
13	59	M	CHB	High	1.78E + 06	–	+	69	97	4.3	0~ 2	–	–	No
14	65	M	CHB	High	1.37E + 06	–	+	60	110	5	0~ 2	–	–	No
15	60	F	CHB	High	8.30E + 05	–	+	171	242	2.8	0~ 2	–	–	Yes
16	42	M	CHB	High	7.47E + 05	–	+	22	24	< 1.3	2~ 5	–	–	Yes
17	55	F	CHB	High	7.25E + 05	+	+	299	424	7.4	0~ 2	–	–	Yes
18	60	M	Cirrhosis	High	4.17E + 05	–	+	64	63	32.8	0~ 2	–	–	No
19	36	M	CHB	High	3.38E + 05	+	+	34	50	4.2	2~ 5	10	–	Yes
20	60	F	CHB	High	3.19E + 05	–	+	99	124	2.6	0~ 2	–	–	No
21	41	M	CHB	High	2.10E + 05	–	+	89	207	6.5	0	–	–	No
22	48	M	CHB	High	1.67E + 05	–	+	31	35	< 1.3	0	–	–	No
23	63	F	CHB	High	1.48E + 05	–	+	43	30	1.9	0~ 2	–	–	No
24	65	F	HCC	High	1.08E + 05	+	+	186	95	2623.1	0~ 2	–	–	No
25	62	M	CHB	High	1.02E + 05	–	+	27	39	3.4	0~ 2	–	–	No
26	48	F	CHB	Low	9.31E + 04	–	+	28	31	3.3	0~ 2	–	–	No
27	46	M	CHB	Low	4.85E + 04	–	+	33	53	2.1	0	–	–	No
28	67	F	CHB	Low	3.93E + 04	–	+	38	27	5	0	–	–	No
29	52	M	CHB	Low	3.82E + 04	–	+	32	37	4.1	0~ 2	–	–	No
30	75	F	CHB	Low	2.75E + 04	–	+	41	30	3.4	2~ 5	–	–	Yes
31	31	M	CHB	Low	2.65E + 04	+	+	38	57	< 1.3	0	–	–	Yes

Table 1 Detailed clinicopathological characteristics of the patient population *(Continued)*

Sample ID	Age	Gender	Liver Disease	Serum Analysis							Urine analysis		Any known kidney disease	Anti-viral therapy
				HBV viral load category	HBV viral Load (IU/mL)	HBeAg (+/−)	HBsAg (+/−)	AST (IU/L)	ALT (IU/L)	AFP (ng/ml)	RBC/ High power field	Urine albumin (mg/dL)		
32	44	M	Cirrhosis	Low	1.74E + 04	+	+	72	95	2.4	> 100	70	–	No
33	48	F	CHB	Low	1.65E + 04	–	+	22	22	< 1.3	0	–	–	No
34	54	M	CHB	Low	1.49E + 04	–	+	40	52	< 1.3	0~ 2	10	–	No
35	51	F	CHB	Low	1.01E + 04	–	+	36	22	1.4	2~ 5	–	NA	No
36	48	M	CHB	Low	9.68E + 03	–	+	38	30	6.7	0~ 2	600	–	No
37	53	F	CHB	Low	6.40E + 03	–	+	46	81	2.1	0~ 2	–	–	No
38	59	M	CHB	Low	4.36E + 03	–	+	44	25	2.1	0~ 2	–	–	Yes
39	46	M	CHB	Low	4.08E + 03	–	+	27	35	5.2	0	–	–	No
40	18	M	CHB	Low	3.18E + 03	+	+	45	78	1.6	0~ 2	10	–	No
41	57	M	CHB	Low	3.00E + 03	–	+	29	38	3.5	0~ 2	–	–	Yes
42	57	F	Cirrhosis	Low	2.93E + 03	–	+	33	44	1.4	0~ 2	–	–	No
43	28	M	CHB	Low	2.68E + 03	–	+	35	48	21.4	0~ 2	30	–	No
44	47	M	CHB	Low	2.42E + 03	–	+	42	82	2.1	2~ 5	10	–	No
45	64	F	CHB	Low	2.24E + 03	–	+	58	67	3.9	0~ 2	–	–	No
46	58	M	CHB	Low	2.02E + 03	–	+	26	28	< 1.3	0~ 2	20	–	No
47	43	F	CHB	Low	1.83E + 03	–	–	26	26	6.2	2~ 5	–	–	No
48	56	F	CHB	Low	1.50E + 03	–	+	26	23	2.4	0~ 2	–	–	No
49	33	F	CHB	Low	1.49E + 03	–	+	28	42	3.2	0~ 2	–	–	No
50	56	F	CHB	Low	1.25E + 03	–	+	34	67	2.6	2~ 5	–	–	Yes
51	38	M	CHB	Low	1.17E + 03	–	+	43	91	5	0~ 2	–	–	No
52	38	M	CHB	Low	1.09E + 03	–	+	38	77	2.4	0~ 2	10	–	No
53	61	M	CHB	Low	1.07E + 03	–	+	26	30	2.1	0~ 2	–	–	No
54	51	M	CHB	Low	1.06E + 03	–	+	21	27	2.8	0	–	–	No
55	28	F	CHB	Low	3.41E + 02	–	+	36	32	2.7	0~ 2	–	–	Yes
56	34	M	CHB	Low	5.40E + 01	–	+	32	53	2.4	0	–	–	Yes
57	36	M	CHB	Low	3.20E + 01	+	+	116	98	3.5	2~ 5	50	–	Yes
58	69	M	HCC	Low	2.00E + 01	–	+	45	21	5060.9	> 100	30	–	No
59	40	M	CHB	Low	2.00E + 01	–	–	41	65	3.8	0	–	–	Yes
60	38	M	CHB	Low	< 20	–	+	46	57	7.7	0~ 2	–	–	Yes

F female, *M* male, *CHB* Chronic hepatitis B infection, *NA* Data not available, *CKD* chronic kidney disease, *FSGS* focal segmental glomerulosclerosis, *CGN* chronic glomerulonephritis
For all patients who received antiviral treatment, the drug received was "Telbivudine," which has no known renal side effects

Table 2 Summary of clinicopathological characteristics of the patient population

Mean Age ± Std Dev (years)	48.45 ± 13.33
Gender (M/F)	35/25
Liver disease (Chronic Hepatitis B/ HBV Cirrhosis/ HBV-HCC)	51/7/2
Serum viral load (Range, IU/L)	< 20–1.7 E+08
HBeAg (Positive/Negative)	17/43
HBsAg (Positive/Negative)	58/2
Mean AST levels ± Std Dev (IU/L)	62.2 ± 66.85
Mean ALT levels ± Std Dev (IU/L)	86.75 ± 141.29
Antiviral therapy (Yes/No)	18/42

Results

Characterization of the study population

Previous studies have suggested that highly viremic HBV carriers may have high titers of HBV DNA in body fluids other than blood, such as urine [13, 14]. In order to investigate whether urine from patients with high viremia contains infectious HBV, we analyzed 25 urine samples from patients that have viral loads ranging from 10^5 to 10^8 IU/mL, designated as the "high viral load" group. In addition, we analyzed urine from 35 CHB patients whose viral loads were below 10^5 IU/mL, designated as the "low viral load" group, as summarized in Table 1 (listed in descending order of their serum HBV viral load). Interestingly, Sample ID #59 was negative for surface antigen with a serum viral load of 20 IU/mL, suggesting an occult HBV infection. The clinicopathological characteristics of the patient population are summarized in Table 2. The mean age of the study population was 48.8 years (SD ± 13.2), consisting of 35 males and 25 females. Seven of the 60 CHB patients had Child Pugh A liver cirrhosis, and two of them were known to have hepatocellular carcinoma. Biomarkers with tested values above the normal range (positive) for any individual in this study cohort are included in Table 1. Immune disease markers (Antinuclear antibody, Rheumatic factor, Cryoglobulin, IgM, IgA, IgE, IgG and IgG4), viral markers (CMV IgM and IgG, EB-VCA IgM and IgG, EBEA and EBNA, HSV IgM) and inflammatory marker (C-reactive protein) were found to be negative in all patients of this study cohort, which suggests this study population has no individual with detectable immune complex deposition.

Detection of HBV DNA in urine of patients with chronic hepatitis B

We employed five quantitative PCR (qPCR) assays and one end-point PCR assay for four different regions of the HBV genome (Fig. 1 and Additional file 1). Our hypothesis was that if the HBV DNA in urine is full-length (3.2 kb genome), any HBV PCR assay should be able to produce amplified product predominantly in both total urine DNA and size-fractionated HMW DNA (> 1 kb). In contrast, if the HBV DNA detected is mostly fragmented, it should be detected predominantly in both total urine DNA and size-fractionated LMW DNA (≤1 kb).

We first performed the five HBV quantitative PCR assays on total urine DNA from all 60 CHB patients. For samples positive for HBV DNA by at least 3 assays, we performed an end-point PCR assay that generates a much larger amplicon (709 bp) in the HBV polymerase/X region (nt. 1108–1816). For samples detecting HBV DNA by at least 1 assay, we performed a fractionation of the total urine DNA into HMW and LMW urine DNA. Both fractions were then retested to determine if the HBV detected was of a full-length or fragmented nature. To control for the amount of DNA in urine, the total DNA was quantified by the *TP53* gene, as described previously [18]. The results are organized into four

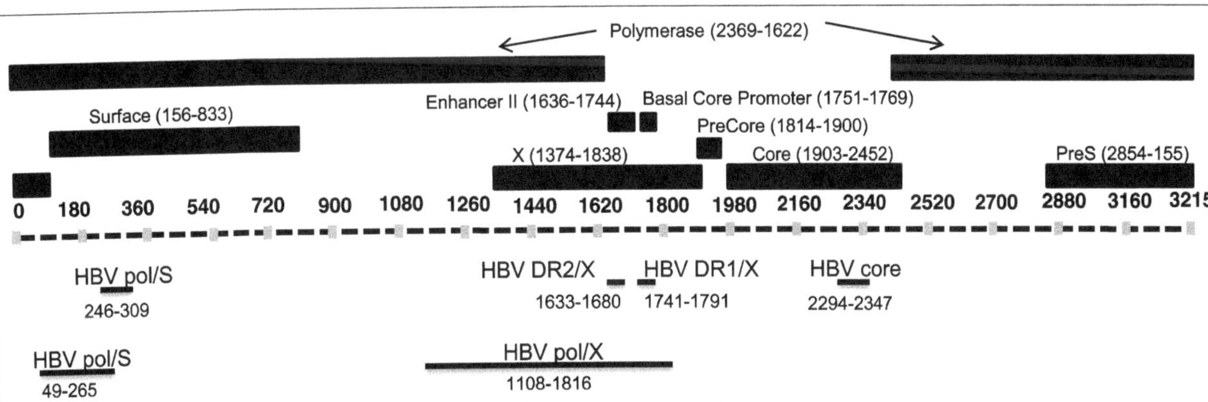

Fig. 1 Diagram of the HBV genome (NC_003977.1), indicating location of primers and the amplicons generated by qPCR assays in this study. Black rectangles represent the following HBV regions: polymerase, enhancer II, basal core promoter, precore, Surface, X, Core, and pre-S gene. These regions correspond to the dashed line representing the HBV genome with vertical gray bars indicating nucleotide location. The black lines below this HBV genome map indicate the amplicon location of each qPCR assay used in the study. The name of the region targeted by the qPCR assay is written above the black line and the exact location of the amplicon is indicated below the black line

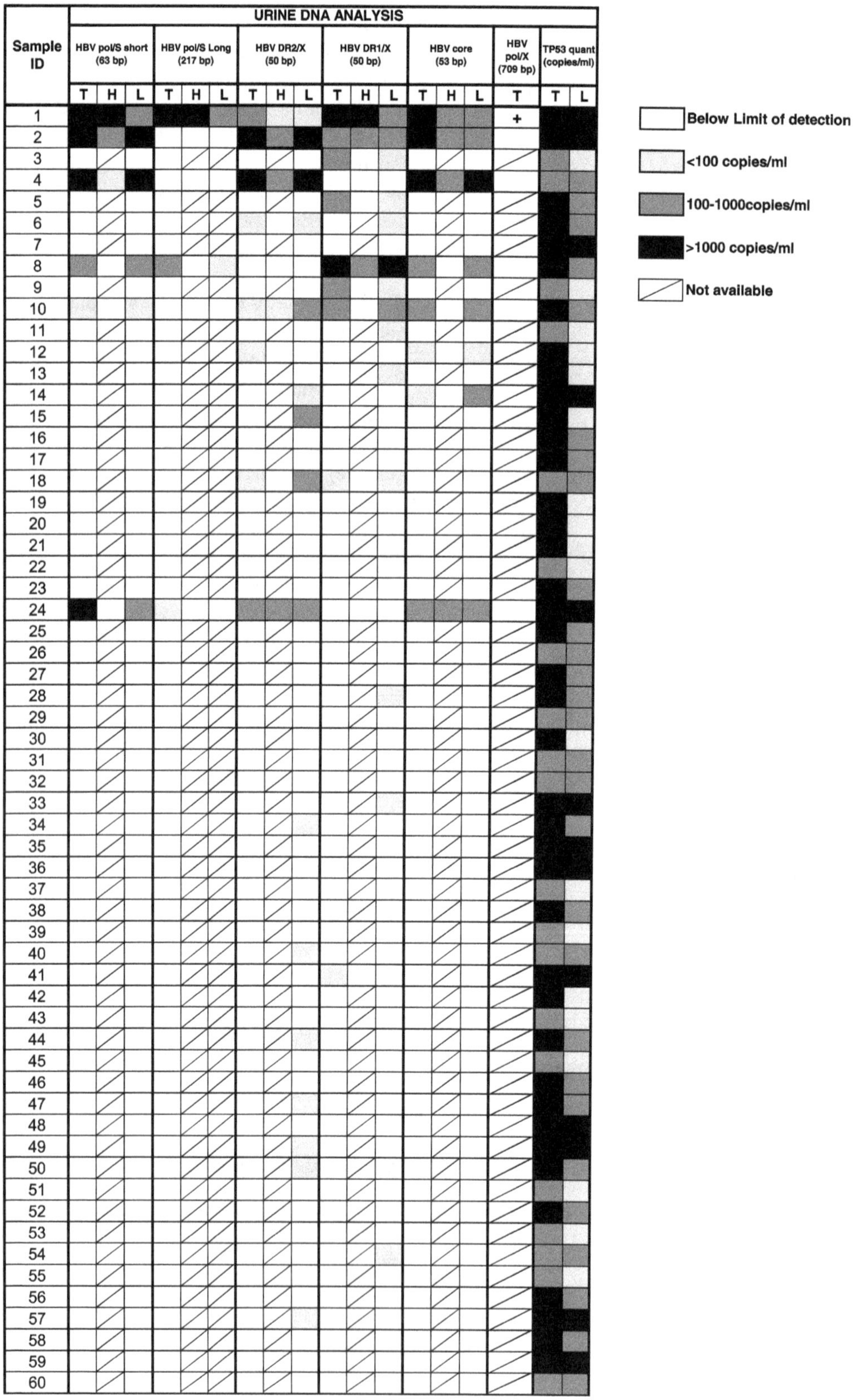

Fig. 2 (See legend on next page.)

(See figure on previous page.)
Fig. 2 Summary of urine DNA analysis by PCR assays targeting multiple locations in the HBV genome. The amount of DNA detected is indicated by patterned boxes as follows: empty box: below the limit of detection; light gray box: less than 100 copies/ml; dark gray box: 100–1000 copies/ml; black box: greater than 1000 copies/ml; box with a slash: Not available, the assay was not run. T: Total urine DNA, H: High molecular weight urine DNA fraction, L: low molecular weight urine DNA fraction

categories based on the quantities of DNA detected in Fig. 2 (illustrated by four patterns).

Thirteen of the 60 patient urine samples tested (Pt. IDs: 1–6, 8–10, 12, 14, 18, and 24) contained detectable HBV DNA in total urine DNA. Six of these patients (Pt. IDs: 1, 2, 4, 8, 10, and 24) contained HBV DNA detected by at least three of the five HBV DNA qPCR assays and only one (Pt. ID #1) produced the 709 bp PCR product, suggesting that the urine from this patient contained full-length HBV DNA. The HBV DNA in the remaining 12 patients is likely all fragmented, unless the amount of full-length DNA is below the limit of detection (20 copies per mL of urine).

To further investigate the size of the HBV DNA detected in the total urine DNA, we performed HBV DNA analysis in both fractionated HMW DNA and LMW DNA. As expected, only the HMW DNA from Pt. ID #1 was found to contain HBV DNA detected by all six assays, including the end-point PCR assay generating a 709 bp PCR product. Note, this patient contained very high serum viral load (10^8 IU/mL) and her clinicopathological information of hematuria and albuminuria (red blood cells and serum albumin in urine) indicated a compromised renal barrier with contamination of blood in urine. Data obtained from the analysis of total urine DNA indicated that fragmented HBV DNA was unevenly distributed across the HBV genome. Among these 13 samples, HBV DNA was detected in: The pol/S region (63 bp amplicon) for six patients, the pol/S region (217 bp amplicon) for three patients, the DR2/X region for eight patients, the DR1/X region for nine patients, and the core region for eight patients.

We and other have shown that the targeted DNA sequence is more readily detectable by PCR when the background DNA in the reaction is reduced [17, 22–26]. Since most of the detectable HBV DNA in urine is less than 1 kb, it was of interest to determine if HBV DNA could be detected in the urine of patients with low serum viral loads, or below the limit of detection in total urine DNA. Hence, total urine DNA from the remaining 47 patients was fractionated to obtain LMW DNA fraction and subjected to the four short (< 100 bp) HBV DNA assays. From this, an additional nine urine samples were found to contain HBV DNA specific for the DR2/X region and six samples specific for the DR1/X assay (Fig. 2).

Association between urine HBV DNA and clinicopathological variables

HBV DNA was detected in the serum from 59 of the 60 CHB patients. Sixteen of 25 urine samples with high viral load (> 10^5 IU/mL) and 11 of 34 urine samples with low viral load (< 10^5 IU/mL) contained detectable HBV DNA in urine. By Fisher's exact test, HBV DNA in urine is significantly associated with high serum viral load ($P = 0.0197$). Fifty-eight of the 60 patients in this study were HBsAg positive and 17 of 60 were HBeAg positive. Twelve of 27 (44.44%) patients with detectable HBV DNA in urine were HBeAg positive as compared to only 5 of 33 (15.15%) patients with no detectable HBV DNA in urine that were HBeAg positive, suggesting a significant association between active viral replication and HBV DNA in urine by Fisher's exact test ($P = 0.0203$). Twelve of 17 (70.58%) of HBeAg positive patients had detectable HBV DNA in urine, whereas only 15 of 43 (34.88%) HBeAg negative patients had detectable HBV DNA in urine. There was no correlation between urinary HBV DNA and age, gender, or AST and ALT levels by Kruskal-Wallis test ($P > 0.05$). While one patient with full length HBV DNA had hematuria and albuminuria, not every patient with compromised kidney barrier/function had detectable HBV DNA in their urine. Statistical analysis was performed using a Mann Whitney U test to assess the association between the number of HBV DNA fragments detected (5 regions of the HBV genome) and liver pathology (51 chronic hepatitis B, 7 cirrhosis). The 2 samples from HCC patients were not included in this analysis. We found no statistically significant liver disease association ($p = 0.170$) with the number of HBV DNA fragments detected.

Discussion

This study investigated the integrity of HBV DNA in the urine of 60 CHB patients, (including 11 of 60 patients with serum viral loads in a range of 10^7–10^8 IU/mL), by employing 6 different PCR assays that target unique regions of the viral genome. Only one patient (ID #1), with an indication of compromised renal barrier (and blood in the urine), was thought likely to contain full-length HBV DNA in the urine. In the remaining patients with detectable HBV DNA in the urine, the DNA was found to be fragmented. We thus conclude that urine from CHB patients with healthy kidney function should not contain full-length HBV DNA, and therefore should not be infectious. To our knowledge this is the first study to investigate the integrity of HBV DNA in a comprehensive manner by examining multiple locations of the HBV genome.

While there are other methods available for detection of HBV virus (such as southern blot or protein analysis), we chose a PCR approach because it is the most sensitive method available. Since we were unable to detect full-length HBV DNA by PCR, less sensitive methods are unlikely to detect intact, infectious viral particles. Although HBV susceptible cell lines (such as HepG2-NTCP cells) are available for direct infectivity testing with cell culture derived virus, they require high multiplicity of infection (MOI > 100) [27, 28]. It has been reported that serum-derived virus is difficult to infect NTCP cells for unknown reasons. For urine samples that are negative for full-length HBV DNA by PCR (with a limit of detection of 20 copies per mL of urine), sufficient levels of virus are simply not available to accurately test cell-culture infectivity. Thus, the infectivity assay was not performed in this study.

Viruria (virus in urine) has only been suggested in viral infections of kidney cells, such as cytomegaloviruses [29], coxsackie viruses [30], adenoviruses [31] etc [32]. Hence, it is not surprising that the full-length HBV virus was is not detected in the urine of the CHB patients, even when serum viral loads reach 10^8 IU/mL, unless there is blood contamination or compromised kidney function. Interestingly, case ID's #2 and #5 showed impaired renal structure with high serum viral load but no sign of blood contamination, which seems to suggest that blood contamination might be the source of full-length HBV DNA detectable in the urine of Pt. ID #1. Urine from Pt. ID #32 (with a serum viral load of 1.7×10^4 IU/mL) and Pt. ID #58 (with a serum viral load of 20 IU/mL) were also contaminated with blood, but no HBV DNA was detected in urine suggesting that high serum viral load might be necessary to have full-length HBV DNA detected above the limit of detection in urine.

According to Knutsson et al. [11], HBV DNA was detected (by PCR) in serum from 46 of 56 CHB patients (82%) and in urine from 28 of 56 patients (50%). Most HBeAg (+) patients had HBV DNA detectable in urine (91%). Robert et al [14] detected HBV DNA from urine in 32% (47/147) of patients with CHB and in 60% (39/65) with HBeAg positive status. In addition to PCR detection, molecular hybridization methods have been used to detect HBV DNA from urine in about 55% of chronic HBV cases that are positive for HBeAg [12]. In the present study, we found that 45% (27/59) of CHB patients with detectable HBV in serum contained detectable HBV DNA in urine. Similar to previous studies [11, 12, 14], 70.58% (12/17) of HBeAg positive patients had detectable HBV DNA in urine, suggesting that active viral replication is associated with HBV DNA in urine.

Interestingly, the HBV DR2 ($n = 17$) and DR1 ($n = 15$) regions were more frequently detected (of the HBV qPCR assays) as compared to the pol/S ($n = 6$) and core region ($n = 8$) of the HBV genome. One would expect a similar frequency of detection regardless the region of the genome if fragmentation of the DNA were random. Our data suggest that the fragmentation of the genome or preservation of the fragmented HBV DNA could be different from region to region. Our previous studies have suggested the LMW DNA in urine is mostly derived from circulation and from cells undergoing cell death. Most of the HBV DNA detected in urine is also detected in the LMW DNA fraction, which suggests the HBV DNA detected in urine is predominantly cell-free DNA likely derived from apoptotic, infected hepatocytes.

Conclusions

In conclusion, this study of HBV DNA integrity in urine suggests that urine is likely not infectious, except in cases of compromised renal structure or blood contamination. Although an infectivity study was not conducted here, the absence of detectable, full-length HBV genomic DNA in urine suggests the risk of HBV infection from urine is very unlikely. This is of particular importance for infection control guidelines to prevent HBV transmission.

Abbreviations

ALT: alanine transaminase; AST: aspartate transaminase; CHB: Chronic HBV infection; CRP: C-reactive protein; HBeAg: Hepatitis B envelope antigen; HBsAg: Hepatitis B surface antigen; HBV: Hepatitis B virus; HMW: HIgh molecular weight; LMW: Low molecular weight; qPCR: Quantitative PCR

Acknowledgements

Not applicable.

Funding

This study is funded by R43CA192507 from the NIH. The funding body has no role in the design of the study and collection, analysis, and interpretation of data and in writing the manuscript.

Authors' contributions

Y-HS, WS, and C-TH conceived the study; SJ, Y-PS, McCloud S, Xue R, Lee TJ, Lin SC, Lin SY and Hu CT generated the data; Jain S, Su YH, Su YP, McCloud S, Song W, Steffen JD and Hu CT analyzed the data; All authors contributed to writing and/or revising the manuscript. All authors read and approved the final manuscript.

Consent for publication

Not applicable.

Competing interests

Jain S, McCloud S and Steffen JD are employees of JBS Science, Inc. Song W is a stockholder of JBS Science, Inc. Steffen JD is an employee of Hepron Molecular Lab, Inc. All other authors have no conflicts of interest.

Author details

[1]JBS Science, Inc., Doylestown, PA 18902, USA. [2]The Baruch S. Blumberg Institute, Doylestown, PA 18902, USA. [3]The Second Hospital of Yuncheng,

Yuncheng, Shanxi Province 044000, China. [4]Buddhist Tzu Chi General Hospital and Tzu Chi University, 707, Sec. 3, Chung-Yang Rd, Hualien 970, Taiwan, R.O.C.. [5]U-Screen Dx Inc., Doylestown, PA 18902, USA. [6]Hepron Molecular Lab, Inc., Doylestown, PA 18902, USA.

References

1. Di Bisceglie AM. Hepatitis B and hepatocellular carcinoma. Hepatology. 2009;49(S5):S56–60.
2. Pungpapong S, Kim W, Poterucha JJ. Natural history of hepatitis B virus infection: an update for clinicians. In: Mayo Clinic Proceedings. Elsevier; 2007;82(8):967–75.
3. El-Serag HB. Epidemiology of viral hepatitis and hepatocellular carcinoma. Gastroenterology. 2012;142(6):1264–73. e1261
4. Lavanchy D. Hepatitis B virus epidemiology, disease burden, treatment, and current and emerging prevention and control measures. J Viral Hepat. 2004; 11(2):97–107.
5. World Health Organization. Hepatitis B (Fact Sheet No. 204). 2017. http://www.who.int/mediacentre/factsheets/fs204/en/. Accessed 9 Mar 2018.
6. Elgouhari HM, TIA-r T, Carey WD. Hepatitis B virus infection: understanding its epidemiology, course, and diagnosis. Cleve Clin J Med. 2008;75(12):881–9.
7. Lok AS, McMahon BJ. Chronic hepatitis B. Hepatology. 2007;45(2):507–39.
8. Komatsu H, Inui A, Sogo T, Tateno A, Shimokawa R, Fujisawa T. Tears from children with chronic hepatitis B virus (HBV) infection are infectious vehicles of HBV transmission: experimental transmission of HBV by tears, using mice with chimeric human livers. J Infect Dis. 2012;206(4):478–85.
9. Lin SY, Jain S, Song W, Hu C-T, Su Y-H. Strategic assay developments for detection of HBV 1762T/1764A double mutation in urine of patients with HBV-associated hepatocellular carcinomas. InTech Hepatocellular Carcinoma - Clinical Research. 2012. p. 139-54. ISBN 978-953-51-0112-3.
10. Davison F, Alexander GJ, Trowbridge R, Fagan EA, Williams R. Detection of hepatitis B virus DNA in spermatozoa, urine, saliva and leucocytes, of chronic HBsAg carriers. J Hepatol. 1987;4(1):37–44.
11. Knutsson M, Kidd-Ljunggren K. Urine from chronic hepatitis B virus carriers: implications for infectivity. J Med Virol. 2000;60(1):17–20.
12. Karayiannis P, Novick DM, Lok AS, Fowler MJ, Monjardino J, Thomas HC. Hepatitis B virus DNA in saliva, urine, and seminal fluid of carriers of hepatitis B e antigen. Br Med J (Clin Res Ed). 1985;290(6485):1853–5.
13. Kidd-Ljunggren K, Holmberg A, Bläckberg J, Lindqvist B. High levels of hepatitis B virus DNA in body fluids from chronic carriers. J Hosp Infect. 2006;64(4):352–7.
14. van der Eijk AA, Niesters HGM, Hansen BE, Pas SD, Richardus JH, Mostert M, Janssen HLA, Schalm SW, de Man RA. Paired, quantitative measurements of hepatitis B virus DNA in saliva, urine and serum of chronic hepatitis B patients. Eur J Gastroenterol Hepatol. 2005;17(11):1173–9.
15. Song BP, Jain S, Lin SY, Chen Q, Block TM, Song W, Brenner DE, Su Y-H. Detection of hypermethylated vimentin in urine of patients with colorectal cancer. J Mol Diagn. 2012;14(2):112–9.
16. Su YH, Wang M, Brenner DE, Norton PA, Block TM. Detection of mutated K-ras DNA in urine, plasma, and serum of patients with colorectal carcinoma or adenomatous polyps. Ann N Y Acad Sci. 2008;1137(1):197–206.
17. Su YH, Wang M, Brenner DE, Ng A, Melkonyan H, Umansky S, Syngal S, Block TM. Human urine contains small, 150 to 250 nucleotide-sized, soluble DNA derived from the circulation and may be useful in the detection of colorectal cancer. J Mol Diagn. 2004;6(2):101–7.
18. Lin SY, Dhillon V, Jain S, Chang T-T, Hu C-T, Lin Y-J, Chen S-H, Yu L, Block TM, Su Y-H. A locked nucleic acid clamp-mediated PCR assay for detection of a p53 codon 249 hotspot mutation in urine. J Mol Diagn. 2011;13(5):474–84.
19. Lichtenstein AV, Melkonyan HS, Tomei D, Umansky SR. Circulating nucleic acids and apoptosis. Ann N Y Acad Sci. 2001;945:239–49.
20. Chan AKC, Chiu RWK, Lo YMD. Cell-free nucleic acids in plasma, serum and urine: a new tool in molecular diagnosis. Ann Clin Biochem. 2003;40(2):122–30.
21. Diaz LA, Bardelli A. Liquid biopsies: genotyping circulating tumor DNA. J Clin Oncol. 2014;32(6):579–86.
22. Su Y-H, Song J, Wang Z, Wang X, Wang M, Brenner DE, Block TM. Removal of high molecular weight DNA by carboxylated magnetic beads enhances the detection of mutated K-ras DNA in urine. Ann N Y Acad Sci. 2008;1137:82–91.
23. Sikora A, Zimmermann G, Rusterholz C, Birri D, Kolla V, Lapaire O, Hoesli I, Kiefer V, Jackson L, Hahn S. Detection of increased amounts of cell-free fetal DNA with short PCR amplicons. Clin Chem. 2010;56(1):136–8.
24. Chan KCA, Leung SF, Yeung SW, Chan ATC, Lo YMD. Quantitative analysis of the transrenal excretion of circulating EBV DNA in nasopharyngeal carcinoma patients. Clin Cancer Res. 2008;14(15):4809–13.
25. Su YH, Wang M, Block TM, Landt O, Botezatu I, Serdyuk O, Lichtenstein A, Melkonyan H, Tomei D, Umansky S. Transrenal DNA as a diagnostic tool: important technical notes. Ann N Y Acad Sci. 2004;1022(1):81–9.
26. Shekhtman EM, Anne K, Melkonyan HS, Robbins DJ, Warsof SL, Umansky SR. Optimization of transrenal DNA analysis: detection of fetal DNA in maternal urine. Clin Chem. 2009;55(4):723–9.
27. Verrier ER, Colpitts CC, Schuster C, Zeisel MB, Baumert TF. Cell culture models for the investigation of hepatitis B and D virus infection. Viruses. 2016;8(9):261.
28. Witt-Kehati D, Bitton Alaluf M, Shlomai A. Advances and challenges in studying hepatitis B virus in vitro. Viruses. 2016;8(1):21.
29. Weller TH, Neva FA. Propagation in tissue culture of cytopathic agents from patients with rubella-like illness. Proc Soc Exp Biol Med. 1962;111(1):215–25.
30. JP U, CF S. Mumps III. Comparison of methods for detection of viruria. Proc Soc Exp Biol Med. 1962;110:841–4.
31. Gutekunst RR, Heggie AD. Viremia and Viruria in adenovirus infections. N Engl J Med. 1961;264(8):374–8.
32. Virus in urine. Br Med J. 1967;1(5533):126–6.

18

Case report: lactic acidosis and rhabdomyolysis during telbivudine and tenofovir treatment for chronic hepatitis B

Yue Ying[†], Yue-Kai Hu[†], Jia-Lin Jin, Ji-Ming Zhang, Wen-Hong Zhang and Yu-Xian Huang[*]

Abstract

Background: Current treatment options for chronic hepatitis B (CHB) are pegylated interferon alpha and nucleoside analogues (NAs). NAs have relatively fewer side effects than interferon alpha, and generally well tolerated. Previously 12.9% of patients on telbivudine treatment were reported to develop severe elevation of serum creatine phosphokinase (CPK) levels, but related clinical disease, like lactic acidosis (LA) and rhabdomyolysis (RM) were rare. The pathophysiology may be mitochondrial toxicity, for the NAs inhibit not only hepatitis B virus (HBV) polymerase, but also the host mitochondrial DNA polymerase γ. As mitochondria are the main sites of oxidative phosphorylation, there will be an increase of pyruvate reduction to lactic acid and insufficient adenosine triphosphate. The accumulation of lactic acid causes LA, while lack of energy leads to cell dysfunction and mitochondria-associated disease, including RM. All five NAs, except tenofovir, have been reported causing LA and RM. Here we report the first case of CHB patients developing fatal LA and RM during telbivudine and tenofovir treatment.

Case presentation: The patient is a 51-year-old man who was hospitalized in November 2015. He had taken telbivudine regularly because of CHB. Later, tenofovir was added to antiviral treatment because of HBV resistance. Then he had myalgia, chest tightness and anorexia. The blood lactate was 12.7 mmol/L. The arterial blood gas analysis showed pH 7.25, base excess 21.1 mmol/L. CPK was 991 U/L, myoglobin was 1745 ng/ml and creatine was 83 μmol/L. Abdomen magnetic resonance revealed cirrhosis. Muscle biopsy revealed myogenic lesion with abnormality of mitochondria and fat metabolism. The patient was diagnosed with Hepatitis B envelope Antigen positive CHB, cirrhosis, LA and RM characterized by myalgia and elevated myoglobin. He was given tenofovir alone as antiviral treatment instead. After hemodialysis and 4 weeks` treatment of corticosteroids, his symptoms recovered, and blood lactate gradually returned to a normal range.

Conclusions: This case shows that tenofovir may trigger muscle damage and fatal RM in combination with telbivudine treatment in CHB patients. Thus, patients receiving tenofovir and telbivudine should be closely monitored for muscular abnormalities, blood lactate level and other mitochondrial toxicity associated side effects.

Keywords: Lactic acidosis, Rhabdomyolysis, Mitochondrial toxicity, Myopathy, Telbivudine, Tenofovir

Background

Current treatment options for chronic hepatitis B (CHB) are pegylated interferon alpha and nucleoside analogues (NAs) including telbivudine. These agents suppress hepatitis B virus (HBV) DNA effectively so that significantly decreasing the risk of hepatocellular carcinoma. NAs have relatively fewer side effects than interferon alpha, and generally well tolerated [1]. Infrequent but serious adverse events have been reported in clinical trials and post-marketing surveillance in individual cases. Previously 12.9% of patients on telbivudine treatment developing severe elevation of serum creatine phosphokinase (CPK) levels [2], but lactic acidosis (LA) and rhabdomyolysis (RM) were rare. These two diseases may due to the same pathophysiology: mitochondrial toxicity. The NAs inhibit HBV polymerase and also have a low level of activity against the host mitochondrial DNA polymerase γ, leading to impaired replication with

* Correspondence: yxhuang@fudan.edu.cn
[†]Equal contributors
Department of Infectious Diseases, Huashan Hospital Affiliated to Fudan University, 12, Middle Wulumuqi Road, Shanghai 200040, China

mitochondrial loss or dysfunction. As mitochondria are the main sites of oxidative phosphorylation, there will be an increase of pyruvate reduction to lactic acid and insufficient ATP. The accumulation of lactic acid causes LA, while lack of energy leads to cell dysfunction and mitochondria-associated disease, including RM. Here we report the first case of CHB patients developing fatal LA and RM during telbivudine and tenofovir treatment.

Case presentation

In November 2015, a 51-year-old man was hospitalized because of myalgia for more than 1 month. He had a history of Hepatitis B envelope Antigen (HBeAg) positive hepatitis B for 13 years without being treated with antiviral drug. Two years before admission, he was diagnosed with hepatitis B and cirrhosis by local hospital, and HBV DNA was $6.5*10^3$ copies/ml. Then he began to take telbivudine regularly and HBV DNA became undetected after some time. However, two months before admission, HBV DNA again reached $7*10^3$ copies/ml. Considering HBV resistance to telbivudine, the antiviral treatment converted to the combination of telbivudine and tenofovir. After taking combination treatment, he began to feel muscle pain, especially in both lower limbs after walking. He also had hypoesthesia in distal limbs. There were no other concurrent symptoms, such as fever, headache, abdominal pain and altered level of consciousness. The symptoms became increasingly heavier. After 1 month of combination treatment, telbivudine and tenofovir were discontinued, and he began to take adefovir instead. However, his symptoms didn't relieve. Ten days before admission, laboratory testing revealed an elevated alanine aminotransferase (ALT, 66 U/L), aspartate transaminase (AST, 129 U/L), lactate dehydrogenase (LDH, 474 U/L) and CPK (1050 U/L). Total bilirubin and indirect bilirubin level were normal. To rule out liver cancer, abdomen magnetic resonance (MRI) was done, which revealed cirrhosis and gallstone. The patient received liver-protecting treatment. Two days before admission, he had chest tightness and short of breath. The blood lactate level was 12.7 mmol/L. The arterial blood gas analysis showed pH 7.25, base excess − 21. 1 mmol/L. The patient received sodium bicarbonate ($NaCO_3$) for the treatment of acidosis and eventually transferred to our hospital diagnosed with LA and RM. On the day of admission, he began to develop chest tightness and palpitation. The blood routine test showed normal white blood cell count and percentage of neutrophils. His urine color was black and urine output was about 200 ml per day. ALT was 77 U/L, total bilirubin was 25.2 μmol/L, CPK was 991 U/L, LDH was 509 U/L, creatine was 83 μmol/L, myoglobin was 1745 ng/ml and lactic acid was 20 mmol/L. The electrolytes test was normal, while uric acid was 1.019 mmol/L. HBV markers showed Hepatitis B surface Antigen (HBsAg), HBeAg and Hepatitis B core Antibody (HBcAb) were positive, while HBV DNA was undetected. Physical examination on admission revealed swelling and tenderness of all his extremities, muscle dumbness and weakness in both lower limbs, which quantitative value was 3 grade without redness and warm skin. Besides chronic hepatitis, the patient denied a past history of significant comorbidities, including diabetes and chronic kidney disease. He had no previous trauma and also denied any other drug, Chinese herb and nutritional supplementary use except antiviral drug for CHB.

Low extremity MRI showed mild atrophy in both lower extremities and increased signal intensity (Fig. 1), consistent with the manifestation of myopathy. Electromyography revealed multiple peripheral neuropathy with predominant motor and sensory axonal injury. Muscle biopsy on left biceps revealed myogenic lesion with abnormality of mitochondria and fat metabolism (Fig. 2). Muscle fibers are of variable size and irregular shape, with scattered atrophy and degeneration. In atrophic fibers, Modified Gomori trichrome (MGT) stain showed red granular changes, with increased succinic dehydrogenase (SDH) activity and negative cytochrome oxidase (COX) activity.

As the patient had myalgia, oliguria and black urine, combining with serum myoglobulin>500μg/L, severe metabolic acidosis and his past medical history, he was diagnosed with RM, LA and HBeAg negative CHB. Without the history of injury, other concurrent drug intake and infection, we concluded that RM was caused by telbivudine and tenofovir.

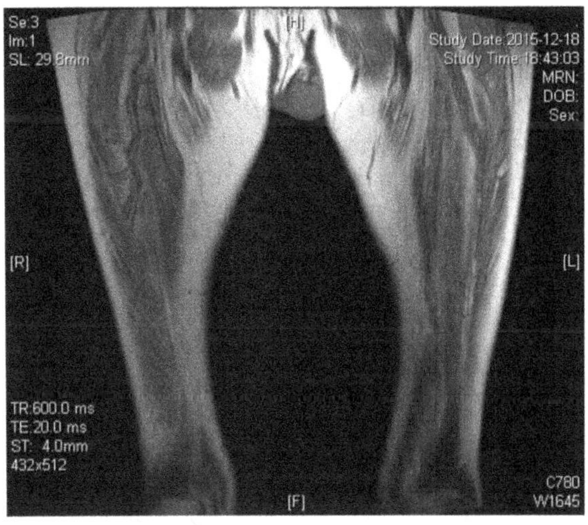

Fig. 1 The low extremity MRI. Mild atrophy of both thigh muscle with uniformly increased signal intensity, which is accordant with the features of myopathy

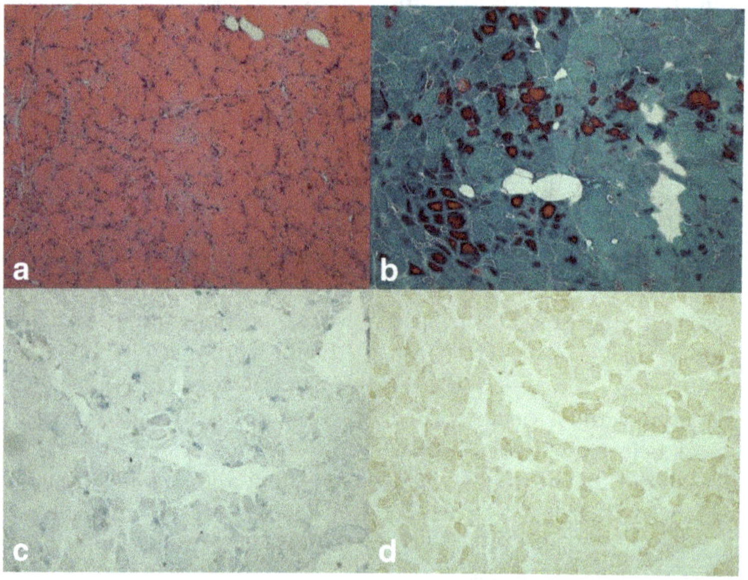

Fig. 2 Microscopic findings of muscle biopsy specimen showed mitochondrial toxicity. **a** Muscle fibers are of variable size and irregular shape, and there are many atrophic and degenerating muscle fibers. (HE, magnification × 200); **b** A lot of red granular changes in atrophic fibers. (modified Gomori trichrome stain, magnification × 200); **c** Increased enzyme activities in many atrophic fibers. (succinic dehydrogenase, magnification × 200); **d** Many muscle fibers are deficient for enzyme activities. (cytochrome oxidase stain, magnification × 200)

After admission, the antiviral treatment converted to entecavir because of its lower reporting portion of muscle-related adverse drug reaction. The patient was given hemodialysis twice. He was also given hydration, alkalization and supplementation treatment. After one week, the blood lactate, myoglobin and CPK dropped rapidly, but the blood lactate level fluctuated between 3 and 5 mmol/L (Fig. 3). His arterial blood gas analysis returned to normal, showing pH between 7.40 and 7.45. Then he received tenofovir disoproxil instead of entecavir and methylprednisolone for 40 mg each day. In the following four weeks, blood lactate reduced to normal range and didn't rebound. Five months later, the patient could walk naturally. His dumbness in distal limbs relieved but still existed. (Table 1) During the whole period from 2015.9 (before taking tenofovir) to 2016.6, the patient's renal function was normal and GFR levels were estimated between 106.1 to 120.2/ml/min/1.73m^2.

Discussion and Conclusions

In basic terms, lactic acid is the product of anaerobic metabolism. The normal blood lactate concentration is 0.5-1 mmol/L. LA is defined as a constant increase in blood lactate levels (usually > 5 mmol/L) in association with metabolic acidosis (usually present as pH < 7.3 and serum bicarbonate < 10 mmol/L) [1]. The LA syndrome presents as steatosis, abnormal mitochondrial appearance and function, pancreatitis, neuropathy, and myopathy. The onset may be abrupt or insidious, which generally begins with nausea, vomiting, and abdominal pain. It will progress to tachypnea, shortness of breath, and hypoxia. Patients with severe LA may subsequently develop renal failure, liver failure, coagulopathy, seizures, arrhythmias, and even death. The patient reported here was a severe LA case with a constant higher lactate level (more than 12 mmol/L) and pH value (about 7.2).

On the other hand, RM is a syndrome characterized by damage of striated muscle cells, which release a large amount of intracellular substance, including myoglobin, potassium ion, CPK, etc. The prognosis of RM is poor, and fatality rate reaches 3%~ 27%. Early symptoms are mild and non-specific, like malaise, muscular weakness and tenderness. The most important clinical manifestations are myoglobinuria and higher specific gravity of urine (> 1.025). The color of urine can change from pale red to deep red, even black. CPK rises rapidly, up to 10,000-20,000 U/L. Blood gas analysis can reveal hypoxemia and metabolic acidosis. The diagnosis criteria are as follows: 1. Serum CPK significantly rise; 2. Blood and urine myoglobulin positive, with myalgia and muscle swollen; 3. Hyperkalemia, hyperphosphatemia, hyperuricemia and hypocalcemia. About 20%~ 33% RM patients will develop acute renal failure. RM is usually caused by trauma or non-trauma factors (like drugs, toxics, ischemia, and infection). Drugs that can induce RM contain statins, theophylline, anti-H1, benzodiazepines, amphotericin B and antidepressants [3].

In this case, the patient developed fatal syndrome LA and RM, after taking telbivudine and tenofovir as antiviral treatment. Without evidence of other causes like infection

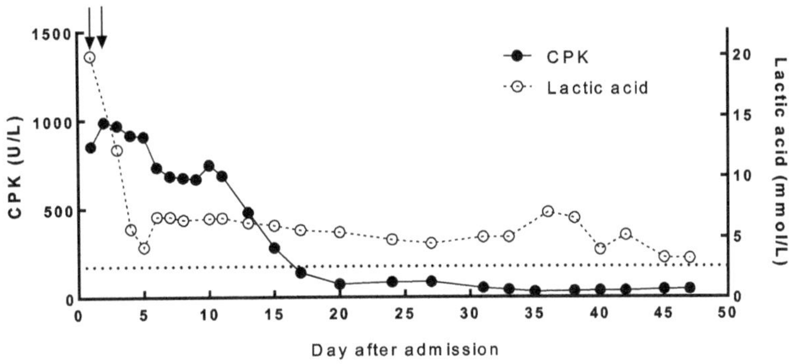

Fig. 3 Progression of serum creatine kinase (CPK) and lactic acid level. The dotted line indicates normal level. Each arrow shows one hemodialysis. The CPK and lactic acid level dropped quickly after hemodialysis

or trauma, telbivudine and tenofovir may be the cause of their complications.

Telbivudine is a potent nucleoside analogue for treatment of chronic hepatitis B, while it was often associated with muscle-related adverse events. During the large, multinational registration trials, telbivudine was reported a significantly higher side effect of grade 3 to 4 CPK elevations (defined as 7 times upper limit of normal) in two years compared to lamivudine [4]. In the phase III GLOBE trial, despite 12.9% of patients on telbivudine developing severe elevation of serum CPK levels, clinical myopathy was reported only in two (0.3%) patients [2]. Another study monitored CPK levels of 200 patients who were treated with telbivudine for chronic hepatitis B, the 3-year cumulative incidence of CPK elevations and myopathy was 84.3% and 5%, respectively. Male, younger age and HBeAg negativity were independent predictors of CPK elevations. CPK elevations usually occurred 21 months after starting treatment. However, no risk factors of myopathy were identified [5]. As a result, although an elevated CPK may be an early indicator of muscle injury, this may be nonspecific and can often be elevated due to strenuous or prolonged exercise.

Table 1 The timeline of the patient's medical history and interventions

Dates	Summaries	Diagnostic Testing	Interventions
2002	Found HBV infection	HBsAg, HBeAg, HBcAb positive	No antiviral treatment
2013	Diagnosed with cirrhosis	HBV DNA: $6.5*10^3$ copies/ml	Telbivudine
2013-2015.9		HBV DNA undetected	Telbivudine
2015.9		HBV DNA: $7*10^3$ copies/ml	Telbivudine and Tenofovir
2015.9-2015.10	Myalgia and hypoesthesia in both lower limbs		Telbivudine and Tenofovir
2015.10	Myalgia and hypoesthesia not relieved		Adefovir
2015.11.17	Myalgia and hypoesthesia not relieved	ALT 66 U/L, LDH 474 U/L, CPK 1050 U/L	Adefovir; liver-protecting treatment
2015.11.25	Myalgia and hypoesthesia not relieved; Chest tightness and short of breath occurred	Blood lactate 12.7 mmol/L, arterial blood gas: pH 7.25, base excess −21.1 mmol/L	Adefovir; liver-protecting treatment
2015.11.27 (Admission)	Myalgia, hypoesthesia, chest tightness, short of breath, palpitation; Swelling and tenderness of all extremities, muscle dumbness and grade 3 strength in both lower limbs	ALT: 77 U/L, TBil: 25.2 μmol/L, CPK: 991 U/L, LDH: 509 U/L, creatine: 83 μmol/L, myoglobin: 1745 ng/ml, blood lactate: 20 mmol/L, HBV DNA undetected	Entecavir; hemodialysis; hydration; alkalization
2015.12.4	Nearly all symptoms relieved gradually	CPK 683 U/L, blood lactate 6.67 mmol/L	Tenofovir, Methylprednisolone 40 mg qd
2016.1.13	Swelling of lower limbs disappeared	CPK 47 U/L, blood lactate 3.21 mmol/L	Tenofovir
2016.6	Walk naturally; Dumbness in distal limbs relieved but still existed	HBV undetected	Tenofovir

HBV Hepatitis B virus, *HBsAg* Hepatitis B surface Antigen, *HBeAg* Hepatitis B envelope Antigen, *HBcAb* Hepatitis B core Antibody, *ALT* Alanine aminotransferase, *LDH* Lactate dehydrogenase, *CPK* Creatine phosphokinase, *TBil* Total Bilirubin

Telbivudine-associated myopathy generally occurred after taking drugs for more than one year, more common in male patients, presenting as myalgia, muscle weakness and elevated CPK [6]. Without any management, it possibly develops to RM. Yi et al. [7] has collected a total of 22 RM cases associated with telbivudine. All the cases were male patients with an average age of (34.5 ± 11.2) years. Half of the patients occurred RM within 6 to 10 months. Clinical manifestations were mostly nausea, vomiting, palpitations, weakness and edema of the lower extremities. After discontinuing telbivudine and getting symptomatic treatments, 4 deaths were still reported.

Long-term telbivudine treatment also make some patients develop resistance. This patient we reported also had a history of telbivudine resistance. At first, we converted antiviral therapy to entecavir because its lower reporting portion of muscle-related adverse drug reaction. As entecavir and telbivudine shared cross-resistance in some HBV variants, it was recommended that tenofovir should be the rescue strategy when telbivudine resistance occurred according to EASL guidelines in 2017 [8]. On the other side, tenofovir disoproxil fumarate was recommended as first-line monotherapy against hepatitis B with a high barrier to resistance [8]. So far, tenofovir was only reported a side effect of rhabdomyolysis during antiretroviral treatment in HIV patients, which combined with other concurrent antiretroviral drugs [9, 10]. In a clinical trial studying the safety of tenofovir monotherapy for 5 years [11], the researchers reported no fatal adverse reaction like LA or RM. So, we thought tenofovir monotherapy was safe. When the patients` condition was steady, we used tenofovir under close monitoring. In another two large trials that have investigated the safety of telbivudine and tenofovir combination therapy in CHB patients during at most 1 year's follow-up, there were no muscle-related severe adverse events reported, like myopathy, LA and RM [12, 13]. For this patient we reported, he took telbivudine for two years and suffered myalgia immediately after addition of tenofovir, so we conjure that tenofovir sometimes may still have a synergistic effect on the development of myopathy after much longer medication time, especially in patients with cirrhosis.

The pathophysiology of NAs associated LA and RM is likely to be the malfunction of mitochondria [14, 15]. For according to muscle biopsy, the mitochondrial damage is identified in both patients. All five of the approved oral antiviral agents for HBV treatment can inhibit the polymerase activity of HBV. At the same time, they also have a low level of activity against the human mitochondrial DNA polymerase gamma and can lead to impaired mitochondrial replication with mitochondrial loss or dysfunction. Mitochondria are the main sites for oxidative phosphorylation and producing adenosine transferase (ATP). There are approximately 300-400 mitochondria in each cell. When mitochondria function is impaired or the number of mitochondria is decreased, there will be an impact on the aerobic metabolism and production of ATP. Lack of aerobic metabolism resulted in the increase of pyruvate reduction to lactic acid. Then the accumulation of lactic acid causes LA. On the other side, the insufficient ATP means lack of energy for cell activities, leading to dysfunction of cells and mitochondria-associated disease. Mitochondria are mainly distributed over organs and tissues which are metabolically active. Thus, the clinical manifestations of mitochondria toxicity vary based on the affected tissues, which may include myopathy, neuropathy, hepatic steatosis, pancreatitis, and nephrotoxicity. All NAs have a "black box" warning regarding potential mitochondrial toxicity in their product labeling.

For all five NAs approved of treatment for hepatitis B, the strength of inhibition of mtDNA polymerase gamma in an in vitro test system is substantially lower than antiretroviral agents like zalcitabine [1]. In particular, entecavir has demonstrated little evidence of mitochondrial toxicity compared to the other available agents at concentrations exceeding 100 times the maximum concentration seen in humans [16]. The impact of drug combinations in causing additive or synergistic mitochondrial toxicity in vitro has not been well studied.

Except drug withdrawal immediately, other management options for this kind of serious adverse reaction may include renal replacement therapy, bicarbonate alkalization and supplementation with L-acetylcarnitine, thiamine, as well as Coenzyme Q 10 to improve mitochondrial function. Most of the LA cases can resolve rapidly after discontinuation of the causative drug. For telbivudine associated myopathy, CPK decrease after 2-4 weeks as the symptoms are improved.

This case shows that tenofovir may trigger rhabdomyolysis in combination with telbivudine treatment in chronic hepatitis B patients. Thus, patients receiving tenofovir and telbivudine should be closely monitored for muscular abnormalities, blood lactate level and other mitochondrial toxicity associated side effects.

Abbreviations

ALT: Alanine aminotransferase; AST: Aspartate transaminase; ATP: Adenosine transferase; CHB: Chronic hepatitis B; COX: Cytochrome oxidase; CPK: Creatine phosphokinase; HBcAb: Hepatitis B core Antibody; HBeAg: Hepatitis B envelope Antigen; HBsAg: Hepatitis B surface Antigen; HBV: Hepatitis B virus; LA: Lactic acidosis; LDH: Lactate dehydrogenase; MGT: Modified Gomori trichrome; MRI: Magnetic resonance; NAs: Nucleoside analogues; RM: Rhabdomyolysis; SDH: Succinic dehydrogenase; TBil: Total Bilirubin

Acknowledgments

Not applicable.

Funding

Project 81670560 supported by National Natural Science Foundation of China. The funders had no role in study design, data collection and analysis, decision to publish, or preparation of the manuscript.

Authors' contributions

YY wrote the manuscript; HYK diagnosed and treated the patient, also designed Fig. 2; JJL helped to draft the manuscript and revised written English; ZJM and ZWH helped diagnose and manage the patients and draft the manuscript; HYX helped to draft the manuscript and revised it critically for important intellectual content; all authors have read and approved the final manuscript, and ensured that this is the case.

Consent for publication

Written informed consent for publication from the patient was obtained.

Competing interests

The authors declare that they have no competing interests.

References

1. Fontana RJ. Side effects of long-term oral antiviral therapy for hepatitis B. Hepatology. 2009;49:S185–95.
2. Liaw YF, Gane E, Leung N, Zeuzem S, Wang Y, Lai CL, Heathcote EJ, Manns M, Bzowej N, Niu J, Han SH, Hwang SG, Cakaloglu Y, Tong MJ, Papatheodoridis G, Chen Y, Brown NA, Albanis E, Galil K, Naoumov NV, GLOBE Study Group. 2-Year GLOBE trial results: telbivudine is superior to lamivudine in patients with chronic hepatitis B. Gastroenterology. 2009;136(2):486–95.
3. Caroleo B, Galasso O, Staltari O, Girofrè C, De Sarro G, Guadagnino V, Gallelli L. Muscular damage during telbivudine treatment in a chronic hepatitis B patient. Muscles, Ligaments and Tendons Journal. 2011;1(2):57–60.
4. Chan HL, Chen YC, Gane EJ, Sarin SK, Suh DJ, Piratvisuth T, Prabhakar B, Hwang SG, Choudhuri G, Safadi R. Randomized clinical trial: efficacy and safety of telbivudine and lamivudine in treatment-naïve patients with HBV-related decompensated cirrhosis. J Viral Hepat. 2012;19:732–43.
5. Zou XJ, Jiang XQ, Tian DY. Clinical features and risk factors of creatine kinase elevations and myopathy associated with telbivudine. J Viral Hepat. 2011;18(12):892–6.
6. Ambang T, Tan JS, Ong S, Wong KT, Goh KJ. Clinicopathological Features of Telbivudine-Associated Myopathy. PLoS One. 2016;11(9):e0162760.
7. Yi ZM, Tang SD, Fang L, Zhai SD, Jiao LG. Evaluation on telbivudine-associated rhabdomyolysis. J Clin Pharm Sci. 2016;25(1):66–72.
8. Lampertico P, Agarwal K, Berg T, Buti M, Janssen HLA, Papatheodoridis G, Zoulim F, Tacke F. EASL 2017 Clinical Practice Guidelines on the management of hepatitis B virus infection. J Hepatol. 2017;67(2):370–98.
9. Suttels V, Florence E, Leys J, Vekemans M, Van den Ende J, Vlieghe E, Kenyon C. A 68-year old male presenting with rhabdomyolysis-associated acute kidney injury following concomitant use of elvitegravir/cobicistat/emtricitabine/tenofovir disoproxil fumarate and pravastatin/fenofibrate: a case report. J Med Case Rep. 2015;9:190.
10. Callens S, De Roo A, Colebunders R. Fanconi-like syndrome and rhabdomyolysis in a person with HIV infection on highly active antiretroviral treatment including tenofovir. J Inf Secur. 2003;47(3):262–3.
11. Marcellin P, Buti M, Krastev Z, de Man RA, Zeuzem S, Lou L, Gaggar A, Flaherty JF, Massetto B, Lin L, Dinh P, Subramanian GM, McHutchison JG, Flisiak R, Gurel S, Dusheiko GM, Heathcote EJ. Kinetics of hepatitis B surface antigen loss in patients with HBeAg-positive chronic hepatitis B treated with tenofovir disoproxil fumarate. J Hepatol. 2014;61(6):1228–37.
12. Piratvisuth T, Komolmit P, Tanwandee T, Sukeepaisarnjaroen W, Chan HL, Pessoa MG, Fassio E, Ono SK, Bessone F, Daruich J, Zeuzem S, Cheinquer H, Pathan R, Dong Y, Trylesinski A. 52-week efficacy and safety of telbivudine with conditional tenofovir intensification at week 24 in HBeAg-positive chronic hepatitis B. PLoS One. 2013;8(2):e54279.
13. Leung NW, Herrmann E, Lau GK, Chan HL, So TM, Zeuzem S, Dong Y, Trylesinski A, Naoumov NV. Early Viral Kinetics with Telbivudine, Tenofovir or Combination of Both in Immunotolerant Patients with Hepatitis B e Antigen-Positive Chronic Hepatitis B. Infect Dis Ther. 2014;3(2):191–202.
14. Johnson AA, Ray AS, Hanes J, Suo Z, Colacino JM, Anderson KS, Johnson KA. Toxicity of antiviral nucleoside analogs and the human mitochondrial DNA polymerase. J Biol Chem. 2001;276:40847–57.
15. Kohler JJ, Lewis W. A brief overview of mechanisms of mitochondrial toxicity from NRTIs. Environ Mol Mutagen. 2007;48(3-4):166–72.
16. Mazzucco CE, Hamatake RK, Colonno RJ, Tenney DJ. Entecavir for treatment of hepatitis B virus displays no in vitro mitochondrial toxicity or DNA polymerase gamma inhibition. Antimicrob Agents Chemother. 2008;52:598–605.

IFI16 is involved in HBV-associated acute-on-chronic liver failure inflammation

Xiuqing Pang[1,2†], Xinhua Li[1,2†], Zhishuo Mo[1,2], Jing Huang[1,2], Hong Deng[1,2], Ziying Lei[1,2], Xingrong Zheng[1,2], Zhiying Feng[3], Dongying Xie[1,2,4*] and Zhiliang Gao[1,2,4*]

Abstract

Background: Hepatitis B virus (HBV) is a hepatotropic DNA virus, and its DNA may be a potent inflammatory molecule. Interferon-inducible protein 16 (IFI16), a newly discovered DNA sensor, plays an important role in the process of inflammation in viral infections. Our study sought to identify a correlation between IFI16 expression and inflammation in patients with chronic hepatitis B (CHB) and HBV-associated acute-on-chronic liver failure (HBV-ACLF).

Methods: We performed flow cytometry to measure IFI16 levels in peripheral blood mononuclear cells (PBMC) and used immunohistochemistry and western blotting to measure IFI16 protein levels in liver tissues. The cellular source of IFI16 was detected using double immunofluorescence. All datum were analyzed using SPSS 13.0 and GraphPad Prism 6.

Results: The number of IFI16+ cells was significantly associated with the degree of inflammation. In detail, the number of IFI16+ cells was higher in livers but lower in PBMCs in HBV-ACLF patients than those in CHB patients and healthy controls. There was no significant difference between CHB patients and healthy controls in numbers of IFI6+ cells in livers and PBMCs. There was no significant relationship between IFI16 expression levels and HBV parameters. Furthermore, IFI16 was expressed in the nucleus of Kupffer cells (KCs), endothelial cells, natural killer cells, dendritic cells, and hepatic stellate cells in healthy donors and CHB patients, but only in the cytoplasm of KCs in the livers of HBV-ACLF patients.

Conclusions: IFI16 was closely related to the degree of inflammation in CHB and HBV-ACLF patients and may serve as a vital contributor to the pathogeneses of liver damage in HBV-ACLF.

Keywords: IFN inducible protein 16 (IFI16), Chronic hepatitis B (CHB), HBV-associated acute-on-chronic liver failure (HBV-ACLF), Inflammation

Background

Hepatitis B virus (HBV) is a non-cytopathic human Hepadnavirus that causes a spectrum of diseases, such as chronic hepatitis B (CHB), liver cirrhosis, primary hepatocellular carcinoma, and liver failure. The pathology of HBV disease is closely associated with chronic inflammation, a dynamic process orchestrated by the complex interplay between virus replication and host immune response. It is widely accepted that adaptive immune responses play major roles in HBV infection [1]; however, the role of innate immunity during HBV infection is not to be well understood. The innate immune system is activated by viruses through pattern-recognition receptors (PRRs) that recognize specific viral structures, such as viral protein, single-stranded RNA and double-stranded RNA. Following recognition, recruitment of distinct adaptor proteins will initiate sequentially signaling cascades to induce inflammation cytokine production in virus-infected cells. Several PRRs, including Toll-like receptors (TLRs), RIG-I-like receptors (RLRs), and NOD-like receptors (NLRs), have been found to play important roles in HBV sensing and the formation of inflammasomes in the liver [2]. Current evidence suggests that a new type of PRRs, named DNA sensors, can detect microbial DNAs and initiate innate responses to provoke inflammation. HBV is a hepatotropic DNA virus, and thus, its DNA may be a potent immune stimulatory molecule.

Interferon inducible protein 16 (IFI16), a newly discovered molecule that senses DNA in cells and stimulates stimulator of IFN genes (STING)-dependent IFN expression

* Correspondence: xdy-gz@163.com; gaozhl@mail.sysu.edu.cn
†Equal contributors
[1]Department of Infectious Diseases, Third Affiliated Hospital of Sun-Yat-SenUniversity, GuangZhou, China

and apoptosis-associated speck-like protein containing caspase recruitment domain (ASC)-dependent inflammation activation [3]. Based on its structure, IFI16 is clustered into the PYHIN family of proteins which is defined by one or two C-terminal DNA binding HIN domains and an N-terminal homotypic protein–protein interactions pyrin domain (PYD). Currently, four members of the PYHIN family have been discovered: absent in melanoma 2 (AIM-2), interferon-inducible protein X (IFIX), Myeloid cell nuclear differentiation antigen (MNDA) and IFI16. Previous studies showed that AIM2 can stimulate inflammasome activation and downstream cleavage of pro-interleukin (IL)1b and pro-IL18 to bioactive cytokines via interactions between the PYD and the inflammasome adaptor protein ASC [4]. Such AIM2-ASC inflammatory signaling pathways activation may occur during HBV infection [5]. To date, IFI16 is the only one member of this family with two HIN domains, termed HIN-A and HIN-B [6], and these two domains potentially increase the DNA-binding ability. Recently, IFI16 was reported to also have the capacity to activate ASC-dependent inflammasomes during HSV-1, Kaposi sarcoma-associated herpes virus (KSHV) or Epstein–Barr virus infection [7–9]. Furthermore, IFI16 was demonstrated to stimulate IFN expression through a mechanism through STING, TANK-binding kinase 1 (TBK1), and interferon regulatory factor-3 (IRF-3) signaling in a DNA-driven manner. Based on its unique structure of HIN domains, IFI16 can bind different nucleotide structures, such as dsDNA, superhelical and cruciform DNA, HIV-Nef DNA. Studies have demonstrated the induction of IFN responses during infection with herpes simplex virus (HSV), Human cytomegalovirus (HCMV), HIV and lentiviruses, as well as with *Listeria monocytogenes* [10–13].

Taken together, IFI16 plays an important role in the process of immune response in viral infections. Therefore, we predicted that IFI16 may play a vital role in the development of HBV sensing and inflammasomes in the liver, although the expression of IFI16 in human HBV infection has not been thoroughly investigated. During HBV infection, peripheral blood mononuclear cells (PBMCs) are very important part of the peripheral immune system. In addition, the liver is well-known to be an immunological organ with a predominant innate immune system. Our laboratory investigated whether IFI16 is expressed in PBMCs and livers in CHB and HBV-ACLF patients and whether HBV DNA is recognized by IFI16.In addition, we examined the correlation between IFI16 expression and the inflammation.

Methods

Patients

All patient samples were collected in our hospital from June 2013 to December 2014. Peripheral blood samples were collected from 31 CHB patients and 13 patients with HBV-associated acute-on-chronic liver failure (HBV-ACLF); 16 sex-matched healthy individuals were enrolled as normal controls. Liver tissue samples were collected from 59 CHB patients who had liver biopsies, 17 HBV-ACLF patients who received a liver transplant, and 19 healthy liver transplant donors. CHB patients were defined as those who were HBsAg-positive for more than 6 months and that exhibited symptoms or signs of hepatitis and abnormal hepatic function on occasion or those that had the disease histologically confirmed. By contrast, the diagnosis of HBV-ACLF was based on clinical evidence of either ≥grade 2 hepatic encephalopathy, abrupt and obvious increase in ascites, spontaneous bacterial peritonitis, or hepatorenal syndrome; these clinical criteria were associated with recent development of jaundice [total bilirubin [TBIL] ≥10. 0 mg/d or rapidly rising levels of TBIL(TBIL≥1.0 mg/dL/ day)] and a prothrombin activity ≤40%. Patients with autoimmune liver diseases or cancer were excluded. All patients were seronegative for markers of hepatitis A, C, D, and E viruses and for HIV virus. The model for end-stage liver disease (MELD) score [14] was used to assess disease severity and prognosis. Alanine aminotransferase (ALT) and aspartate aminotransferase (AST)levels, bilirubin levels, international normalized ratio (INR), creatinine, HBV DNA load, and MELD score were measured. The study protocol was approved by the ethics committee of our hospital and written informed consent was obtained from each subject. The basic characteristics of the enrolled subjects are listed in Tables 1 and 2.

Antibodies

Mouse anti-human IFI16 monoclonal antibody (sc-137,970) was obtained from Santa Cruz Biotechnology Inc., Santa Cruz, CA, USA. Kupffer cell (KC) marker rabbit anti-human CD68 (clone F7.2.38) polyclonal antibody, Natural killer (NK) cell marker rabbit anti-human CD56 (EP2567Y) , liver sinusoidal endothelial cell (LESC) marker rabbit anti-human CD299 (EPR11211), dendritic cell (DC) marker rabbit anti-human CD11c (EP1347Y), and hepatic stellate cell (HSC) marker rabbit anti-human SMA (E184) monoclonal antibodies were purchased from ABclonal Biotech Co., Ltd. (Woburn, MA, USA) and Abcam's RabMAb®technology (Cambridge, UK), respectively. Alexa Fluor® 488 Goat Anti-Mouse IgG and Alexa Fluor® 555 Goat Anti-Rabbit IgG antibodies were obtained from Life Technologies (Grand Island, NY,USA).

PBMC isolation and flow cytometry

PBMCs were purified from EDTA-treated blood using a Ficoll density gradient. For intranuclear IFI16 staining, PBMCs (200 μL) were incubated in 800 μL of RPMI 1640 medium. The cells were treated with Human TruStain FcX, Nuclear Factor Fixation Buffer, and Nuclear

Table 1 Clinical characteristics of the populations with PBMCs enrolled in the study

group	NC	CHB	HBV-ACLF
case	16	31	13
sex(M/F)	12/4	25/6	12/1
age(years)	29.5(26-63)	36(21-61)	44(37-67)
ALT(U/L)	21.5(11-34)	50(11-217)	90(46-245)
AST(U/L)	22(12-34)	46(21-222)	117(58-158)
Tbil(umol/L)	ND	12.6(4.0-119.9)	473.8(51.9-720)
INR	ND	1.04(0.88-1.23)	2.87(2.01-4.68)
PTA(%)	ND	94(72-128)	26(16-39)
Log10 (HBV DNA)	ND	5.17(1.30-8.23)	3.25(1.51-8.19)
HBsAg-positive	0	31	13
HBsAb-positive	16	0	0
HBeAg-positive	0	13	3
HBeAb-positive	0	18	10
HBcA-bpositive	0	31	13
MELD score	ND	ND	28.2±1.22

Data are shown as median and range
ACLF, acute on chronic liver failure; CHB, chronic hepatitis B; ALT, alanine aminotransferase; AST, aspartate aminotransferase; Tbil, total bilirubin;HBcAb, hepatitis B c antibody; HBeAb, hepatitis B e antibody; HBeAg, hepatitis B e antigen; HBsAb, hepatitis B s antibody; HBsAg,hepatitis B s antigen; HBV, hepatitis B virus; ND, not determined; NC,normal control; PTA, prothrombin time activity; MELD Model for end-stage liver disease

Table 2 Clinical characteristics of the populations with liver tissues enrolled in the study

group	NC	CHB	HBV-ACLF
case	19	59	17
sex(M/F)	ND	46/13	16/1
age(years)	ND	37(23-65)	41(29-61)
ALT(U/L)	ND	50(7-570)	40(11-156)
AST(U/L)	ND	37(15-256)	92(40-202)
Tbil(umol/L)	ND	12.1(2.6-119.9)	600.6(238-809)
INR	ND	1.03(0.87-1.35)	2.88(2.11-5.83)
PTA(%)	ND	95(63-128)	21(11-35)
Log10 (HBV DNA)	ND	5.42(0-8.54)	2(0.83-8.05)
HBsAg-positive	ND	59	17
HBsAb-positive	ND	0	0
HBeAg-positive	ND	24	2
HBeAb-positive	ND	35	15
HBcA-bpositive	ND	59	17
MELD score	ND	ND	33.33±2.02

Data are shown as median and range
ACLF, acute on chronic liver failure; CHB, chronic hepatitis B; ALT, alanine aminotransferase;AST, aspartate aminotransferase; Tbil, total bilirubin; HBcAb, hepatitis B c antibody; HBeAb, hepatitis B e antibody;HBeAg, hepatitis B e antigen; HBsAb, hepatitis B s antibody; HBsAg, hepatitis B s antigen; HBV, hepatitis B virus; ND, not determined; NC, normal control; PTA, prothrombin time activity. MELD Model for end-stage liver disease.

Factor Permeabilization Buffer (Biolegend, San Diego, CA, USA) and stained with the IFI16 antibody and Alexa Fluor® 488 Goat Anti-Mouse IgG. Data collection was performed on a BDFACSCantoII (BD Biosciences, San Jose, CA, USA), and data files were analyzed using FlowJo software (FlowJo, LLC, Ashland, OR, USA). Statistical analysis was based on IFI16 staining of at least 10,000 gated cells.

Liver pathology

The liver biopsy specimens were considered reliable when the liver specimen length was ≥1.5 cm. The liver biopsy specimens were fixed in formaldehyde, embedded in paraffin, cut into 4-μm sections, and conventionally stained with hematoxylin and eosin. Images were acquired using an Olympus Leica DM4000B microscope. According to the Scheuer scoring system, hepatic inflammation activity grade (G) was divided into G0 (no hepatic necroinflammation) and G1-G4 and hepatic fibrosis stage was divided into F0 (no hepatic fibrosis) and F1-F4. The degree of hepatic inflammation and fibrosis was graded using the modified histology activity index (HAI) [14] described by Scheuer. Liver specimens were interpreted by experienced liver pathologists. Sections of liver tissue were scored in a blinded fashion to assess their histological diagnoses.

Immunohistochemistry

Immunohistochemistry was carried out using standard techniques [15]. The expression of IFI16-positive cells was determined by image analysis of the histological sections. Ten sections from each sample were randomly selected, and photomicrographs were obtained under high-power fields (0.625 mm^2) and captured for analysis using Image Pro-Plus 6.0 software (Media Cybernetics, Silver Spring, MD, USA). The number of IFI16-positive cells per high-power field was counted and expressed as the mean + the standard error of the mean (SEM).

Immunofluorescence double staining

For immunofluorescence double staining, paraffin-embedded tissue blocks were cut into 3.5-μm sections. After dewaxing and rehydration, antigen retrieval was performed with EDTA (pH 8.0). Then, sections were incubated at 4 °C overnight with primary anti-IFI16 (1:50) and cell type-specific marker antibodies anti-CD68 (1:100), anti-CD11c (1:50), anti-CD56 (1:50), anti-CD299 (1:100), and anti-SMA (1:1000). The sections were then incubated with Alexa Fluor® 488 Goat Anti-Mouse IgG and Alexa Fluor® 555 Goat Anti-Rabbit IgG Antibodies (1:1000) for 1 h. Finally, the sections were incubated with 1 μg/ml Hoechst 33,342 (Sigma-Aldrich, St. Louis, MO, USA) to stain the nuclei. Sections incubated with the PBS control primary antibodies and fluorescently labeled secondary antibodies were used as negative controls. The results were analyzed using fluorescence microscopy (Leica Corp.).

Western blotting analysis

Cells were lysed in radioimmunoprecipitation assay (RIPA) buffer supplemented with protease inhibitor cocktail (Sigma-Aldrich), sonicated, and clarified by centrifugation. Equal amounts of protein were separated by SDS-PAGE and electrophoretically transferred to nitrocellulose membranes. Membranes were incubated with primary antibodies and secondary antibodies conjugated to horseradish peroxidase (KPL, Gaithersburg, MD, USA). Immunoreactive bands were visualized using an ECL western blotting substrate (Pierce Chemical, Rockford, IL, USA). Blots were scanned using FluorChemFC2 software with the AlphaImager system (Alpha Innotech Corp., San Leandro, CA, USA). Figures shown are representative of three or more experiments each.

Statistical analysis

All datum were analyzed using the SPSS version 13.0 software (SPSS Inc., Chicago, IL, USA) or GraphPad Prism 6 (GraphPad, La Jolla, CA, USA) and summarized as the means and standard errors (SEs) or medians and range. Differences invariables were analyzed using ANOVA and Student's t-tests (for normally distributed data) or the Kruskal–Wallis and Mann–Whitney U-tests (for non-normally distributed data), as appropriate. Correlation analysis was evaluated by the Spearman rank correlation test. A two-sided P value < 0.05 was considered statistically significant.

Results

Expression of IFI16 in PBMCs of HBV patients and healthy controls

We first examined the expression of IFI16 in PBMCs from 31 patients with CHB,13 patients with ACLF, and 16 healthy controls using flow cytometry. The number of IFI16-positive cells in patients with ACLF was significantly lower than the number in patients with CHB and in healthy controls (median [25th percentile; 75th percentile], 82.80 [62.53, 90.95] vs 93.00 [87.95, 95.00], and 91.63 [87.95, 95.00], $P < 0.001$ and $P < 0.05$; Fig. 1a). There was no difference between CHB patients and healthy controls($P > 0.05$). Then, we tested for a relationship between IFI16 expression levels and HBV parameters. There was no significant difference between the HBeAg(+) and HBeAg(−) groups ($P = 0.43$),and no statistically significant relationships were found between IFI16 expression levels and HBV DNA load ($r = 0.104$, $P = 0.501$; Fig. 1 b-c). In addition, we tested for a relationship between IFI16 expression levels and HBV DNA load only in chronic HBV infected patients, there was no statistically significant relationships ($r = 0.335$, $P = 0.065$). To further identify whether IFI16 expression contributed to the severity of CHB and ACLF, we evaluated the correlations between IFI16 and clinical parameters, including serum ALT, AST, TBIL, prothrombin time activity (PTA), and INR, in patients with HBV. IFI16 expression levels were positively correlated with PTA ($r = 0.336$, $P = 0.026$; Fig. 1g) and negatively correlated with AST ($r = -0.334$, $P = 0.027$), INR ($r = -0.339$, $P = 0.025$), and TBIL ($r = -0.449$, $P = 0.002$) (Figs. 1d–f). No statistically significant relationships were found between IFI16 expression levels and ALT ($r = -0.027$, $P = 0.861$). These results suggest the possibility that aberrant expression of IFI16 might be involved in the development of CHB and ACLF, especially in ACLF patients, and may be closely associated with disease severity.

Expression of intrahepatic IFI16 protein in CHB and ACLF patients

Furthermore, we evaluated the intrahepatic expression of IFI16 protein in 59 patients with CHB, 17 HBV-ACLF patients who received a liver transplant, and 19 healthy liver transplant donors. To measure the expression of IFI16 in the livers of CHB and ACLF patients, we used immunohistochemistry with anti-IFI16 to probe sections of paraffin-embedded livers. First, we saw different degrees of damage to the liver tissue from CHB and HBV-ACLF patients, as demonstrated by H&E staining (Fig. 2a). IFI16 expression that was observed in the livers of healthy donors and patients with HBV was mainly in non-parenchymal liver cells, especially the inflammatory cells in the livers of HBV patients. Furthermore, intrahepatic IFI16 expression gradually increased in accord with elevations in the grade of liver inflammation (Fig. 2a). Then, a semi-quantitative analysis of IFI16 expression in liver tissues was conducted using the software Image-Pro-Plus 6.0 to measure the number of IFI16-positive cells. The number of IFI16-positive cells in patients with ACLF was significantly higher than that in those with CHB or healthy controls (median [25th percentile; 75th percentile], 435.3 [372.9496.5] vs 199.6 [188.0, 307.1] vs160.8 [142.0, 218.0], both $P < 0.0001$; Fig. 2b). There was also no difference between the CHB patients and healthy controls ($P > 0.05$). In detail, the intrahepatic IFI16 expression in patients with inflammation grade 4 was significantly higher than in those with inflammation grade 0,1, or 2 ($P < 0.0001$; Fig. 2c). Moreover we found the intrahepatic IFI16 expression in patients with fibrosis stage 4 was also significantly higher than in those with fibrosis stage 0,1, or 2 (P < 0.0001; Fig. 2h). To further confirm our results obtained from the semi-quantitative immunohistochemistry, the protein level of IFI16 was analyzed by a western blotting analysis of cell extracts from liver tissues isolated from the different groups.

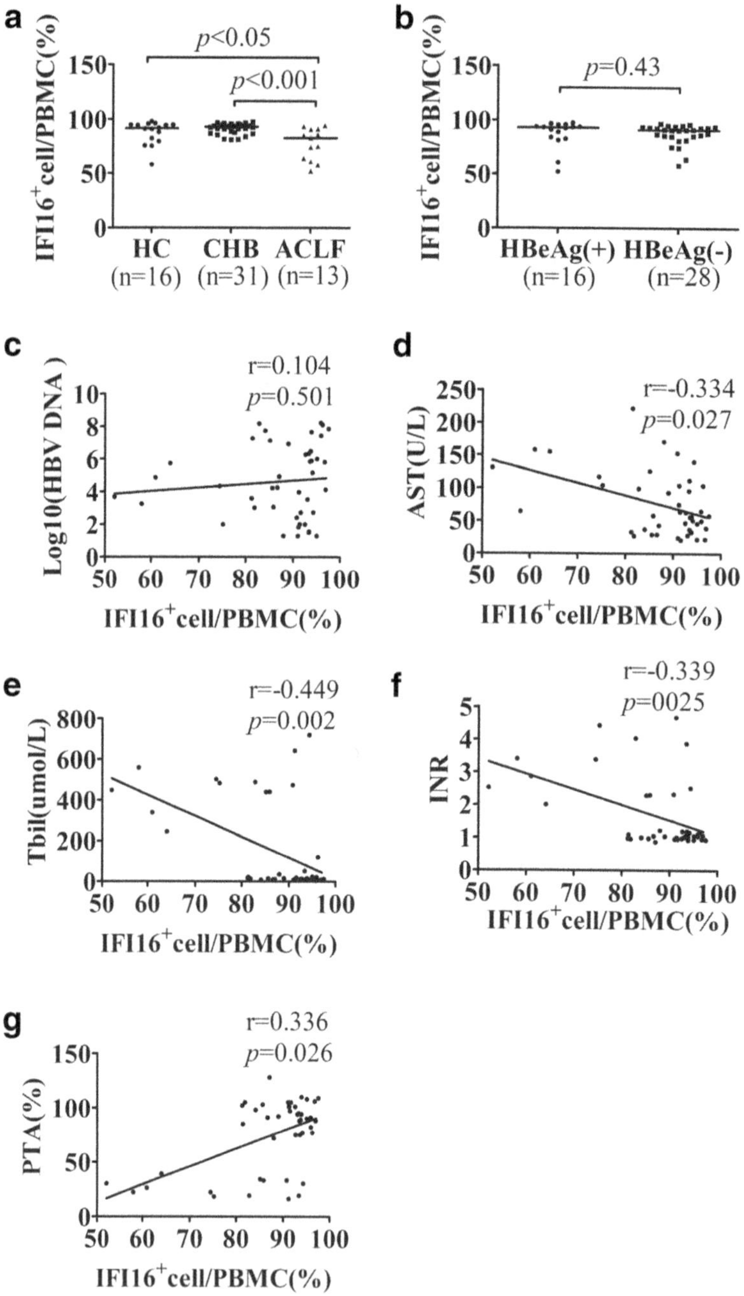

Fig. 1 IFI16 expression levels in PBMCs from patients with ACLF, CHB, and healthy controls. There was a significant increase in IFI16 expression in ACLF patients compared with CHB patients and healthy controls (**a**). No significant difference was found between the HBeAg (+) and HBeAg (–) groups (**b**). No significant correlations were found between the IFI16 level and HBV DNA load (**c**). The expression of IFI16 was significantly negatively correlated with aspartate aminotransferase (AST) (**d**), serum total bilirubin (TBIL) (**e**), and the international normalized ratio(INR) (**f**), and positively correlated with prothrombin time activity (PTA) (**g**). AST aspartate aminotransferase, CHB chronic hepatitis B, ACLF acute-on-chronic liver failure, HBeAg hepatitis B e antigen, HBV hepatitis B virus, PBMCs peripheral blood mononuclear cells, TBIL total bilirubin, PTA prothrombin time activity, INR international normalized ratio

As shown in Fig. 2d, the protein level of IFI16 in the HBV-ACLF group was remarkably higher than in the CHB($P = 0.006$) and normal control groups ($P = 0.001$), and there is no difference between CHB and normal control groups ($P > 0.05$; Fig. 2e). In particular, this finding was consistent with the semi-quantitative immunohistochemistry levels for all groups. Then, we evaluated the correlations between IFI16 and clinical parameters, including HAI, serum AST, TBIL, PTA, and INR, in patients with HBV. IFI16 expression

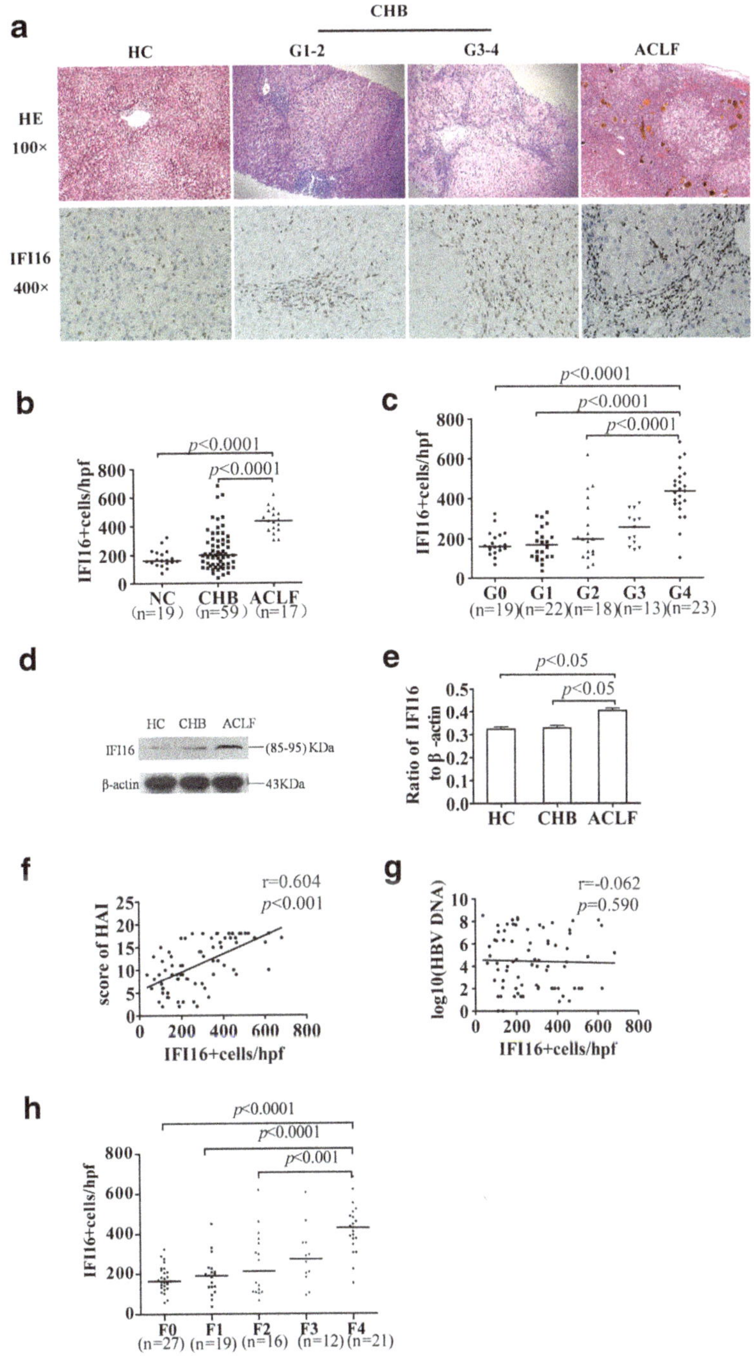

Fig. 2 IFI16 expression levels in livers from patients with ACLF, CHB, and healthy controls. Different degrees of damage can be observed in the liver tissue from CHB and HBV-ACLF patients, as demonstrated by H&E staining. IFI16 expression was observed in the livers of healthy donors and patients with HBV and was mainly detected in liver non-parenchymal cells, especially the inflammatory cells in the livers of HBV patients(**a**). There was a significant increase in IFI16 expression in ACLF patients compared with CHB patients and healthy controls (**b**). In detail, the intrahepatic IFI16 expression in patients with inflammation grade 4 was significantly higher than those with inflammation grade 0, 1, 2, or 3 (**c**). The expression of IFI16 protein is shown by western blotting (**d**). The protein level of IFI16 in the HBV-ACLF group was remarkably higher than that of the CHB and normal control groups (**e**). The expression of IFI16 was significantly positively correlated with HAI (**f**). No significant correlations were found between the IFI16 level and HBV DNA load (**g**). The intrahepatic IFI16 expression in patients with fibrosis stage 4 was also significantly higher than in those with fibrosis stage 0,1, or 2 (**h**)

levels were positively correlated with HAI ($r = 0.604$, $P < 0.001$) (Fig. 2f), AST ($r = 0.468$, $P < 0.001$), INR ($r = 0.562$, $P < 0.001$), and TBIL ($r = 0.515$, $P < 0.001$) and negatively correlated with PTA ($r = -0.564$, $P < 0.001$). We also found that there was no significant difference between the HBeAg (+) and HBeAg (−) groups ($P = 0.773$), and no statistically significant relationships were found between IFI16 expression levels and HBV DNA load ($r = -0.062$, $P = 0.590$; Fig. 2g). Moreover, there was no statistically significant relationships were found between IFI16 expression levels and HBV DNA load only in chronic HBV infected patients ($r = 0.169$, $P = 0.198$).

The distribution of IFI16 in common liver innate cells

The liver is well-known to be an immunological organ with a predominant innate immune system. The phenotypes of IFI16+ cells in liver tissues were further examined by immune fluorescence double staining. From these analyses, the expression of IFI16 in healthy donors and CHB patients was observed in the nucleus of $CD299^+$ endothelial cells, $CD68^+$KCs, $CD56^+$ NK cells, $CD11c^+$DCs, α-SMA^+HSCs (Fig. 3), but this expression was completely absent from $CD299^+$ endothelial cells, $CD56^+$ NK cells, $CD11c^+$DCs, and α-SMA^+HSCs in HBV-ACLF patients. To our surprise, we found that IFI16 was expressed in the cytoplasm of $CD68^+$KCs in HBV-ACLF patients (Fig. 4).

Discussion

IFI16 was first reported in 1992, and subsequently research found its expression was associated with human myeloid cell differentiation [16]. Dawson and Trapani first discovered a DNA binding domain in IFI16 protein [17], and Leonie Unterholznerl identified IFI16 as an intracellular DNA sensor that mediates the induction of IFN [18]. Recent evidences show that IFI16 is involved in viral infection procedure and specifically serve as an inhibitor to viral infections. In addition, IFI16 mediates IFN-γ induction and stimulates inflammatory activation in certain cell types during infection with KSHV [8],HSV-1 [7] and HIV [19]. IFI16 may also act as a possible target in autoimmune diseases [20] and can be found in human fibroblasts, endothelial cells, and B cells. We hypothesized that IFI16 contributes to HBV infection and HBV-associated liver inflammation.

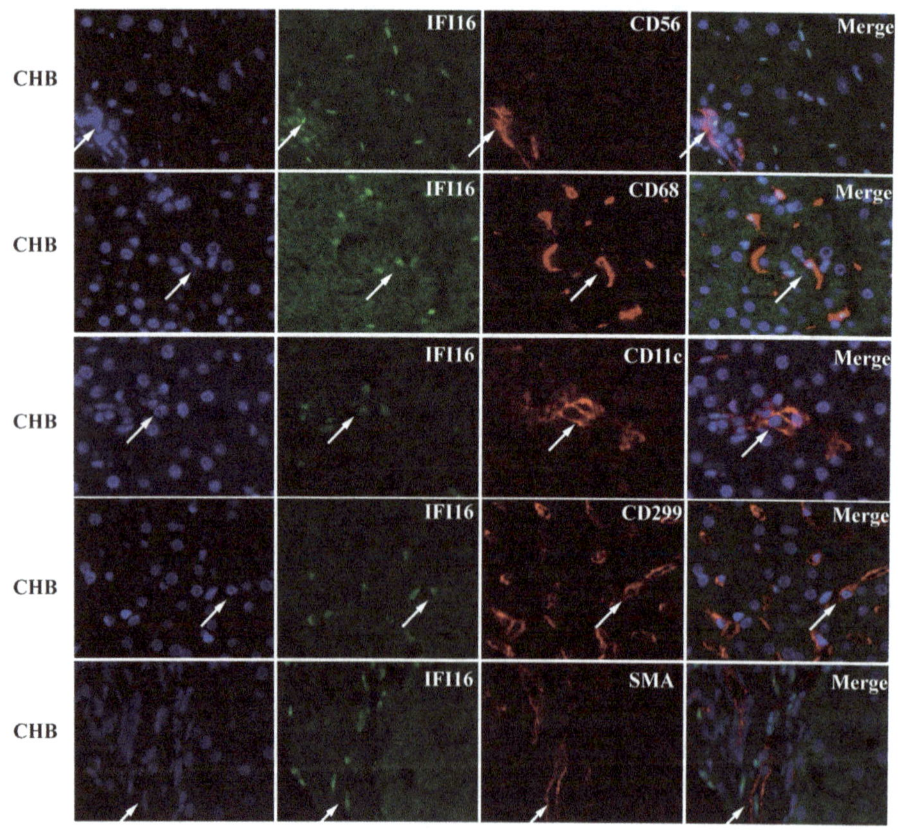

Fig. 3 The morphology of $IFI16^+$ cells in liver tissues from healthy donors and CHB patients was detected by immunofluorescence double staining. Immunofluorescence double staining revealed that IFI16 was expressed by $CD299^+$ endothelial cells, $CD68^+$ macrophages, $CD56^+$ NK cells, $CD11c^+$dendritic cells, and α-SMA^+ hepatic stellate cells. Arrows indicate positive cells. The nuclei were stained with Hoechst33342, and the scale bar indicates 20 μm

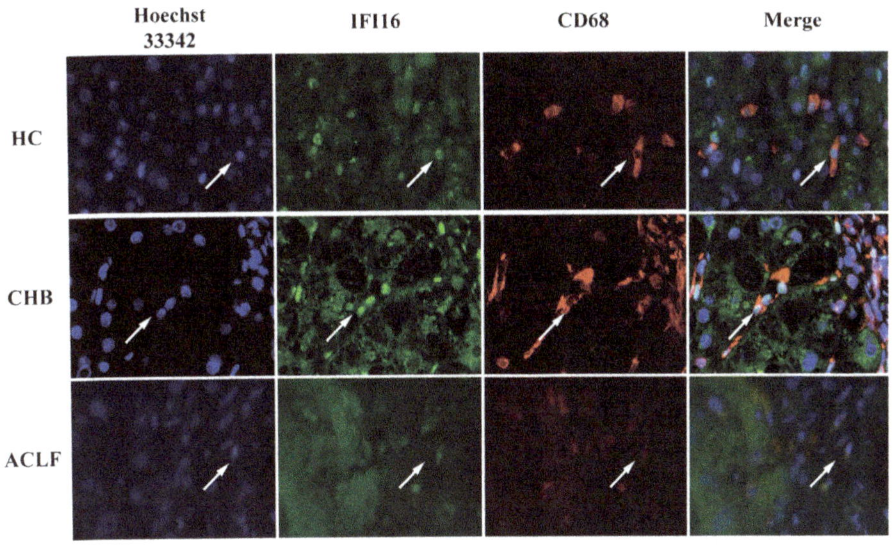

Fig. 4 The localization of IFI16+ cells in CD68+ macrophages from the livers of healthy donors, CHB patients, and ACLF patients was detected by immunofluorescence double staining. Immunofluorescence double staining revealed that IFI16 was localized in the nucleus of CD68+ macrophages in healthy donors and CHB patients but in the cytoplasm of HBV-ACLF patients. Arrows indicate positive cells

Here, we show for the first time that IFI16 expression levels are associated with liver inflammation in HBV-liver diseases. In particular, the number of IFI16+ PBMCs in HBV-ACLF patients was significantly lower than that in CHB patients and healthy controls. In contrast, the number of IFI16+ cells in livers of HBV-ACLF patients was significantly higher than that in CHB patients and healthy controls. In livers and PBMCs, there was no significant difference between CHB patients and healthy controls. Together, these results imply that the expression of IFI16 may predict the development of HBV-associated ACLF and that IFI16 may play an important role in disease pathogenesis. Though the precise mechanisms involved in HBV-associated ACLF have yet to be clarified, the host immune response and the inflammatory cascade are critical in this syndrome. The role that cytokines, including tumor necrosis factor-α (TNF-α), IL-1, and IFNs, play in HBV-ACLF remains a key unresolved point in our understanding of the pathogenesis of the inflammatory response. The rise in cytokine levels can be related to necrotic liver cells, decreased hepatic clearance, or the activation of PRRs [2]. Hyperactivation of the PRR signaling pathway is involved in liver injury [21]. IFI16 has now been identified as one of the PRRs. The receptor can sense DNA, then induce STING-dependent IFN expression and stimulate ASC-dependent inflammatory activation, such as the activation of caspase-1, which cleaves pro-IL-1β and pro-IL-18 to generate their active forms. Overexpression of IFI16 in the liver contributes to the injury, but the expression of IFI16 in PBMCs was lower in ACLF patients. We hypothesize that peripheral IFI16+ cells are selectively recruited to the liver, where they will mature and initiate a destructive immune response, leading to liver injury. This hypothesis will be tested in further studies.

IFI16 is categorized as one of the PYHIN family of proteins that are defined by an N-terminal PYD and one or two C-terminal DNA-binding HIN domains. According to its crystal structures, IFI16 can bind directly to different types of DNA via the C-terminal HIN-200 domain [18]. We speculated that IFI16 may sense HBV DNA to trigger the innate immune response, but our study did not uncover a statistically significant relationship between IFI16 expression levels and HBV parameters. In addition, there was no significant difference in the protein levels between CHB patients and healthy controls in livers or in PBMCs. This result suggests that HBV DNA cannot directly bind to IFI16. One possibility is that HBV DNA may have evolved mechanisms to counteract the actions of IFI16. Some studies have found that viruses have evolved mechanisms to counteract the actions of IFI16. For example, HSV-1 E3 ubiquitin ligase ICP0 targets IFI16 for degradation in human fibroblasts, thus impairing virus-induced expression of IFN-γ and IFN-stimulated genes [22].Human cytomegalovirus tegument protein pUL83 inhibits IFI16-mediated DNA sensing for immune evasion [11]. Another possibility is that IFI16 may only sense HBV DNA under special conditions. While DNA recognition by IFI16 can occur in both the nucleus and cytoplasm, acetylation at two different sites on the nuclear localization signal, situated in the N-terminal region of IFI16, has been recently discovered to regulate the nucleo-cytoplasmic localization of IFI16 [23].

Through further study, we identified the phenotypes of IFI16+ cells in liver tissues by immunofluorescence double staining. We found that IFI16 was localized in the nucleus of Kupffer cells (KCs), endothelial cells, natural killer (NK) cells, dendritic cells (DCs), and hepatic stellate cells(HSCs)in healthy donors and CHB patients, but in the liver of HBV-ACLF patients IFI16 was only localized in the cytoplasm of KCs. IFI16 was first described as a strictly nuclear protein, but more recent studies have indicated IFI16 can be found in the cytoplasm of many cell types [6]. For example, viral and DNA transfection modulates subcellular localization of IFI16 related to IFN induction and vesicle sorting pathways [23, 24]. Furthermore, UV–light treatment of epithelial cells driven IFI16 moving from the nucleus to back the cytoplasm [25]. This modulation of the localization of IFI16 is likely to impact the protein function. In this study, we found that IFI16 was only localized in the cytoplasm of KC which are cells that play a key role in liver injury by internalizing ligands, activating signaling cascades, and inducing transcription of proinflammatory cytokines and superoxide agents, thereby contributing to microcirculatory dysfunction. KCs are able to activate NK cells and natural killer T(NKT) cells, both of which are present at relatively high numbers in the liver, via the production of proinflammatory cytokines [26].In the future, we aim to understand how modulation of the subcellular localization of IFI16 in KCs contributes to the pathological mechanism of HBV-ACLF.

There are some limitations to the present study. First, we determined the IFI16 protein levels in only a small number of patients from a single unit. We cannot rule out the interference of age and believe that repeating the study in a community-based population or large cohort dataset would be helpful to understand the value of this marker. Second, other diseases that occur during the progression of HBV infection, including cirrhosis, should be included to explore the comprehensive role of IFI16 in the complete progression of HBV infection. However, it is hard to collect the samples from these patients. Actually, we found the intrahepatic IFI16 expression in patients of F4 was significantly higher than in F0 to F2. This is similar to what we found the relationship between IFI16 and inflammation. Researches show that chronic liver inflammation may lead to fibrosis and cirrhosis through IL-1signaling [27].And IFI16 can stimulate cleavage of pro-IL1b and pro-IL18 to the bioactive cytokines [6].So IFI16 may play a role in the pathogenesis of liver cirrhosis, next step we can further investigate it. Third, in future studies the effects of silencing the IFI16 gene in cell lines and HBV transgenic mice will be comprehensively investigated to understand the interplay between IFI16 and HBV.

Conclusion

Our study revealed that the expression of IFI16 in HBV-ACLF patients was higher in livers but lower in PBMCs and that IFI16 was only localized in the cytoplasm of KCs. These results suggest that IFI16 might contribute to the pathogenesis of HBV-associated ACLF; however, the function of IFI16 during HBV infection remains to be determined. Further work is needed to elucidate the role of IFI16 in the liver and the importance of its subcellular localization in KCs.

Abbreviations

AIM-2: absent in melanoma 2; ALT: alanine amino transferase; ASC: apoptosis-associated speck-like protein containing a caspase recruitment domain; AST: aspartate aminotransferase; CHB: chronic hepatitis B; DC: dendritic cell; EBV: Epstein–Barr virus; HBV-ACLF: HBV-associated acute-on-chronic liver failure; HCMV: human cytomegalovirus; HSC: hepatic stellate cell; HSV-1: herpes simplex virus 1; IBD: inflammatory bowel disease; IFI16: IFN inducible protein 16; IL-1: interleukin-1; ISGs: IFN-stimulated genes; KC: Kupffer cell; KSHV: Kaposi's sarcoma-related herpesvirus; LESC: liver sinusoidal endothelial cell; MELD: Model for end-stage liver disease; NK: Natural Killer; NKT: natural killer T.; NLRs: NOD-like receptors; NLS: nuclear localization signal; PBMCs: peripheral blood mononuclear cells; PRRs: pattern-recognition receptors; PTA: prothrombin time activity; PYD: pyrin domain; RLRs: RIG-I-like receptors; STING: stimulate stimulator of IFN genes; Tbil: total bilirubin; TLRs: Toll-like receptors; TNF-α: tumor necrosis factor-α

Acknowledgements

The authors thank all patients, study-site staff, and participating consultants for their contributions, which made this study possible.

Funding

This study was funded by National Science and Technology Major Project (2016ZX10002003, 2016ZX10002008, 2016ZX10002009) and Natural Science Fund of Guangdong Province(2015A030313022).

Authors' contributions

XP and XL designed the experiments, analyzed the statistics, and were major contributors in writing the manuscript. ZM and JH analyzed and interpreted the patient data regarding the disease. ZL and XZ collected the samples of patients. HD and ZF performed the histological examination. DX and ZG proposed the conception and provided funding. All authors read and approved the final manuscript.

Competing interests

XP, XL, ZM, JH, HD, ZL, XZ, ZF, DX and ZG declare that they have no competing interest.

Author details

[1]Department of Infectious Diseases, Third Affiliated Hospital of Sun-Yat-SenUniversity, GuangZhou, China. [2]GuangDong Provincial Key Laboratory of Liver Disease, Third Affiliated Hospital of Sun-Yat-Sen University, GuangZhou, China. [3]Department of Pathology, Third Affiliated Hospital of Sun-Yat-Sen University, GuangZhou, China. [4]GuangZhou, China.

References:

1. Bertoletti A, Ferrari C. Innate and adaptive immune responses in chronic hepatitis B virus infections: towards restoration of immune control of viral infection. Gut. 2012;61:1754–64.
2. Han Q, Zhang C, Zhang J, Tian Z. The role of innate immunity in HBV infection. Semin Immunopathol. 2013;35:23–38.
3. Connolly DJ, Bowie AG. The emerging role of human PYHIN proteins in innate immunity: implications for health and disease. Biochem Pharmacol. 2014;92:405–14.

4. Hornung V, Ablasser A, Charrel-Dennis M, Bauernfeind F, Horvath G, Caffrey DR, Latz E, et al. AIM2 recognizes cytosolic dsDNA and forms a caspase-1-activating inflammasome with ASC. Nature. 2009;458:514–8.
5. Pan X, Xu H, Zheng C, Li M, Zou X, Cao H, Xu Q. Human hepatocytes express absent in melanoma 2 and respond to hepatitis B virus with interleukin-18 expression. Virus Genes. 2016;52:445–52.
6. Jakobsen MR, Paludan SR. IFI16: at the interphase between innate DNA sensing and genome regulation. Cytokine Growth Factor Rev. 2014;25:649–55.
7. Johnson KE, Chikoti L, Chandran B. Herpes simplex virus 1 infection induces activation and subsequent inhibition of the IFI16 and NLRP3 inflammasomes. J Virol. 2013;87:5005–18.
8. Kerur N, Veettil MV, Sharma-Walia N, Bottero V, Sadagopan S, Otageri P, Chandran B. IFI16 acts as a nuclear pathogen sensor to induce the inflammasome in response to Kaposi sarcoma-associated herpesvirus infection. Cell Host Microbe. 2011;9:363–75.
9. Ansari MA, Singh VV, Dutta S, Veettil MV, Dutta D, Chikoti L, Lu J, et al. Constitutive interferon-inducible protein 16-inflammasome activation during Epstein-Barr virus latency I, II, and III in B and epithelial cells. J Virol. 2013;87: 8606–23.
10. Horan KA, Hansen K, Jakobsen MR, Holm CK, Soby S, Unterholzner L, Thompson M, et al. Proteasomal degradation of herpes simplex virus capsids in macrophages releases DNA to the cytosol for recognition by DNA sensors. J Immunol. 2013;190:2311–9.
11. Li T, Chen J, Cristea IM. Human cytomegalovirus tegument protein pUL83 inhibits IFI16-mediated DNA sensing for immune evasion. Cell Host Microbe. 2013;14:591–9.
12. Jakobsen MR, Bak RO, Andersen A, Berg RK, Jensen SB, Tengchuan J, Laustsen A, et al. IFI16 senses DNA forms of the lentiviral replication cycle and controls HIV-1 replication. Proc Natl Acad Sci U S A. 2013;110:E4571–80.
13. Hansen K, Prabakaran T, Laustsen A, Jorgensen SE, Rahbaek SH, Jensen SB, Nielsen R, et al. Listeria monocytogenes induces IFNbeta expression through an IFI16-, cGAS- and STING-dependent pathway. EMBO J. 2014;33: 1654–66.
14. Schaff Z. The value of liver biopsy in chronic hepatitis. Orv Hetil. 2011;152: 856–8.
15. Lei Z, Mo Z, Zhu J, Pang X, Zheng X. Soluble ST2 plasma concentrations predict mortality in HBV-related acute-on-chronic liver failure. 2015;2015: 535938.
16. Trapani JA, Dawson M, Apostolidis VA, Browne KA. Genomic organization of IFI16, an interferon-inducible gene whose expression is associated with human myeloid cell differentiation: correlation of predicted protein domains with exon organization. Immunogenetics. 1994;40:415–24.
17. Dawson MJ, Trapani JA. The interferon-inducible autoantigen, IFI 16: localization to the nucleolus and identification of a DNA-binding domain. Biochem Biophys Res Commun. 1995;214:152–62.
18. Unterholzner L, Keating SE, Baran M, Horan KA, Jensen SB, Sharma S, Sirois CM, et al. IFI16 is an innate immune sensor for intracellular DNA. Nat Immunol. 2010;11:997–1004.
19. Monroe KM, Yang Z, Johnson JR, Geng X, Doitsh G, Krogan NJ, Greene WC. IFI16 DNA sensor is required for death of lymphoid CD4 T cells abortively infected with HIV. Science. 2013;
20. Gugliesi F, Bawadekar M, De Andrea M, Dell'Oste V, Caneparo V, Tincani A, Gariglio M, et al. Nuclear DNA sensor IFI16 as circulating protein in autoimmune diseases is a signal of damage that impairs endothelial cells through high-affinity membrane binding. PLoS One. 2013;8:e63045.
21. Ojiro K, Ebinuma H, Nakamoto N, Wakabayashi K, Mikami Y, Ono Y, Po-Sung C, et al. MyD88-dependent pathway accelerates the liver damage of Concanavalin A-induced hepatitis. Biochem Biophys Res Commun. 2010;399: 744–9.
22. Orzalli MH, DeLuca NA, Knipe DM. Nuclear IFI16 induction of IRF-3 signaling during herpesviral infection and degradation of IFI16 by the viral ICP0 protein. Proc Natl Acad Sci U S A. 2012;109:E3008–17.
23. Li T, Diner BA, Chen J, Cristea IM. Acetylation modulates cellular distribution and DNA sensing ability of interferon-inducible protein IFI16. Proc Natl Acad Sci U S A. 2012;109:10558–63.
24. Dell'Oste V, Gatti D, Gugliesi F, De Andrea M, Bawadekar M, Cigno IL, Biolatti M, et al. Innate nuclear sensor IFI16 translocates into the cytoplasm during early stage of in vitro HCMV infection and is entrapped in the egressing virions during late stage. J Virol. 2014;
25. Costa S, Borgogna C, Mondini M, De Andrea M, Meroni PL, Berti E, Gariglio M, et al. Redistribution of the nuclear protein IFI16 into the cytoplasm of ultraviolet B-exposed keratinocytes as a mechanism of autoantigen processing. Br J Dermatol. 2011;164:282–90.
26. Boltjes A, Movita D, Boonstra A, Woltman AM. The role of Kupffer cells in hepatitis B and hepatitis C virus infections. J Hepatol. 2014;61:660–71.
27. Szabo G, Csak T. Inflammasomes in liver diseases. J Hepatol. 2012;57:642–54.

20

A case series evaluating the impact of Hepatitis C eradication using direct acting antivirals on primary biliary cholangitis-associated autoimmunity

Henry H. Nguyen[1], Abdullah Khathlan[1], Marvin J. Fritzler[2] and Mark G. Swain[1,3*]

Abstract

Background: Chronic Hepatitis C Virus (HCV) infection has been commonly linked to the development of autoimmunity, in part through activation of B cells. B cells are also postulated to play a pathogenic role in the autoimmune liver disease Primary Biliary Cholangitis (PBC). Patients with concurrent PBC and HCV infection carry an increased risk of more progressive disease, although the mechanism underlying this effect is poorly understood. Utilizing a case series of patients with concurrent PBC and HCV, the aim of this study was to evaluate for the potential impact of HCV eradication upon autoimmunity/autoantibody production.

Case presentation: A case series evaluating three patients with co-existing PBC-HCV infection receiving non-interferon based HCV treatments with direct-acting antivirals (DAA). One of three patient received Ursodeoxycholic acid (UDCA; 13 mg/kg/day) during the treatment period. Sustained virological response (SVR) to DAA's was assessed using a HCV Quantitative Nucleic Acid Test (Abbott). Autoantibodies associated with autoimmune liver diseases (including PBC) and liver biochemistry, were measured before, during and after DAA treatment (Mitogen Advanced Diagnostics Laboratory, Calgary, Canada).

All patients achieved an SVR, as determined by negative HCV RNA test 12 weeks post-DAA therapy. Titres of anti-mitochondrial antibodies (AMA-M2), anti- branched-chain 2-oxo-acid dehydrogenase complex and 2-oxo glutarate dehydrogenase complex (anti-3E-BPO), and anti- tripartite motif-containing protein 21 (TRIM21/Ro52) remained unchanged, despite successful HCV eradication. Two of the three patients exhibited a transient decrease in some autoantibody titres during DAA treatment, but these returned to baseline levels post-DAA therapy.

Conclusions: Within the limitations of a case series, our results suggest that HCV co-infection may not be a significant driver of PBC-related autoimmunity/autoantibody production. However, a larger n-value is required to truly assess for the effect of HCV eradication on autoantibody production.

Keywords: Primary biliary cholangitis, Hepatitis C virus, Autoimmunity, Autoantibodies

Background

The effects of HCV infection can extend beyond the liver. Specifically, HCV has been implicated as driving a number of extrahepatic manifestations that are characterized by autoimmunity including mixed cryoglobulinemia, glomerulonephritis, thyroid disease, Sjogren's syndrome (SS), systemic sclerosis (SSc), and autoimmune liver disease [1, 2]. These associations suggest a close interplay between HCV and the host immune response, with HCV augmenting immune responses. How HCV infection drives autoimmunity remains unclear; however, HCV appears to be capable of directly and indirectly augmenting B cell responses [1, 3]. In general, HCV-associated autoimmune manifestations are thought to be mediated, at least in part, by autoantibodies. Antinuclear antibody

* Correspondence: swain@ucalgary.ca
[1]Division of Gastroenterology and Hepatology, University of Calgary Liver Unit, Calgary, Canada
[3]Teaching Research & Wellness Centre, 3280 Hospital Drive NW, Calgary, AB T2N 4N1, Canada

(ANA), anti-smooth muscle antibody (ASMA), anti-liver kidney microsome type 1 (anti-LKM1), and anti-mitochondrial antibody (AMA) have all been previously identified in the sera of patients with chronic HCV [1, 4, 5]. Moreover, the presence of ANA, ASMA, and anti-LKM1 in HCV patients have been associated with clinical and biochemical evidence suggestive of increased liver injury [1, 6, 7]. Given the potential interactions between HCV, B cell activation and autoantibody production, defining the potential impact of HCV on coexisting autoimmune disease is of interest.

Although not common, patients with primary biliary cholangitis (PBC) and concurrent HCV infection (PBC-HCV) have been previously described [8, 9]. PBC-HCV patients appear to have more aggressive liver disease, as demonstrated by an increased risk of developing cirrhosis [8] and hepatocellular cancer (HCC), compared to patients with HCV alone [9]. Despite this increased risk, avoidance of treatment with interferon based regimens in PBC-HCV patients has been recommended due to the potential (and documented) risk of immune stimulation with drugs such as interferon exacerbating PBC [10]. With the increasing availability of direct-acting antivirals (DAA) this theoretical risk can now be circumvented. Inhibiting and/or eradicating HCV viral replication with DAA's would remove HCV-specific stimulation of host immunity, thereby allowing for the determination of the true impact of HCV replication on driving underlying autoimmune processes; including autoantibody production associated with PBC.

Therefore, we treated three PBC-HCV patients with DAA's and determined whether HCV replication suppression and eradication impacted PBC-related autoimmunity, as reflected by treatment-induced declines in serum levels of a number of autoantibodies associated with the diagnosis and clinical progression of PBC.

Case presentations

Three patients with coexisting PBC and HCV were treated with interferon free DAA regimens between the years 2014 and 2015. All three patients were followed in the University of Calgary Liver Unit (UCLU) (Calgary, Alberta, Canada) which is a tertiary referral center serving Southern Alberta (~ 1.5 million people). HCV viral loads were determined before, during and after DAA treatment (ledipasvir + sofosbuvir (Harvoni®) for genotype 1a infected patients, and sofosbuvir + ribavirin for the genotype 4 infected patient) using a using Hepatitis C Virus Quantitative Nucleic Acid Test (HCV NAT; Abbott GmbH & Co., Wiesbaden, HE, Germany) performed by the Alberta Provincial Laboratory (Calgary AB, Canada). HCV-NAT were assessed at either 12 or 24 weeks post-HCV treatment to define Sustained Virologic Response (SVR). A spectrum of auto-antibodies reported to occur in the context of PBC and/or autoimmune liver diseases in general, were measured in serum samples obtained before, during and after DAA therapy. Autoantibodies targeting the following antigens were assessed: mitochondrial antibodies M2 (AMA-M2), branched-chain 2-oxo-acid dehydrogenase complex and 2-oxo glutarate dehydrogenase complex (3E-BPO), tripartite motif-containing protein 21 (TRIM21/Ro52), glycoprotein 210 (gp210), sp100 nuclear antigen (sp100), soluble liver antigen (SLA), promyelocytic leukemia cell antigen (PML), and liver cytosolic-1 antigen (LC-1). These autoantibodies were analyzed using a Line Immunoassay (Mitogen Advanced Diagnostic Laboratory, Calgary, AB Canada). Liver stiffness was measured using a Fibroscan® (carried out by experienced operators) as an indirect measure of the degree of liver fibrosis. Comparison of the patients autoantibody profiles and serum biochemistry were made against established guidelines by international liver associations for the diagnosis of PBC [11, 12].

Table 1 summarizes the patient demographics along with respective autoantibody, serological, and virological profiles. On initial assessment at the UCLU, Patient 1 tested positive for AMA in the setting of a normal serum Alkaline Phosphatase (AP) levels. Diagnostic criteria for PBC, which requires concurrent elevation in serum AP levels and a positive AMA (if no liver biopsy is performed), was therefore not met. However, Patient 1 subsequently fulfilled the diagnostic criteria for PBC with the development of cholestasis (i.e. elevated serum AP level). Treatment with Ursodeoxycholic acid (UDCA; 13 mg/kg/day) was initiated at that time and continued throughout the concurrent treatment period for HCV with DAA. Serum AP normalized with UDCA therapy and remained normal throughout the DAA treatment period.

Patient 2 fulfilled diagnostic criteria for PBC on initial clinic evaluation, having both an elevated serum AP level and AMA positivity. UDCA (13 mg/kg/day) therapy was initiated but was subsequently discontinued due to intolerable side effects. The patient was not taking UDCA during the treatment period for HCV with DAA, as reflected by persistently elevated serum AP levels during the pre- and post-HCV treatment period.

Patient 3 had a positive AMA on initial investigation in the setting of a normal serum AP level, therefore failing to meet classical diagnostic criteria for PBC. Therefore, this patient was not treated with UDCA during the HCV treatment period.

In all three patients serum IgG and IgM levels were within normal range on initial clinical assessment. No liver biopsies were obtained from any of the patients. All 3 patients achieved a SVR with DAA therapy. Serum alanine aminotransferase (ALT) levels demonstrated a

Table 1 Characteristics of patients with positive anti-mitochondrial antibody and Hepatitis C Virus infection

Characteristics	Patient 1	Patient 2	Patient 3
Demographics			
Age, yrs	67	63	64
Sex, M/F	M	F	F
Anti-Mitochondrial Antibody			
Titer by IF at diagnosis	1:40	1:160	1:160
Liver Enzymes at diagnosis			
AP (N<145 IU/L)	67	134	71
GGT (N<35)	130	330	41
Hepatitis C Virus			
Duration HCV+ status, yrs	19	19	15
Genotype	1a	1a	4
Treatment Naive	Yes	No	Yes
Treatment Regimen	LDV + SOF	LDV + SOF	SOF +RBV
RNA NAT, weeks post tx	<12 IU/ml (12)	ND (24)	ND (24)
Autoantibody Profile (Mitogen)	AMA-M2+, Anti-3E-BPO+	Anti-3E-BPO+, Anti-Ro52+	AMA-M2+, Anti-3E-BPO+
Fibroscan (fPa)			
Pre-treatment with DAA	37.4	15.1	14.1
Post-treatment with DAA	19.8	12.3	No data
Ursodeoxycholic acid treatment	Yes	No (discontinued)	No

Abbreviations: *AP* alkaline phospate, *AMA* anti-mitochondrial antibody, *DAA* direct –acting antivirals, *F* females, *GGT* gamma glutamyl-transferase, *HCV* Hepatitis C Virus, *IF* immunoflourescence, *LDV* ledispavir, *M* male, *ND* not detected, *Post-tx* post treatment, *RNA NAT* Ribonucleic acid quantitative nucleic acid test, *RBV* ribravin, *SOF* sofosbivur, *yrs* years, *IF* immunoflourescence

robust early and sustained decrease in association with DAA therapy in all three patients (Fig. 1). Serum alkaline phosphatase, GGT, and total bilirubin levels remained within the normal range during DAA treatment for both Patient 1 and Patient 3 (Normal range of Alkaline Phosphatase 35–125 IU/L; GGT < 61; Bilirubin < 20 umol/L). Patient 2 had cholestatic liver enzymes with serum AP ranging from 130 to 150 IU/L and GGT 220–250 U/L during the treatment period with DAA. In 2 of 3 patients there was documented improvement in the

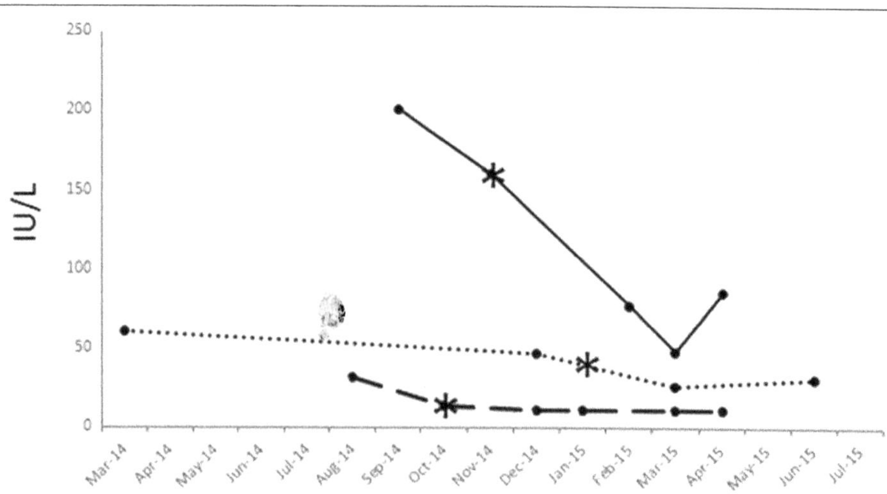

Fig. 1 Serum alanine aminotransferase (ALT) levels of all three patients during HCV treatment. Patient 1 (solid line) was treated with ledipasvir + sofosbuvir X 12 weeks between the dates of November 29, 2014 to February 20, 2015. Patient 2 (dotted line) was treated with ledipasvir + sofosbuvir X 24 weeks between the dates of January 15, 2015 to July 2, 2015. Patient 3 (dashed line) was treated with sofosbuvir + ribavirin X 24 weeks between the dates of October 23, 2014 to April 8, 2015. Treatment initiation dates with DAA are indicated by a black asterisk (*). ALT levels were measured at different time points as shown in the X-Axis

Fibroscan® score post-HCV treatment. In one patient, a Fibroscan® assessment could not be done post-HCV treatment as the patient had left the country after finishing treatment. Serum autoantibody titres were measured for each patient before, during and after HCV treatment, and results are shown in Fig. 2. In all three patients, pre- and post-DAA treatment autoantibody titres for anti-3E-BPO, TRIM21/Ro52, and AMA (M2) were similar. In Patient 2 (Fig. 2b), the titre of anti-3E BPO exhibited a transient decrease during DAA treatment, followed by a rebound to baseline levels post-DAA therapy. This trend was also noted in Patient 3 for both AMA-M2 and anti-3E BPO titre levels (Fig. 2c).

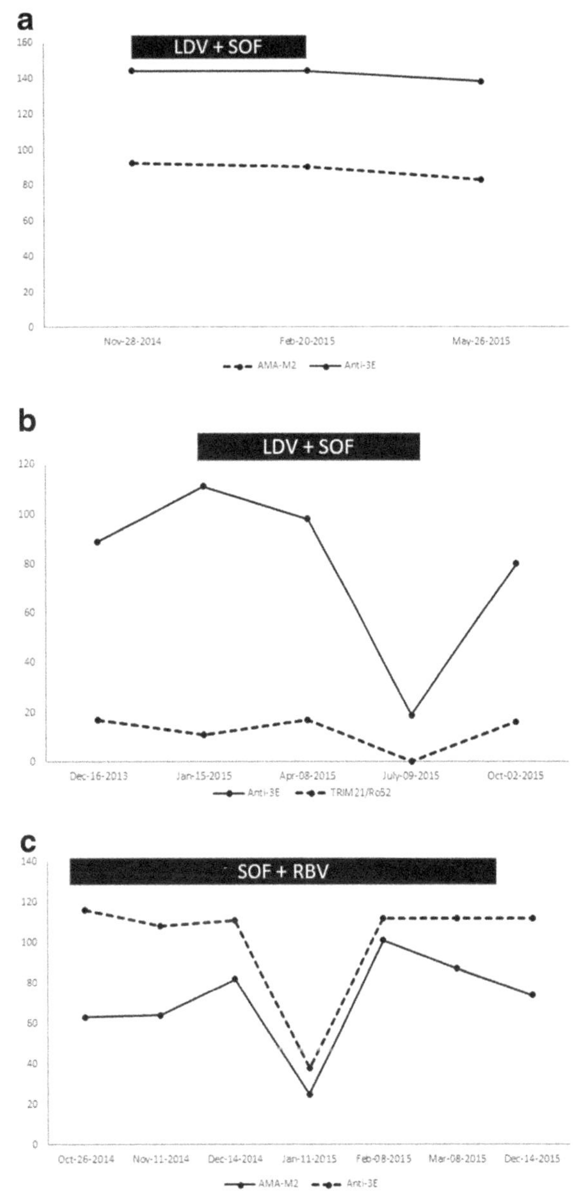

Fig. 2 a Titres of anti-mitochondrial antibody M2 (AMA-M2) and anti-3E-BPO during HCV therapy with ledipasvir (LDV) and sofosbuvir (SOF) X 12 weeks in Patient 1. LDV + SOF therapy was given between the dates of November 29, 2014 to February 20, 2015 (black box). Antibody titres were measured at three different time points as shown in the X-Axis. **b** Titres of anti-TRIM21/Ro52 and anti-3E-BPO during HCV therapy with ledipasvir (LDV) + sofosbuvir (SOF) X 24 weeks in Patient 2 LDV + SOF was given between the dates January 15, 2015 to July 2, 2015 (black box). Autoantibody titres were measured at various time points as shown in the X-Axis. **c** Titres of anti-mitochondrial antibody (AMA-M2) and anti-3E-BPO during HCV therapy with Sofosbuvir (SOF) and Ribavirin (RBV) X 24 weeks in Patient 3 SOF + RBV therapy was given between the dates of October 23, 2014 to April 8, 2015 (black box). Autoantibody titres were measured at various time points as shown in the X-Axis

Discussion and conclusion

HCV was successfully eradicated by DAA treatment in all 3 of our HCV patients. However, in these successfully treated patients, serum titres of the PBC-related autoantibodies AMA (M2), anti-3E BPO and/or anti-Ro52 were similar in the pre-treatment and post-treatment serum samples. These findings suggests that ongoing HCV replication is not a significant driver of autoantibody production in PBC.

The diagnostic criteria for PBC requires both AMA positivity and concurrent elevation in serum AP levels [11]. Two patients met these diagnostic criteria, one on initial presentation (Patient 2) and the other who developed cholestatic liver enzymes in follow up (Patient 1). Only one patient did not fulfill classical diagnostic criteria for PBC; exhibiting normal serum AP levels before, during, and after HCV eradication in the setting of AMA positivity (Patient 3). Despite failure to meet diagnostic criteria, the presence of AMA at high titer (by immunofluorescence) in this patient is highly suggestive of an underlying diagnosis of PBC. AMA is a highly specific biomarker for PBC, found in up to 95% of patients, and is widely considered a hallmark autoantibody for this condition [13]. In fact, it has been shown that the majority of AMA positive patients with normal liver enzymes at baseline, will ultimately progress over time to develop overt clinical and biochemical features of PBC [14, 15]. Moreover, AMA-M2 and Anti-3E-BPO autoantibodies were also detected in this patient (Patient 3). Both of these autoantibodies have been previously described to be both prevalent in, and specific for, the diagnosis of PBC [16–18]. Taken together, this constellation of autoantibodies in Patient 3 is highly suggestive of the underlying diagnosis PBC, despite the absence of cholestatic serum biochemistry.

AMA is non-organ specific, targeting ATPase-associated antigens located on the inner mitochondrial membrane [19, 20]. There are four principal mitochondrial antigens targeted in PBC, collectively classified as the M2 subtype. These include the E2 subunits of the pyruvate dehydrogenase complex, the branched chain 2-oxo-acid dehydrogenase complex, the ketoglutaric acid dehydrogenase complex, and the dihydrolipoamide dehydrogenase-binding protein [21–23]. Despite being highly specific for PBC, AMA is one of many autoantibodies that have been documented in patients with chronic HCV infection. It is estimated that up to 8% of patients with HCV are AMA+ [4, 5, 9]. However, it is difficult to ascertain from these studies whether AMA positivity was secondary to previously undiagnosed PBC, or HCV- mediated seroconversion. AMA seroconversion has been documented in one case report of a patient with HCV, but this was in the unique setting of treatment with PEGylated interferon [24]. In our case, with 2 of 3 patients fulfilling diagnostic criteria for PBC and all three patients harboring highly specific autoantibodies for PBC, it is inferred that this is more likely a reflection of underlying PBC rather than a sequelae of seroconversion due to chronic HCV infection. However, given the established association of chronic HCV infection and autoimmune disease/ autoantibody production, larger prospective studies would be required to further define the role of HCV infection in mediating AMA seroconversion.

Contrary to its utility in diagnosing PBC, the role of AMA titers for monitoring disease activity and in defining disease prognosis in PBC appears to be of limited value [25, 26]. Anti-Ro52 is an autoantibody associated with a wide range of autoimmune conditions, including autoimmune myositis, SS, SSc, and systemic lupus erythematosus (SLE) [27]. In PBC patients, the most frequently detected extractable nuclear antigen (ENA) is that of TRIM21/Ro52 [28]. The presence of anti-TRIM21/Ro52 at the time of PBC diagnosis is associated with elevated serum IgM and bilirubin levels, and advanced liver fibrosis stage [28]. Anti-Ro52 has also been associated with increased risk of cirrhosis and hepatic death or liver transplantation in the setting of autoimmune hepatitis [29]. One of our patients had detectable serum anti-TRIM21/Ro52 before HCV treatment. Contrary to previous studies, this patient did not have an associated elevation in serum IgM or bilirubin level, despite having a positive anti-TRIM21/Ro52 level. In addition, there was no overall sustained change in the titre of anti-TRIM21/Ro52 in this patient during their successful HCV treatment.

There are however limitations to this study that warrants further discussion. In addition to the inherent biases associated with the retrospective nature of a case series, the limited sample size does not allow for generalization of our findings to all patients with HCV and PBC. A larger n-value of patients are needed to truly evaluate the effects of HCV eradication on autoimmunity/autoantibody production. Ideally, a prospectively designed study with measurements of autoimmune liver disease associated autoantibodies before and after HCV treatment are needed. This however may be challenging due the fact that patients with concurrent HCV and PBC are not common.

In conclusion, the outcome of our case series highlights that HCV eradication does not significantly impact PBC-related autoantibody production in PBC-HCV patients. The findings in our case series may suggest that HCV infection is not a significant driver of autoimmunity in PBC patients, and cannot explain previous reports suggesting more aggressive clinical disease in HCV infected PBC patients. Currently there are no therapeutic guidelines on the management of PBC-HCV patients. Our case series suggests that DAA treatment is safe and effective in this group of patients, but does not alter underlying PBC-related autoimmunity. Further studies are however needed to better elucidate the association between HCV treatment and underlying autoantibody production as well as evaluate the safety of using DAAs in patients with concurrent HCV and PBC.

Abbreviations

3E-BPO: Branched-chain 2-oxo-acid dehydrogenase complex and 2-oxo glutarate dehydrogenase complex; AMA-M2: Antimitochondrial antibody; ANA: Antinuclear antibody; anti-LKM1: Anti-liver kidney microsome type 1; ASMA: Anti-smooth muscle antibody; DAA: Direct-acting antivirals; gp210: Glycoprotein 210; HCV NAT: Hepatitis C Virus Quantitative Nucleic Acid Test; HCV: Hepatitis C virus; LC-1: Liver cytosolic-1 antigen; PBC: Primary Biliary Cholangitis; PML: Promyelocytic leukemia cell antigen; SLA: Soluble liver antigen; sp100: sp100 nuclear antigen; SS: Sjogren's syndrome; SSc: Systemic sclerosis; TRIM21/Ro52: Tripartite motif-containing protein 21

Acknowledgements

We would like to show our gratitude to Haiyan (Teresa) Hou, Laboratory Manager at Mitogen Advanced Diagnostics Laboratory for her help in retrieving stored serological information used in this study. We would also like to thank Alberta Provincial Laboratory (ProvLab) for their assistance with the HCV Quantitative Nucleic Acid Test utilized in our study.

Grant Support: 1) Canadian Institutes of Health Research (CIHR) operating and Team Grant. 2) Cal Wenzel Family Foundation Chair in Hepatology.

Funding

This research work was completed under the supervision of Dr. Mark G Swain. He receives research funding from the Canadian Institutes of Health Research (CIHR) and holds the Cal Wenzel Family Foundation Chair in Hepatology. The funding bodies listed above were not involved in the design of the study, collection/analysis/interpretation of data, or the writing of the manuscript.

Authors' contributions

MGS is the Primary Investigator and was responsible for critical revisions of the manuscript. HHN and AK were responsible for data acquisition/analysis along with drafting of the manuscript. MJF was responsible for assessment of patient serum for autoantibodies and critical revision of manuscript. All authors have read and approved the manuscript prior to submission.

Consent for publication

Consent for publication was obtained from all patients in this study.

Competing interests

MJF has been a consultant to Inova Diagnostics (San Diego, CA), Werfen International (Barcelona, Spain) and BioRad (Hercules, CA, USA). He has also received gifts in kind from Euoimmun GmbH (Luebeck, Germany).
MGS has served as a speaker and/or advisory board member and/or has received research support from Allergan, Genfit, Bristol Myers Squibb, Gilead Sciences, CymaBay Therapeutics, Abbott, Intercept Pharmaceuticals, Genkyotex, Novartis, Glaxo Smith Kline, Abbvie and Merck. He has served as a data and safety monitoring committee member in clinical trials for Gilead Sciences and GRI Bio Inc. MGS also holds the Cal Wenzel Family Foundation Chair in Hepatology. HHN and AK have no disclosures or competing interests to declare.

Author details

[1]Division of Gastroenterology and Hepatology, University of Calgary Liver Unit, Calgary, Canada. [2]University of Calgary, Calgary, AB, Canada. [3]Teaching Research & Wellness Centre, 3280 Hospital Drive NW, Calgary, AB T2N 4N1, Canada.

References

1. Vergani D, Mieli-Vergani G. Autoimmune manifestations in viral hepatitis. Semin Immunopathol. 2013;35:73–85.
2. Cacoub P, Renou C, Rosenthal E, Cohen P, Loury I, Loustaud-Ratti V, et al. Extrahepatic manifestations associated with hepatitis C virus infection. A prospective multicenter study of 321 patients. The GERMIVIC. Groupe d'Etude et de Recherche en Medecine interne et maladies Infectieuses Sur le virus de l'Hepatite C. Medicine (Baltimore). 2000;79:47–56.
3. Zignego AL, Gragnani L, Piluso A, Sebastiani M, Giuggioli D, Fallahi P, et al. Virus-driven autoimmunity and lymphoproliferation: the example of HCV infection. Expert Rev Clin Immunol. 2015;11:15–31.
4. Ramos-Casals M, Pares A, Jara L-J, Solans R, Viñas O, Vázquez P, et al. Antimitochondrial antibodies in patients with chronic hepatitis C virus infection: description of 18 cases and review of the literature. J Viral Hepat. 2005;12:648–54.
5. Marconcini ML, Fayad L, Shiozawa MBC, Dantas-Correa EB, Schiavon L, De L, et al. Autoantibody profile in individuals with chronic hepatitis C. Rev Soc Bras Med Trop. 2013;46:147–53.
6. Lenzi M, Bellentani S, Saccoccio G, Muratori P, Masutti F, Muratori L, et al. Prevalence of non-organ-specific autoantibodies and chronic liver disease in the general population: a nested case-control study of the Dionysos cohort. Gut. 1999;45:435–41.
7. Gregorio GV, Pensati P, Iorio R, Vegnente A, Mieli-Vergani G, Vergani D. Autoantibody prevalence in children with liver disease due to chronic hepatitis C virus (HCV) infection. Clin Exp Immunol. 1998;112:471–6.
8. Chen H-W, Huang H-H, Lai C-H, Chang W-E, Shih Y-L, Chang W-K, et al. Hepatitis C virus infection in patients with primary biliary cirrhosis. Ann Hepatol. 2013;12:78–84.
9. Floreani A, Baragiotta A, Leone MG, Baldo V, Naccarato R. Primary biliary cirrhosis and hepatitis C virus infection. Am J Gastroenterol. 2003;98:2757–62.
10. Maeda T, Onishi S, Miura T, Iwamura S, Tomita A, Saibara T, et al. Exacerbation of primary biliary cirrhosis during interferon-alpha 2b therapy for chronic active hepatitis C. Dig Dis Sci. 1995;40:1226–30.
11. European Association for the Study of the Liver. EASL clinical practice guidelines: management of cholestatic liver diseases. J Hepatol. 2009;51:237–67.
12. Lindor KD, Gershwin ME, Poupon R, Kaplan M, Bergasa NV, Heathcote EJ, et al. Primary biliary cirrhosis. Hepatol Baltim Md. 2009;50:291–308.
13. Miyakawa H, Tanaka A, Kikuchi K, Matsushita M, Kitazawa E, Kawaguchi N, et al. Detection of antimitochondrial autoantibodies in immunofluorescent AMA negative patients with primary biliary cirrhosis using recombinant autoantigens. Hepatol Baltim Md. 2001;34:243–8.
14. Metcalf JV, Mitchison HC, Palmer JM, Jones DE, Bassendine MF, James OF. Natural history of early primary biliary cirrhosis. Lancet Lond Engl. 1996;348:1399–402.
15. Zeman MV, Hirschfield GM. Autoantibodies and liver disease: uses and abuses. Can J Gastroenterol. 2010;24:225–31.
16. Stinton LM, Swain M, Myers RP, Shaheen AA, Fritzler MJ. Autoantibodies to GW bodies and other autoantigens in primary biliary cirrhosis. Clin Exp Immunol. 2011;163:147–56.
17. Hu S, Zhao F, Wang Q, Chen W-X. The accuracy of the anti-mitochondrial antibody and the M2 subtype test for diagnosis of primary biliary cirrhosis: a meta-analysis. Clin Chem Lab Med. 2014;52:1533–42.
18. Xiao H, Chen J, Xie X, Liu Y, Li F. Diagnostic significance of autoantibodies in patients with primary biliary cirrhosis. Beijing Da Xue Bao. 2012;44:209–14.
19. Fussey SP, Guest JR, James OF, Bassendine MF, Yeaman SJ. Identification and analysis of the major M2 autoantigens in primary biliary cirrhosis. Proc Natl Acad Sci U S A. 1988;85:8654–8.
20. Leung PS, Coppel RL, Ansari A, Munoz S, Gershwin ME. Antimitochondrial antibodies in primary biliary cirrhosis. Semin Liver Dis. 1997;17:61–9.
21. Kaplan MM, Gershwin ME. Primary biliary cirrhosis. N Engl J Med. 2005;353:1261–73.
22. Nakamura M. Clinical significance of autoantibodies in primary biliary cirrhosis. Semin Liver Dis. 2014;34:334–40.
23. Carey EJ, Ali AH, Lindor KD. Primary biliary cirrhosis. Lancet. 2015;386:1565–75.
24. Marquez-Azalgara V, Hussaini T, Erb SR, Yoshida EM. Antimitochondrial antibody serocoversion post-liver transplant during hepatitis C treatment with peginterferon α, ribavirin and telaprevir. Ann Hepatol. 2014;13:565–7.
25. Van Norstrand MD, Malinchoc M, Lindor KD, Therneau TM, Gershwin ME, Leung PS, et al. Quantitative measurement of autoantibodies to recombinant mitochondrial antigens in patients with primary biliary cirrhosis: relationship of levels of autoantibodies to disease progression. Hepatology. 1997;25:6–11.
26. Tana MM, Shums Z, Milo J, Norman GL, Leung PS, Gershwin ME, et al. The significance of autoantibody changes over time in primary biliary cirrhosis. Am J Clin Pathol. 2015;144:601–6.
27. Menéndez A, Gómez J, Escanlar E, Caminal-Montero L, Mozo L. Clinical associations of anti-SSA/Ro60 and anti-Ro52/TRIM21 antibodies: diagnostic utility of their separate detection. Autoimmunity. 2013;46:32–9.
28. Granito A, Muratori P, Muratori L, Pappas G, Cassani F, Worthington J, et al. Antibodies to SS-A/Ro-52kD and centromere in autoimmune liver disease: a clue to diagnosis and prognosis of primary biliary cirrhosis. Aliment Pharmacol Ther. 2007;26:831–8.
29. Montano-Loza AJ, Shums Z, Norman GL, Czaja AJ. Prognostic implications of antibodies to Ro/SSA and soluble liver antigen in type 1 autoimmune hepatitis. Liver Int Off J Int Assoc Study Liver. 2012;32:85–92.

21

Efficacy and safety of tenofovir in preventing mother-to-infant transmission of hepatitis B virus: a meta-analysis based on 6 studies from China and 3 studies from other countries

Wenhui Li[1], Li Jia[1], Xin Zhao[1], Xiaoyuan Wu[1] and Hongxia Tang[2*]

Abstract

Background: The vertical transmission of HBV from mothers to their infants at birth or in early infancy has a significant role in the endemicity of HBV infection. Tenofovir is one of the most potent anti-HBV agents with a high genetic barrier to resistance. The study is to evaluate the efficacy of tenofovir in preventing perinatal HBV transmission, as well as monitoring safety for mothers and infants.

Methods: PubMed, Embase, Web of Science, and CNKI (National Knowledge Infrastructure, China) database were systematically reviewed for studies that compared the efficacy and safety of tenofovir with other treatments. Pooled estimates were expressed with weight mean difference (WMD) with 95% confidence intervals (95% CIs) and risk ratio (RR) with 95% CIs.

Results: Nine studies involving 1046 pregnant patients met the inclusion criteria and were included in this meta-analysis. Compared with other treatments, tenofovir significantly reduced maternal HBV DNA levels (WMD = 2.33 $\log_{10}$ IU/mL, 95% CI: 1.01, 3.64; $P < 0.001$), infant HBsAg positivity rate (RR = 0.25, 95% CI: 0.16, 0.38; $P < 0.001$), infant HBeAg positivity rate (RR = 0.26, 95% CI: 0.14, 0.48; $P < 0.001$), infant HBV DNA positivity rate (RR = 0.15, 95% CI: 0.07, 0.31; $P < 0.001$), and immunoprophylaxis failure rate (RR = 0.31, 95% CI: 0.13, 0.73; $P = 0.008$). Moreover, maternal and infant safety profiles, including ALT, CK, and Cr were comparable between tenofovir and other treatment groups.

Conclusion: Based on the current evidence, our study suggested that tenofovir significantly reduced the rate of vertical transmission of HBV, as well as the HBV DNA levels in HBV-infected mothers. Moreover, tenofovir was safe and tolerable for both mothers and their infants.

Keywords: Hepatitis B, Tenofovir, Vertical transmission, Meta-analysis

* Correspondence: opv3ht@163.com
[2]Department of Neurology, Children's Hospital of Hebei Province, 133 South Jianhua Street, Shijiazhuang 050031, Hebei, China

Background

Chronic hepatitis B virus (HBV) infection is a serious threat to public health and is associated with cirrhosis and liver cancer [1, 2]. Although the universal infant immunization reduces 80–90% of chronic HBV infection, the active/passive immunoprophylaxis has not eradicated mother-to-infant HBV transmission [3–5]. The vertical transmission of HBV from mothers to their infants at birth or in early infancy has a significant role in the endemicity of HBV infection [6]. Moreover, after immunoprophylaxis, children with HBV infection have a higher risk of developing hepatocellular carcinoma [7, 8].

HBV immunoprophylaxis failure is influenced by maternal hepatitis B e antigen (HBeAg) positivity and viral load [9, 10]. Several studies have demonstrated a positive correlation between high maternal serum HBV DNA levels and an increased risk for vaccination breakthrough [11, 12]. Thus, these data have introduced the idea of antiviral therapy in pregnant women with high HBV DNA levels to help achieve the goal of global eradication of HBV infection.

Three oral anti-HBV agents have been approved by United States Food and Drug Administration for the preventing of mother-to-infant transmission. These agents included lamivudine, telbivudine, and tenofovir. Lamivudine has been reported to reduce 72–78% risk of vertical transmission compared with passive/active immunization alone [13, 14]. However, it could lead to the emergence of lamivudine-resistant mutants because of its lower genetic barrier to resistance [15]. Telbivudine has been proven to prevent immunoprophylaxis failure in all cases treated; however, the increased risk of resistance limited its prolonged therapy [6, 16].

Tenofovir is one of the most potent anti-HBV agents with a high genetic barrier to resistance [17]. A small but growing body of evidence has suggested that tenofovir may reduce the risk of mother-to-child transmission, however, their results remain inconsistent [6, 13, 16, 18–20]. To increase power and precision, we conducted this meta-analysis based on relevant studies to assess the efficacy of tenofovir in reducing perinatal HBV transmission, as well as monitoring safety for mothers and infants.

Methods

Literature search

We conducted this meta-analysis in accordance with the Preferred Reporting Items for Systematic Reviews and meta-analysis (PRISMA) criteria [21]. PubMed, Embase, Web of Science, and CNKI (National Knowledge Infrastructure, China) database from inception to January 16, 2018 were searched to identify relevant studies. The search was limited to human subject, and no language restriction was imposed. Search terms were as follows: ("hepatitis b virus" [MeSH Terms] OR "hepatitis b virus" [All Fields]) AND ("infectious disease transmission, vertical"[MeSH Terms] OR ("infectious" [All Fields] AND "disease" [All Fields] AND "transmission" [All Fields] AND "vertical" [All Fields]) OR "vertical infectious disease transmission"[All Fields] OR ("mother" [All Fields] AND "child" [All Fields] AND "transmission" [All Fields]) OR "mother to child transmission" [All Fields]) AND ("telbivudine" [Supplementary Concept] OR "telbivudine" [All Fields]). In addition, we also searched the lists of included studies and reviews to identify other potentially eligible studies.

Review strategy

We used Endnote (version X, Thomson Reuters, Inc., Philadelphia, PA) bibliographic software to create an electronic library of citations identified in the literature search. PubMed, Embase, and Web of Science searches were performed using Endnote, and duplicate records were deleted. Two independent investigators were trained to conduct the abstract review and full-text review thereafter. Disagreements between them were resolved by discussion and consensus. The inter-reviewer agreements were calculated using the Cohen K statistic [22].

Study inclusion and exclusion criteria

Studies were included in this meta-analysis if they met the following inclusion criteria: (1) study design: randomized controlled trial (RCT), or case-control study, or cohort study; (2) study population: pregnant women 20 to 35 years of age who had chronic HBV infection, were HBeAg-positive; (3) comparison intervention: tenofovir and other treatments; (4) outcome measure: mother to child transmission rate, maternal HBV DNA levels, maternal and infant safety outcomes. If several publications were from the same clinical trial, we only included the most informative article or the longest follow-up study to avoid duplication of information.

Studies were excluded in this meta-analysis if they were published with the study type of editorials, comments, reviews, letters or unrelated with our topics.

Data extraction and quality assessment

We used a standardized data-extraction sheet to extract the following information: first author, year of publication, number of patients in each arm, age of the pregnant women, population characteristics, study design, and the outcome of interest.

We assessed the risk of bias in RCT using the method recommended by Cochrane Collaboration [23]. This method consisted five items to evaluate the quality of study, including blinding, method of randomization, allocation concealment, follow-up, and intention-to-treat analysis [23]. Each study was considered to be high, low, or unclear risk of bias according to the above-mentioned criteria.

The quality of non-randomized studies was assessed using a modified Newcastle-Ottawa scale (NOS) [24]. This scale consisted three items that descried patient selection, comparability of the tenofovir and other treatment groups, and outcome assessment. The total scale ranged from 0 to 9 points. Study with a scale of more than 5 points was considered as high quality [24].

Statistical analysis

We calculated weight mean difference (WMD) with 95% confidence interval (95% CI) for continuous outcomes, and risk ratio (RR) with 95% CI for dichotomous outcomes. Before the data were pooled, we first tested the heterogeneity between the included studies, using I^2 statistic and Cochrane Q chi-square test [25]. A value of I^2 more than 50%, or the value of P less than 0.10 indicated significant heterogeneity across the included studies [25]. When significant heterogeneity was identified, a random-effects model (DerSimonian-Laird method) [26] was used to summary the estimates; otherwise, a fixed-effects model (Mantel-Haenszel method) [27] was applied. When considerable heterogeneity was found, sensitivity analysis was performed by omitting one study in each turn to explore the influence of a single study on the overall estimate. Publication bias was evaluated by Begg [28] and Egger's [29] test. A P value less than 0.05 was judged as statistically significant, except where otherwise specified. All statistical analyses were performed using STATA, version 12.0 (Stata Corporation, College Station, TX, USA).

Results

Identification of eligible studies

A total of 623 relevant records were identified from the database search. Of these, 479 studies were excluded because of duplicate records, and 129 studies were excluded after a review of title/abstract. Then remaining 15 studies were scrutinized for full-text information review, however, 6 of them were excluded because 2 were single-arm study design [30, 31], 3 did not provide outcomes of our interest [32–34], and one was a study protocol [35]. Finally, nine studies [20, 36–43] that met the inclusion criteria were included in this meta-analysis (Fig. 1). The Cohen statistic K for agreement on study inclusion was 0.91.

Characteristics of eligible studies

The main characteristics of included studies were presented in Table 1. These studies were published between 2013 and 2017. The sample size ranged from 40 to 153. Among these studies, six were conducted in China [36, 37, 40–43], each one in Austria [20], Turkey [38] and Canada [39], respectively. Of the included studies, eight were cohort studies [20, 36, 38–43], and one was RCT [37]. All the pregnant women had HBV DNA ≥6.0 $\log_{10}$ IU/mL. The tenofovir was administrated with a dosage of 300 daily. The timing of pregnancy when tenofovir was started varied greatly across the included studies, with 18–32 weeks of gestation in seven studies [20, 36–41], and 6 or 8 weeks in two studies [42, 43]. All the studies [20, 36–43] compared tenofovir with no medication or usual medical care without antiviral therapy, and two studies compared it with lamivudine [20] and telbivudine [40] additionally. Since these two studies provided two sets of data: tenofovir versus no therapy, tenofovir versus lamivudine/ telbivudine, we extracted all these data for data analysis.

Quality of included studies

The quality of cohort studies was assessed by the modified NOS. The scores of these studies ranged from 6 to 9, indicating that these cohort studies were of high quality (Table 1). For the only one RCT [37], since the blinding of participants and personnel and blinding of outcome assessors were not reported, it was classified as being at unclear risk of bias.

Maternal effects

Maternal HBV DNA suppression

Six studies reported the data of maternal HBV DNA suppression [36–39, 42, 43]. The pooled estimate demonstrated that tenofovir was associated with an improvement in the maternal HBV DNA suppression rate (RR = 7.93, 95% CI: 2.51, 24.99; $P < 0.001$) (Fig. 2). The test for heterogeneity was significant ($P < 0.001$, $I^2 = 89.1\%$). Therefore, we conducted sensitivity analysis to explore the potential sources of heterogeneity. When we excluded the study with outlier [39], the pooled estimate changed a little (RR = 13.70, 95% CI: 3.45, 54.30; $P < 0.001$), but the heterogeneity was still observed ($P < 0.001$, $I^2 = 82.9\%$). When we excluded the two trials [38, 43] that had a relatively small sample size ($N < 50$), the overall estimates did not change substantially (RR = 10.61, 95% CI: 1.46, 76.87; $P = 0.019$), but the heterogeneity was still present ($P < 0.001$, $I^2 = 92.9\%$). We also further excluded any single study; however, this did not materially alter the overall estimate (data not shown).

Maternal HBV DNA level reduction

Four studies reported the data of maternal HBV DNA level reduction [20, 36, 40, 41]. The aggregated result suggested that, tenofovir was associated with a significant reduction in maternal HBV DNA level (WMD = 2.33 $\log_{10}$ IU/mL, 95% CI: 1.01, 3.64; $P < 0.001$) (Fig. 3). There was significant heterogeneity among the included

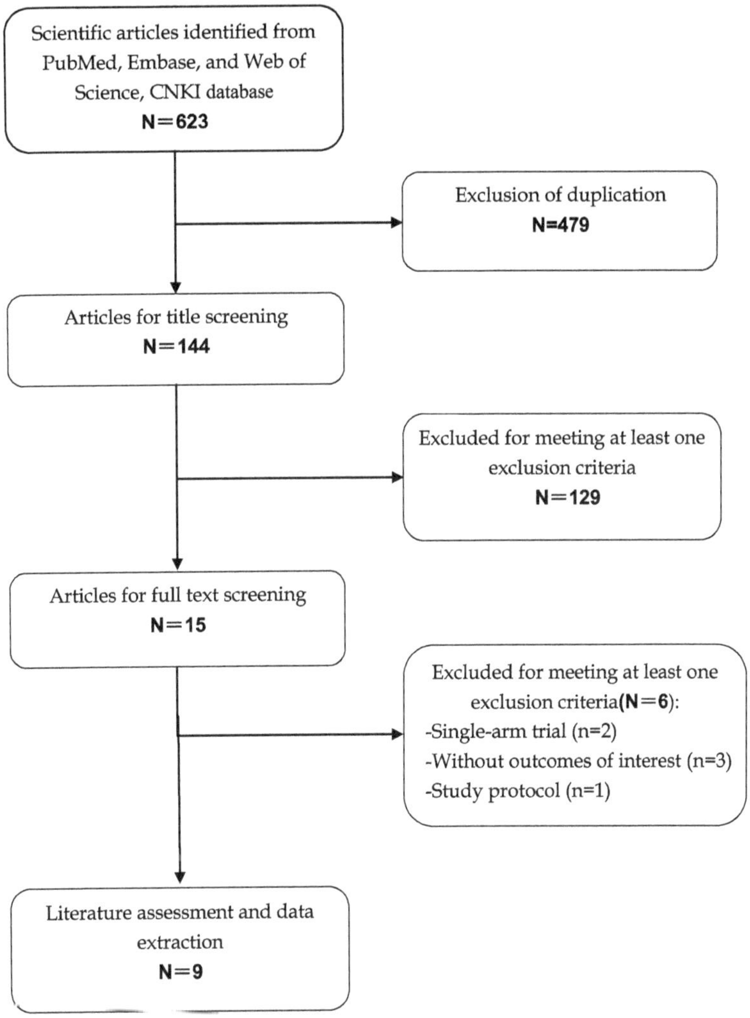

Fig. 1 Eligibility of studies for inclusion in meta-analysis

studies ($P < 0.001$, $I^2 = 99.1\%$). Therefore, we conducted sensitivity. When we excluded the study with outlier [36], the pooled estimate did not change substantially (WMD = 2.69 $\log_{10}$ IU/mL, 95% CI: 1.41, 3.96; $P < 0.001$), however, the heterogeneity was still present ($P < 0.001$, $I^2 = 99.1\%$). When we excluded the study with small sample size ($N = 74$) [[40]], the pooled result did not alter substantially (WMD = 2.59 $\log_{10}$ IU/mL, 95% CI: 1.45, 3.73; $P < 0.001$), but the evidence of heterogeneity was still observed among the remaining studies ($P < 0.001$, $I^2 = 97.7\%$).

Maternal HBeAg seroconversion

Two studies reported the data of maternal HBeAg seroconversion [36, 37]. The pooled estimate showed that tenofovir had a similar maternal HBeAg seroconversion rate with other treatments (RR = 2.87, 95% CI: 0.45, 18.49; $P = 0.266$). The test for heterogeneity was not significant ($P = 0.369$, $I^2 = 0.0\%$).

Maternal ALT, CK and Cr elevation

Six studies reported the data of ALT, CK, and Cr elevation [36–39, 42, 43]. The pooled estimate demonstrated that patients treated with tenofovir had a comparable ALT elevation than those with other treatments (RR = 0.56, 95% CI: 0.25, 1.25; $P = 0.157$) (Fig. 4). Moreover, the ALT levels in the two groups were not significant difference (WMD = 9.37 U/L, 95% CI: -13.50, 32.24; $P = 0.130$).

The CK and Cr levels in the two groups were also comparable. Patients treated with tenofovir developed a similar CK (WMD = 4.45 mg/dL, 95% CI: -1.51, 10.41; $P = 0.143$) and Cr (WMD = – 0.08 mg/dL, 95% CI: -0.23, 0.07; $P = 0.316$) levels as those treated with other treatment.

Infant effects

Infant HBsAg positivity

Five studies reported the data of infant HBsAg positivity [20, 36, 37, 40, 41]. The pooled result suggested that,

Table 1 Baseline characteristics of patients in the trials included in the meta-analysis

Study	Country	Study design	Treatment regimen	No. of patients	Pregnancy time when tenofovir was started (w)	Age (mean ± SD, y)	HBV DNA (log10 IU/ml)	NOS score
Greenup AJ [20]	Austria	Cohort	Tenofovir 300 mg daily	58	30–32	30 ± 8.5	7.94 ± 0.78	7
			Lamivudine 100 mg daily	52		28 ± 5.3	7.72 ± 0.61	
			No medication	20		28 ± 5	8 ± 0.04	
Chen HL [36]	China	Cohort	Tenofovir 300 mg daily	62	32	32.41 ± 3.12	8.25 ± 0.45	9
			No medication	56		32.45 ± 3.2	8.24 ± 0.35	
Pan CQ [37]	China	RCT	Tenofovir 300 mg daily	97	30–32	27.4 ± 3.0	8.2 ± 0.5	NA
			Usual care	100		26.8 ± 3.0	8.0 ± 0.7	
Celen MK [38]	Turkey	Cohort	Tenofovir 300 mg daily	21	18–27	28.2 ± 4.1	8.28	6
			Untreated	24		26.9 ± 2.9	8.31	
Kochaksaraei GS [39]	Canada	Cohort	Tenofovir 300 mg daily	23	28 (21–32)	30(28–34)	7.7(3.2–8.1)	6
			Untreated	138		32(29–36)	2.3(1.6–3.1)	
Chen WJ [40]	China	Cohort	Tenofovir 300 mg daily	30	23.9 ± 1.9	28.67 ± 5.71	≥6.0	7
			Telbivudine 600 mg daily	79		31.13 ± 6.27	≥6.0	
			Untreated	44		29.86 ± 5.05	≥6.0	
Wan JY [41]	China	Cohort	Tenofovir 300 mg daily	74	28	28.5 ± 4.2	7.69 ± 0.54	8
			Untreated	42		27.9 ± 4.0	7.57 ± 0.48	
Qi LW [42]	China	Cohort	Tenofovir 300 mg daily	54	6	27.5 ± 3.6	7.01 ± 0.98	7
			Untreated	32		26.4 ± 3.1	6.51 ± 1.03	
Deng J [43]	China	Cohort	Tenofovir 300 mg daily	20	10	26.15 ± 2.56	NR	7
			Untreated	20		28.32 ± 2.45	NR	

Abbreviation: *SD* standard deviation, *NR* not reported, *NA* not available, *NOS* Newcastle-Ottawa scale

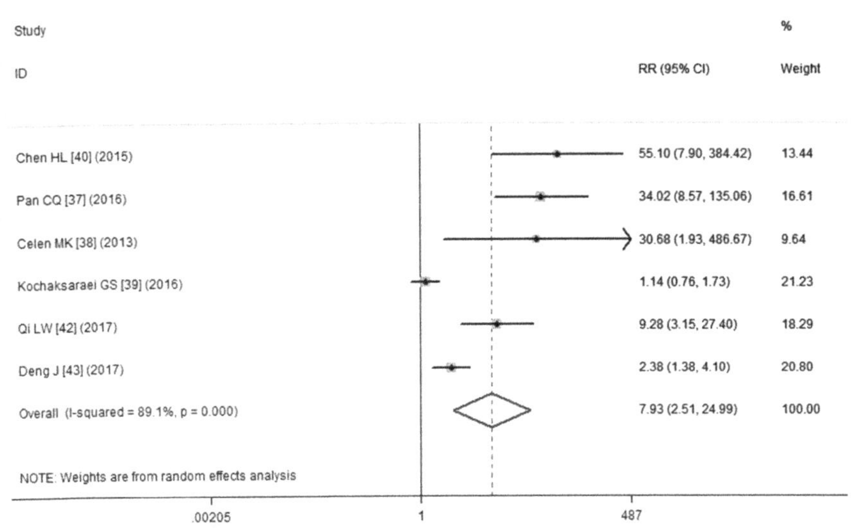

Fig. 2 Forest plot showing the effect of tenofovir on the maternal HBV DNA suppression

infants in the tenofovir group had a significant lower rate of HBsAg positivity compared with the control group (RR = 0.25, 95% CI: 0.16, 0.38; $P < 0.001$) (Fig. 5).

Subgroup analysis based on the infant age showed that, tenofovir was associated with a significant lower rate of infant HBsAg positivity than other treatments when the infants were at the time of birth (RR = 0.28, 95% CI: 0.17, 0.48; $P < 0.001$), 6 months of age (RR = 0.16, 95% CI: 0.05, 0.52; $P = 0.002$), or 12 months of age (RR = 0.22, 95% CI: 0.08, 0.62; $P = 0.004$) (Fig. 5).

Infant HBeAg positivity

Five studies reported the data of infant HBeAg positivity [20, 36, 37, 40, 41]. The pooled estimate demonstrated that, infants in the tenofovir group had a significant

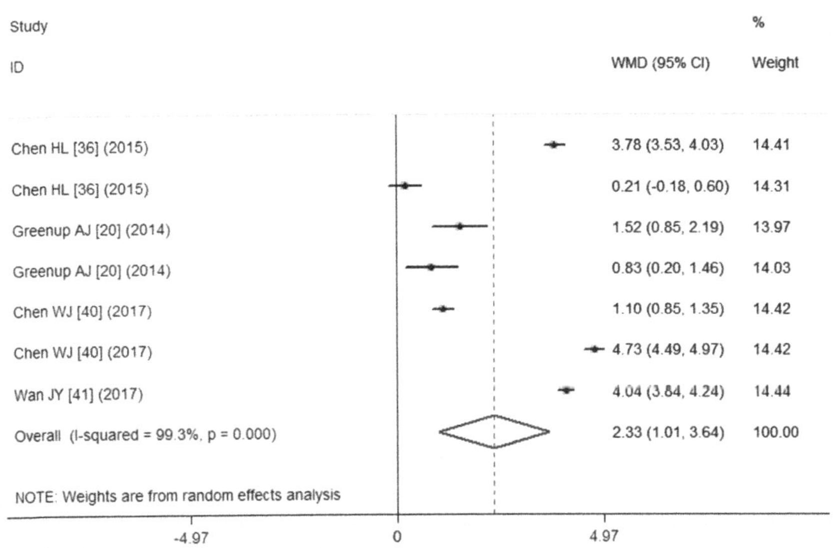

Fig. 3 Forest plot showing the effect of tenofovir on the maternal HBV DNA level reduction

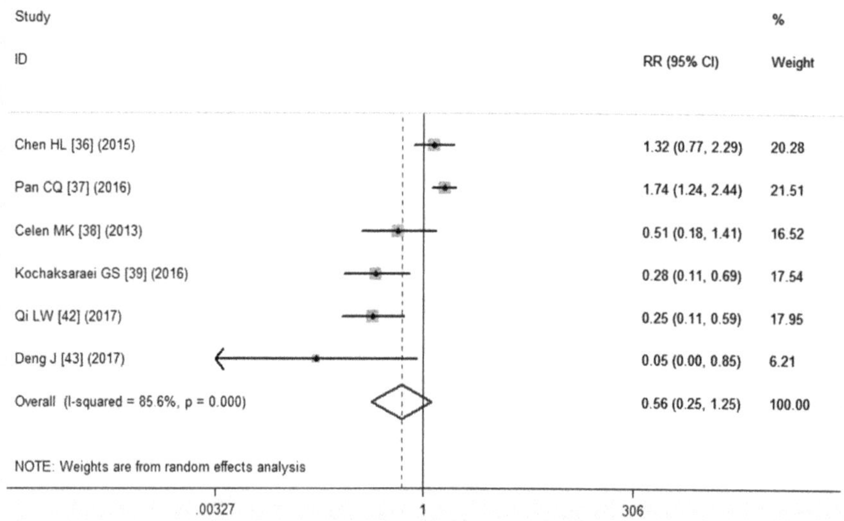

Fig. 4 Forest plot showing the effect of tenofovir on the maternal ALT elevation

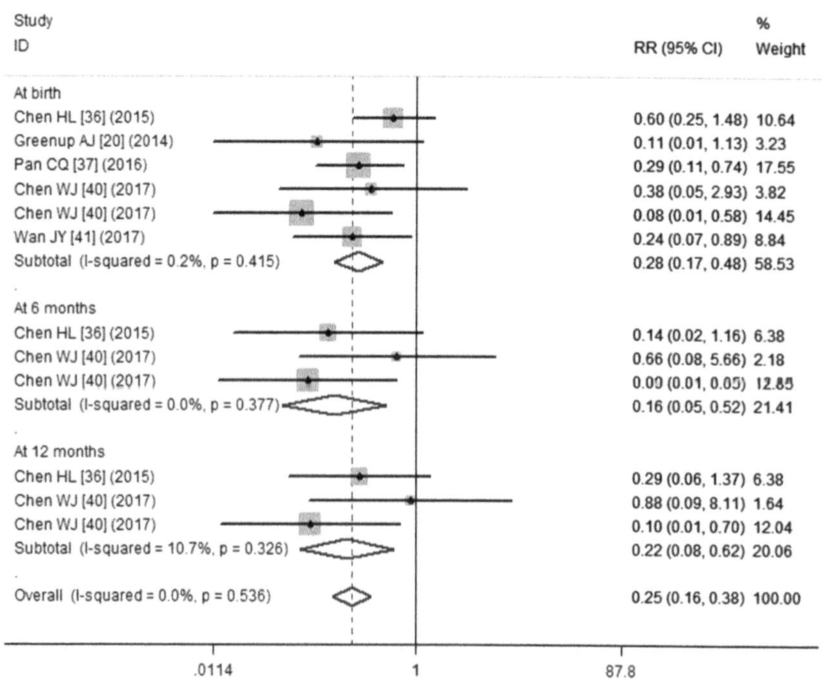

Fig. 5 Forest plot showing the effect of tenofovir on the infant HBsAg positivity

lower rate of HBeAg positivity compared with the control group (RR = 0.26, 95% CI: 0.14, 0.48; $P < 0.001$).

Subgroup analysis based on the infant age suggested that, tenofovir was associated with a significant lower rate of infant HBeAg positivity than other treatments when the infants were at the time of birth (RR = 0.39, 95% CI: 0.18, 0.86; $P = 0.020$), 6 months of age (RR = 0.17, 95% CI: 0.04, 0.66; $P = 0.010$), or 12 months of age (RR = 0.18, 95% CI: 0.04, 070; $P = 0.013$).

Infant HBV DNA positivity

Three studies reported the data of infant HBV DNA positivity [36, 40, 41]. The pooled result showed that, the infants in the tenofovir group had a significant lower rate of HBV DNA positivity compared with the control group (RR = 0.15, 95% CI: 0.07, 0.31; $P < 0.001$).

Subgroup analysis based on the infant age indicated that, tenofovir was associated with a significant lower rate of infant HBV DNA positivity than other treatments when the infants were at the time of birth (RR = 0.39, 95% CI: 0.08, 0.39; $P = 0.020$), 6 months of age (RR = 0.13, 95% CI: 0.02, 0.88; $P = 0.036$), or 12 months of age (RR = 0.06, 95% CI: 0.00, 0.83; $P = 0.043$).

Immunoprophylaxis failure

Three studies reported the data of immunoprophylaxis failure [37–39]. The pooled estimate demonstrated that there was a significant lower rate of immunoprophylaxis failure in infants whose mothers received tenofovir compared with these whose mothers received other treatments (RR = 0.31, 95% CI: 0.13, 0.73; $P = 0.008$).

Maternal safety and infant safety outcomes

All the included studies reported the data of maternal and infant safety outcomes [20, 36–43]. The maternal and infant adverse events were summarized in Table 2. Pooled estimate showed that the incidences of maternal or infant adverse events were not significant difference between the tenofovir and other treatment groups.

Table 2 Summarized risk ratios (RR) with 95% confidence intervals (95% CIs) for adverse events

Adverse events	RR (95% CIs)	*P* value
Maternal adverse events		
Fatigue	1.03 (0.65, 16.25)	0.586
Cough	1.42 (0.60, 3.39)	0.983
Diarrhea	3.61 (0.75, 17.41)	0.424
Fever	1.56 (0.40, 6.17)	0.110
Nausea	2.06 (0.19, 22.37)	0.523
Pruritus	0.41 (0.08, 2.08)	0.552
Palpitation	0.34 (0.01, 8.33)	0.283
Dyspepsia	3.09 (0.13, 74.99)	0.511
Rash	0.95 (0.28, 3.19)	0.488
Insomnia	3.09 (0.13, 74.99)	0.928
Dizziness	0.52 (0.05, 5.59)	0.488
Abdominal pain	3.09 (0.13, 74.98)	0.586
Upper respiratory infection	0.34 (0.04, 3.25)	0.731
Gestational diabetes	3.41 (0.15, 79.47)	0.351
Arrhythmia	3.25 (0.28, 46.72)	0.612
Infant adverse events		
Hypospadias	2.78 (0.12, 67.39)	0.529
Torticollis	1.85 (0.17, 20.08)	0.612
Umbilical hernia	2.78 (0.12, 67.39)	0.529
Pneumonia	4.64 (0.23, 95.24)	0.470
Bronchitis	0.31 (0.01, 7.49)	0.948
Birth weight < 2500 g	1.10 (0.07, 16.43)	0.185
Fetal growth retardation	0.79 (0.15, 21.34)	0.546
Congenital malformation	2.34 (0.25, 64.7)	0.445

Publication bias

We used the Begg and Egger's test to evaluate the publication bias. The results showed that there was no evidence of significant publication bias (Egg test, $P = 0.625$; Begg test, $P = 0.458$).

Discussion

This study is a meta-analysis with the objective of assessing the efficacy of tenofovir in reducing mother-to-infant HBV transmission, as well as monitoring safety for mothers and infants. Our study suggested that tenofovir was associated with significant reductions in maternal HBV DNA levels, infant HBsAg/HBeAg positivity, infant HBV DNA positivity, and immunoprophylaxis failure. Moreover, tenofovir induced a similar incidence of ALT, CK, and Cr elevation with other treatments. This study indicated that tenofovir was effective and safe for both mother and infant in the prevention of vertical transmission of HBV.

In this meta-analysis, we found that tenofovir significantly reduced the maternal HBV DNA levels. This finding was in consistent with the results of other studies available about the efficacy of tenofovir in preventing vertical transmission [20, 36, 40, 41]. In a prospective, multicenter trial conducted in China [36], the authors enrolled 118 pregnant patients who had chronic HBV and HBV DNA levels ≥7.5 $\log_{10}$ IU/ mL. These patients received tenofovir 300 mg daily ($N = 62$, HBV DNA 8.18 ± 0.47 $\log_{10}$ IU/mL), or no medication ($N = 56$, HBV DNA 8.22 ± 0.39 $\log_{10}$ IU/mL) [36]. At the time of delivery, the mean reduction of HBV DNA in the two groups were 3.89 ± 0.87 and 0.11 ± 0.51 $\log_{10}$ IU/mL, respectively [36], which indicated that tenofovir had a greater reduction in maternal HBV DNA than no medication. Similarly, in another multi-center, prospective opt-in observational study from Austria [20], the authors also reported greater decrease of HBV DNA in the tenofovir group. In that study, pregnant women with high viral load (>7 log IU/mL) were treated with tenofovir ($N = 58$), lamivudine ($N = 52$), or no therapy ($N = 20$). The mean reduction of HBV DNA in tenofovir group was 3.64 ± 0.9 log IU/mL, compared with 2.81 ± 1.33 in the lamivudine group [20]. This result indicated that tenofovir had a significant greater reduction of HBV DNA levels than lamivudine.

However, the advantage effect of tenofovir over other treatments in reducing HBV DNA levels was not observed in a prospective cohort study conducted in China [40]. In that study, 153 chronic HBV infectious mothers were assigned into the tenofovir group ($N = 30$) and telbivudine group ($N = 79$) [40]. At the time of delivery, the reductions of HBV DNA levels in these groups were 4.64 ± 0.5 and 3.54 ± 0.8 log IU/mL, respectively. Although tenofovir seemed to have a greater reduction in HBV DNA levels than telbivudine, the difference was not significant. Owning to the limited available data, we did not perform subgroup analysis to explore whether tenofovir had superior effect than telbivudine in reducing the HBV DNA levels.

In this meta-analysis, our results suggested that tenofovir significantly reduced the mother-to-infant transmission compared with other treatments. The use of tenofovir significantly reduced the risk of infant HBsAg positivity by 75% (RR = 0.25, 95% CI: 0.16, 0.38), the infant HBeAg positivity by 74% (RR = 0.26, 95% CI: 0.14, 0.48), and the infant HBV DNA positivity by 85% (RR = 0.15, 95% CI: 0.07, 0.31). Our results were in consistent with the study conducted by Chen WJ, et al. [40]. In that study, 3.3 and 10.0% of infants in tenofovir group had HBsAg and HBeAg positivity, as compared with 40.9 and 43.2% of infants in the control group, respectively. Similarly, other studies also reported the reduced rates of HBsAg/HBeAg positivity by tenofovir. In one prospective trial in China, the rates of HBsAg and HBV DNA positivity in tenofovir group were 1.5 and 6.15%, as compared with 10.7 and 31.48% in the control group, respectively [36]. In another multicenter, open-label, randomized, parallel-group trial in China [37], a striking decline in HBsAg positivity rate was seen from the tenofovir treatment. According to that study, 5.2% (5/97) of infants in the tenofovir group had HBsAg positivity, as compared with 18% (18/100) of infants in the control group ($P = 0.007$). These results indicated that tenofovir was effective in reducing the risk of HBV transmission from their mothers.

Regarding the immunoprophylaxis failure, our study showed that infant in the tenofovir group had a lower immunoprophylaxis failure rate than that in the control group. This result was also observed among the included studies. In a multicenter, open-label RCT, the rate of immunoprophylaxis failure in tenofovir group was 5.2%, as compared with 18% in the control group, which indicated that tenofovir therapy could reduce the immunoprophylaxis failure rate [37]. In another two cohort studies [20, 39] that evaluated the efficacy and safety of tenofovir use in pregnant HBV women, none of the infants of the tenofovir-treated mothers had immunoprophylaxis failure; whereas, 2 of 23 (8.7%) and 1 of 73 (1.4%) of infants in the control group had immunoprophylaxis failure [20, 39].

When the potential benefit of tenofovir is evaluated, the adverse effects of that also should be taken into consideration. These adverse effects include maternal ALT, CK, and Cr flares, and infant congenital malformation. Our results suggested that these adverse events were comparable between the tenofovir and control groups. There were several studies [18, 44] reporting data on ALT flares during and after the antiviral treatment in pregnant women; however, their results remained inconsistent. In the study that used telbivudine or lamivudine for the treatment of late pregnancy women [18], it was reported that 17.1% of the mothers in the treated group had severe hepatitis flare (ALT> 10 times the ULN) compared with 6.3% in the untreated mothers [18]. In another study that used lamivudine or tenofovir, the incidences of postpartum ALT flare (> 95 U/L) in the treatment and no-treatment groups were 40–50 and 29%, respectively [44]. The highly variable and conflicting results could be explained by the different criteria for the definition of ALT flares, different follow-up protocols, different antiviral agents, and lack of controls [44].

This meta-analysis has several potential limitations that should be considered. First, substantial heterogeneity was identified among the included studies. However, it should not be surprising given the differences in maternal age at delivery, gestational age, gravidity, HBV DNA levels, and baseline ALT. These factors may account for the heterogeneity and have an impact on the treatment effect. Second, some of the included studies have a relatively small sample size ($N < 50$). Compared with larger trials, studies with small sample size are more likely to overestimate the treatment effect. Third, among the nine included studies, only one was RCT, and the remaining seven were cohort studies. Despite the cohort studies can reflect the "real-world" and further support the conclusion, the cohort data may be inclined to bias because of the patient selection. Fourth, most of the included studies were conducted in China. Thus, these findings were not representative of experts' prescribing practices all around world. Therefore, physicians should interpret our results with caution when applying them into the clinical practice.

Conclusion

In conclusion, the current meta-analysis suggested that, tenofovir was effective in preventing the vertical transmission of HBV, as well as reducing the HBV DNA levels in HBV-infected mothers. Moreover, tenofovir was safe and tolerable for both mothers and their infants. However, considering the potential limitations in this study, more large-scale, well-designed RCTs are needed to verify these findings.

Abbreviations

CI: Confidence interval; HBeAg: Maternal hepatitis B e antigen; HBsAg: Hepatitis B surface antigen; HBV: Chronic hepatitis B virus; RCT: Randomized controlled trial; RR: Risk ratio; WMD: Weight mean difference

Authors' contributions

HT contributed to the study design. WL, LJ, XZ and XW collected the data and performed the data analysis. All authors prepared the manuscript. All authors read and approved the final manuscript.

Consent for publication

Not applicable.

Competing interests

The authors declare that they have no competing interests.

Author details

[1]Department of Infectious Disease, Children's Hospital of Hebei Province, 133 South Jianhua Street, Shijiazhuang 050031, Hebei, China. [2]Department of Neurology, Children's Hospital of Hebei Province, 133 South Jianhua Street, Shijiazhuang 050031, Hebei, China.

References

1. EASL clinical practice guidelines. Management of chronic hepatitis B virus infection. J Hepatol. 2012;57:167–85.
2. Pan CQ, Zhang JX. Natural history and clinical consequences of hepatitis B virus infection. Int J Med Sci. 2005;2:36–40.
3. Stevens CE, Beasley RP, Tsui J, Lee WC. Vertical transmission of hepatitis B antigen in Taiwan. New Engl J Med. 1975;292:771–4.
4. Beasley RP, Hwang LY, Stevens CE, Lin CC, Hsieh FJ, Wang KY, et al. Efficacy of hepatitis B immune globulin for prevention of perinatal transmission of the hepatitis B virus carrier state: final report of a randomized double-blind, placebo-controlled trial. Hepatology (Baltimore, Md). 1983;3:135–41.
5. Smits LJ, Derikx LA, de Jong DJ, Boshuizen RS, van Esch AA, Drenth JP, et al. Clinical outcomes following a switch from Remicade(R) to the biosimilar CT-P13 in inflammatory bowel disease patients: a prospective observational cohort study. J Crohns Colitis. 2016;10:1287–93.
6. Han GR, Cao MK, Zhao W, Jiang HX, Wang CM, Bai SF, et al. A prospective and open-label study for the efficacy and safety of telbivudine in pregnancy for the prevention of perinatal transmission of hepatitis B virus infection. J Hepatol. 2011;55:1215–21.
7. Chang MH, Chen TH, Hsu HM, Wu TC, Kong MS, Liang DC, et al. Prevention of hepatocellular carcinoma by universal vaccination against hepatitis B virus: the effect and problems. Clin Cancer Res. 2005;11:7953–7.
8. Chang MH, You SL, Chen CJ, Liu CJ, Lee CM, Lin SM, et al. Decreased incidence of hepatocellular carcinoma in hepatitis B vaccinees: a 20-year follow-up study. J Natl Cancer I. 2009;101:1348–55.
9. Chen HL, Lin LH, Hu FC, Lee JT, Lin WT, Yang YJ, et al. Effects of maternal screening and universal immunization to prevent mother-to-infant transmission of HBV. Gastroenterology. 2012;142:773-81. e2
10. Song YM, Sung J, Yang S, Choe YH, Chang YS, Park WS. Factors associated with immunoprophylaxis failure against vertical transmission of hepatitis B virus. Eur J Pediatr. 2007;166:813–8.
11. Burk RD, Hwang LY, Ho GY, Shafritz DA, Beasley RP. Outcome of perinatal hepatitis B virus exposure is dependent on maternal virus load. J Infect Dis. 1994;170:1418–23.
12. Jonas MM. Hepatitis B and pregnancy: an underestimated issue. Liver Int. 2009;29(Suppl 1):133–9.
13. Xu WM, Cui YT, Wang L, Yang H, Liang ZQ, Li XM, et al. Lamivudine in late pregnancy to prevent perinatal transmission of hepatitis B virus infection: a multicentre, randomized, double-blind, placebo-controlled study. J Viral Hepatitis. 2009;16:94–103.
14. van Zonneveld M, van Nunen AB, Niesters HG, de Man RA, Schalm SW, Janssen HL. Lamivudine treatment during pregnancy to prevent perinatal transmission of hepatitis B virus infection. J Viral Hepatitis. 2003;10:294–7.
15. Chayama K, Suzuki Y, Kobayashi M, Kobayashi M, Tsubota A, Hashimoto M, et al. Emergence and takeover of YMDD motif mutant hepatitis B virus during long-term lamivudine therapy and re-takeover by wild type after cessation of therapy. Hepatology (Baltimore, Md). 1998;27:1711–6.
16. Pan CQ, Han GR, Jiang HX, Zhao W, Cao MK, Wang CM, et al. Telbivudine prevents vertical transmission from HBeAg-positive women with chronic hepatitis B. Clin Gastroenterol H. 2012;10:520–6.
17. Buti M, Tsai N, Petersen J, Flisiak R, Gurel S, Krastev Z, et al. Seven-year efficacy and safety of treatment with tenofovir disoproxil fumarate for chronic hepatitis B virus infection. Digestive Dis Sci. 2015;60:1457–64.
18. Zhang H, Pan CQ, Pang Q, Tian R, Yan M, Liu X. Telbivudine or lamivudine use in late pregnancy safely reduces perinatal transmission of hepatitis B virus in real-life practice. Hepatology (Baltimore, Md). 2014;60:468–76.
19. Pan CQ, Mi LJ, Bunchorntavakul C, Karsdon J, Huang WM, Singhvi G, et al. Tenofovir disoproxil fumarate for prevention of vertical transmission of hepatitis B virus infection by highly viremic pregnant women: a case series. Digestive Dis Sci. 2012;57:2423–9.
20. Greenup AJ, Tan PK, Nguyen V, Glass A, Davison S, Chatterjee U, et al. Efficacy and safety of tenofovir disoproxil fumarate in pregnancy to prevent perinatal transmission of hepatitis B virus. J Hepatol. 2014;61:502–7.
21. Moher D, Liberati A, Tetzlaff J, Altman DG. Preferred reporting items for systematic reviews and meta-analyses: the PRISMA statement. BMJ (Clinical research ed). 2009;339:b2535.
22. Sim J, Wright CC. The kappa statistic in reliability studies: use, interpretation, and sample size requirements. Phys Ther. 2005;85:257–68.
23. Higgins JP, Altman DG, Gotzsche PC, Juni P, Moher D, Oxman AD, et al. The Cochrane Collaboration's tool for assessing risk of bias in randomised trials. BMJ (Clinical research ed). 2011;343:d5928.
24. Wells G, Shea B, O'connell D, Peterson J, Welch V. The Newcastle-Ottawa scale (NOS) for assessing the quality of nonrandomized studies in meta-analyses. In: 3rd Symposium on Systematic Reviews: Beyond the Basics; 2000. p. 3–5.
25. Higgins JP, Thompson SG, Deeks JJ, Altman DG. Measuring inconsistency in meta-analyses. BMJ (Clinical research ed). 2003;327:557–60.
26. DerSimonian R, Laird N. Meta-analysis in clinical trials. Control Clin Trials. 1986;7:177–88.
27. Mantel N, Haenszel W. Statistical aspects of the analysis of data from retrospective studies of disease. J Natl Cancer I. 1959;22:719–48.
28. Begg CB, Mazumdar M. Operating characteristics of a rank correlation test for publication bias. Biometrics. 1994;50:1088–101.
29. Egger M, Davey Smith G, Schneider M, Minder C. Bias in meta-analysis detected by a simple, graphical test. BMJ (Clinical research ed). 1997;315:629–34.
30. Sellier PO, Maylin S, Bercot B, Chopin D, Lopes A, Simoneau G, et al. Prospective interventional study of tenofovir in pregnancy to prevent vertical transmission of hepatitis B in highly viremic women. Eur J Gastroenterol Hepatol. 2017;29:259–63.
31. Wang J, Liu J, Qi C, Yan T, Cao F, Jin L, et al. Efficacy of tenofovir disoproxil fumarate to prevent vertical transmission in mothers with lamivudine-resistant HBV. Antiviral Ther. 2015;20:681–7.
32. Chamroonkul N, Piratvisuth T. Hepatitis B during pregnancy in endemic areas: screening, treatment, and prevention of mother-to-child transmission. Paediatric Drugs. 2017;19:173–81.
33. Heathcote EJ, Marcellin P, Buti M, Gane E, De Man RA, Krastev Z, et al. Three-year efficacy and safety of tenofovir disoproxil fumarate treatment for chronic hepatitis B. Gastroenterology. 2011;140:132–43.
34. Virine B, Osiowy C, Gao S, Wang T, Castillo E, Martin SR, et al. Hepatitis B virus (HBV) variants in untreated and Tenofovir treated chronic hepatitis B (CHB) patients during pregnancy and post-partum follow-up. PLoS One. 2015;10:e0140070.

35. Jourdain G, Ngo-Giang-Huong N, Cressey TR, Hua L, Harrison L, Tierney C, et al. Prevention of mother-to-child transmission of hepatitis B virus: a phase III, placebo-controlled, double-blind, randomized clinical trial to assess the efficacy and safety of a short course of tenofovir disoproxil fumarate in women with hepatitis B virus e-antigen. BMC Infect Dis. 2016;16:393.
36. Chen HL, Lee CN, Chang CH, Ni YH, Shyu MK, Chen SM, et al. Efficacy of maternal tenofovir disoproxil fumarate in interrupting mother-to-infant transmission of hepatitis B virus. Hepatology (Baltimore, Md). 2015;62:375–86.
37. Pan CQ, Duan Z, Dai E, Zhang S, Han G, Wang Y, et al. Tenofovir to prevent hepatitis B transmission in mothers with high viral load. New Engl J Medicine. 2016;374:2324–34.
38. Celen MK, Mert D, Ay M, Dal T, Kaya S, Yildirim N, et al. Efficacy and safety of tenofovir disoproxil fumarate in pregnancy for the prevention of vertical transmission of HBV infection. World J Gastroenterol. 2013;19:9377–82.
39. Samadi Kochaksaraei G, Castillo E, Osman M, Simmonds K, Scott AN, Oshiomogho JI, et al. Clinical course of 161 untreated and tenofovir-treated chronic hepatitis B pregnant patients in a low hepatitis B virus endemic region. J Viral Hepatitis. 2016;23:15–22.
40. Chen WJ, Song SR, He H, Liang Q. Efficacy and safety of tenofovir, telbivudine in pregnancy to prevent perinatal transmission of hepatitis B virus. Shandong Med J. 2017;57:73–5.
41. Wan JY, Cai QE, Wang M. Efficacy and safety of tenofovir on blocking mother to child transmission of hepatitis B virus in virus high load pregenant women. China Tropical Med. 2017;17:828–30.
42. Qi WY, Zhao ZJ, Liu JQ. Clinical study on the effectiveness of tenofovir on blocking mother to child transmission of hepatitis B virus in pregnant women with chronic hepatitis B. Chinese J Med Guide. 2017;19:176–7.
43. Deng J, Chen Y, Jia G. Curative effect of tenofovir disoproxil in the treatment of hepatitis B pregnant women and its effect on blocking mother to child transmission of hepatitis B virus. China Modern Doctor. 2017;55:24–6.
44. Nguyen V, Tan PK, Greenup AJ, Glass A, Davison S, Samarasinghe D, et al. Anti-viral therapy for prevention of perinatal HBV transmission: extending therapy beyond birth does not protect against post-partum flare. Aliment Pharm Therap. 2014;39:1225–34.

22

Development and external validation of a prognostic nomogram for acute decompensation of chronic hepatitis B cirrhosis

Fangyuan Gao[1†], Xiaoshu Li[1†], Gang Wan[2†], Yuxin Li[1], Qun Zhang[1], Yao Liu[1], Huimin Liu[1], Hai Li[3*] and Xianbo Wang[1*]

Abstract

Background: Acute decompensation (AD) has been shown to be associated with a high mortality rate for cirrhosis patients. This study aimed to develop a prognostic nomogram to evaluating the individual prognosis for AD of cirrhosis in chronic hepatitis B (CHB).

Methods: The nomogram was developed using data from a retrospective study on 509 patients hospitalized for AD of CHB cirrhosis from October 2008 to February 2014 at the Beijing Ditan Hospital, Capital Medical University. The predictive accuracy, discriminative ability, and clinical net benefit were evaluated by concordance index (C-index), calibration curves, and decision curve analysis (DCA). The results were validated on 620 patients consecutively enrolled from January 2005 to December 2010 at the Renji Hospital, Shanghai Jiao Tong University,.

Results: On multivariate analysis of the derivation cohort, independent factors included in the nomogram were age, previous decompensation, bacterial infection, hepatic encephalopathy, and total bilirubin. The calibration curve for the probability of survival showed good agreement between the nomogram and actual observation. The nomogram had a C-index of 0.897, which was statistically higher than the C-index values of CTP (0.793), MELD (0. 821), SOFA (0.868), or the Chronic Liver Failure Consortium AD (CLIF-C AD) (0.716) scores ($p < 0.001$ for all). Using DCA, the nomogram also demonstrated superior net benefits over other score models. The results were confirmed in the validation cohort.

Conclusions: The proposed nomogram enables more-accurate individualized prediction of survival than MELD, CTP, SOFA, or CLIF-C AD scores for AD of CHB cirrhosis patients.

Keywords: Chronic liver disease, Chronic hepatitis B, Nomogram, Prognosis

Background

Hepatitis B virus (HBV) infection is a critical global health threat, particularly in Asia. In the natural history of chronic HBV infection, partial patients remain asymptomatic until an episode of acute decompensation (AD), which is featured by the rapid development of one or more major complications of liver disease. AD is the common cause of hospital admission and is associated with a high mortality rate for cirrhosis patients. AD of cirrhosis occurs in as many as 15% of cirrhosis patients each year, and the frequency and severity will increase with the progressively deterioration of liver reserve function. The course of illness during a patient's early hospital phase has been related to eventual prognosis. Therefore, early recognition and aggressive treatment are important to improving survival [1–4].

Recently, the CANONIC research team built the Chronic Liver Failure Consortium AD (CLIF-C AD),

* Correspondence: wangxb@ccmu.edu.cn; haili_17@126.com
†Fangyuan Gao, Xiaoshu Li and Gang Wan contributed equally to this work.
[3]Department of Gastroenterology, Ren Ji Hospital, School of Medicine, Shanghai Jiao Tong University, Shanghai, China
[1]Center of Integrative Medicine, Beijing Ditan Hospital, Capital Medical University, Beijing, China

which was demonstrated to be superior to the Model for End-stage Liver Disease (MELD), MELD-Na, and Child-Turcotte-Pugh (CTP) assessments in predicting mortality due to AD [5]. However, the current score models were built primarily base on populations with alcoholism issues and/or hepatitis C virus infections [5]. To date, no reports of a model have been found to assess the prognosis of AD of chronic hepatitis B (CHB) cirrhosis. CHB cirrhosis is deemed as the leading cause of AD in the Asia-Pacific region [6]. Therefore, it is necessary to create a risk model that can predict the prognosis for AD of CHB cirrhosis.

The nomogram is a graphical calculating and two-dimensional diagram, which could offer more precise and individualized prediction relative to the traditional models for multiple illness [6–9]. The specific objective of the study was to determine the risk factors for short-term death of AD with CHB cirrhosis, develop a prognostic nomogram to estimate the individual prognosis, and promote the implementation of preventive measures.

Patients and methods

Derivation cohort

In total, 1781 patients hospitalized at Beijing Ditan Hospital (Beijing, China), which is affiliated with the Capital Medical University, between October 2008 and February 2014 with CHB cirrhosis were screened, and 509 patients with AD of CHB cirrhosis were enrolled for model derivation. All patients were limited to age ≥ 18 years in this study, and patients with the following diseases would be excluded: (1) infected with hepatitis virus (including A, C, D, and E), human immunodeficiency virus, or other viruses; (2) autoimmune hepatitis, drug-induced liver injury, alcohol-induced liver disease, Wilson's disease, liver cancer, or hemolytic diseases; (3) other fatal disease, or gestation; or (4) liver operation or liver transplantation. The Ethics Committee from Beijing Ditan Hospital has approved this study protocol.

Validation cohort

2610 patients hospitalized with CHB cirrhosis at Renji Hospital, Shanghai Jiao Tong University, from January 2005 to December 2010 were screened, and 620 patients with AD of CHB cirrhosis were enrolled for external validation of the model. Only patients meeting the inclusion and exclusion standard and having sufficient data were registered. The research was supported by the Ethics Committee from Renji Hospital.

Cirrhosis was confirmed by previous hepatic pathology or clinical signs and results of laboratory detection, radiologic and endoscopic presentation.

AD of cirrhosis was defined as the rapid development of one or more major complications (ie, large ascites, hepatic encephalopathy (HE), gastrointestinal hemorrhage and bacterial infection) of liver disease [10–14]. Cirrhosis patients with grade 2 to 3 ascites within 2 weeks could be diagnosed with the acute development of large ascites [10]. Acute HE was characterized by the development of the acute confusional status in patients with previously normal conscious state and no evidence of the neurological deficit [11]. Cirrhosis patients with occurrence of upper or lower gastrointestinal bleeding could be diagnosed with acute gastrointestinal hemorrhage [12]. Bacterial infection was defined to include spontaneous bacterial peritonitis (SBP), pneumonia, cellulitis, urinary system infection and spontaneous bacteremia [13].

Definitions of organ failures were as follows [15]: the definition of liver failure was the total bilirubin (TBil) ≥ 12.0 mg/dL; the definition of kidney failure was the serum creatinine (Cr) ≥ 2.0 mg/dL or the use of renal replacement therapy; cerebral failure was defined by grade III-IV HE; the definition of coagulation failure was an international normalized ratio (INR) ≥ 2.5; the definition of circulatory failure was the use of vasoconstrictors; the definition of respiratory failure was $PaO_2/FiO_2 \leq 200$ or $SpO_2/FiO_2 \leq 214$.

The MELD, CTP, SOFA and CLIF-C AD scores were calculated according to previously published criteria [5, 16–18]. All definitions and prognostic scores were applied at baseline.

Treatment

Standard medical therapies were used for all patients after diagnosis, such as bed rest, liver-protecting therapy, antiviral treatment, nutritional support, vitamins supplements, plasma and albumin transfusion, maintenance treatment of water-electrolyte and acid-base balance, control and prevention of complications.

Clinical predictors

Possible variables associated with short-term survival of AD of CHB cirrhosis were collected, including age; sex; mean arterial pressure; decompensation history; occurrences of organ failures or clinic complications; biochemical parameters, including alanine aminotransferase (ALT), aspartate aminotransferase (AST), γ-glutamyl transpeptidase (GGT), albumin (ALB), TBil, Cr, serum Na, INR, white blood cell (WBC) count, absolute neutrophil count (NC), absolute platelet count (PLT), and HBV deoxyribonucleic acid (DNA) levels. Baseline data were obtained at the first diagnosis of AD of CHB cirrhosis. The 7-, 14- and 28-day survival rates were gained by searching the medical records.

Statistical analysis

Statistical analysise were conducted using SPSS version 20.0 (IBM, Armonk, NY, USA). Patient characteristics were compared by the Fisher's exact or χ^2 tests (categorical variables) and the Mann-Whitney *U* or *t* test (continuous variables). Univariate risk factors that reached $p < 0.05$ were subjected to Cox regression analysis.

The nomogram was built in terms of results of Cox regression analyses using R version 3.0.2 with the rms package [19]. According to the Akaike information criterion, backward step-down selection process was applied to the selection of final model [20]. The discrimination of the models were assessed in terms of the concordance index (C-index). Bootstraps with 1000 resamples were drawn to correct the C-index. Comparisons between nomogram and other models were carried out by using the rcorrp.cens in the Hmisc package [21]. Calibration curves were also drawn to evaluate the concordance between predicted and observed probabilities. Decision curve analyses (DCA) were used to compare the benefits and improved performance of different models [22]. All tests were two-sided and were considered statistically significant when $p < 0.05$.

Results

Patient characteristics and outcomes

In total, 509 and 620 patients from the derivation and external validation cohorts, respectively, were included for analyses. The baseline data of enrolled patients were summarized in Table 1. In both sets, the average age was 51–52 years, and the patients were predominantly men. 410 patients (80.6%) were treated with nucleotide analogs (NUCs) and 99 patients (19.4%) didn't received NUCs after hospital admission in the derivation cohort. 372 patients (60.0%) were treated with NUCs and 248 patients (40.0%) didn't receive antiviral therapy in the validation cohort. The most common complication was ascites, followed by HE (I-IV) and gastrointestinal hemorrhage at admission. Liver failure was the most frequent organ failure, which was followed by coagulation and cerebral failure.

When comparing the demographic and clinical characteristics between the derivation and validation sets, we found that patients in the derivation set had lower rates of previous decompensation and hyponatremia, and higher rates of complications (ascites, bacterial infection, gastrointestinal hemorrhage, HE) at the time of admission ($p < 0.05$). Moreover, the validation set had lower Na levels and higher ALT, AST, GGT, TBil, Cr, INR, WBC, and HBV DNA levels ($p < 0.05$). The validation set had higher 7-, 14- and 28-day risk of death than those of the derivation set ($p < 0.05$).

Univariate and multivariate analyses

Univariate analysis showed that age, male sex, previous decompensation, hyponatremia, ascites, bacterial infection, gastrointestinal hemorrhage, HE III-IV, SBP, hepatorenal syndrome, organ failure (liver, kidney, cerebral, coagulation, circulatory, and lung), AST, ALB, TBil, Cr, Na, INR, WBC, and NC were significantly associated with poor prognosis of AD of CHB cirrhosis in the derivation set ($p < 0.05$, Table 2).

These variables were subjected to the Cox regression analyses. The results showed that only age (HR = 1.057, 95% confidence interval [CI]: 1.032–1.082, $p < 0.001$), previous decompensation (HR = 2.449, 95% CI: 1.351–4.438, $p = 0.002$), bacterial infection (HR = 5.325, 95% CI: 3.015–9.405, $p < 0.001$), HE III–IV (HR = 4.660, 95% CI: 3.115–6.972, $p < 0.001$), and TBil (HR = 1.053, 95% CI: 1.030–1.078, $p < 0.001$) were independent risk factors for outcomes (Table 2).

Derivation of the prognostic nomogram

The nomogram was established on the basis of the coefficients gained from multivariate analysis, which included age, previous decompensation, bacterial infection, HE, and TBil (Fig. 1). Each value of the factors was allocated the score in the point scale axis. By summing each single score and using that value in the total point scale axis, the total score could be easily calculated to assign the probability of survival for individual patients.

Validation of the prognostic nomogram

The C-index of the nomogram was 0.897 (95% CI: 0.850–0.943) in the derivation cohort. To more effectively validate the practicability of the nomogram, we adopted an external cohort with AD of CHB cirrhosis for model validation. When the validation set was estimated by the established nomogram, the C-index was 0.839 (95% CI: 0.811–0.867), suggesting that the nomogram is suitable for estimating the short-term outcome for AD of CHB cirrhosis.

The calibration curves were plotted showing that good agreements between the nomogram predictions and observed probabilities for the 7-, 14-, and 28-day outcomes in the primary (Figs. 2A-C) and external validation cohort (Figs. 2D-F).

Performance of the nomogram compared with other models

Futhermore, we compared the C-indexes for evaluating the concordance of these models. The corrected C-index of our nomogram was 0.897, which was significantly higher than that of the MELD (0.820), CTP (0.793), SOFA (0.868), and CLIF-C ADs (0.716) in the primary set ($p < 0.001$, Table 3). Meanwhile, the nomogram also had the highest C-index (0.839) in the validation set, with statistical significance in comparison with MELD (0.826), CTP (0.741), SOFA (0.837), and CLIF-C ADs (0.569) ($p < 0.001$ for all).

On DCA, our nomogram provided superior net benefit and improved performance for the 7-, 14-, and 28-day prognostic evaluation in the primary (Figs. 3A-C) and validation (Figs. 3D-F) cohorts relative to MELD, CTP, SOFA, and CLIF-C AD score models. This represents superior clinical usefulness of the nomogram over other score models.

Table 1 Baseline characteristics in enrolled acute decompensation of CHB cirrhosis patients in the derivation and external validation cohort

Characteristic	Derivation cohort $N = 509$	External validation cohort $N = 620$	P value
Age (yr)	51.9 ± 11.8	51.4 ± 11.3	0.540
Male sex	359 (70.5)	463 (74.7)	0.119
Mean arterial pressure (mm Hg)	87.3 ± 10.7	87.3 ± 12.2	0.997
Previous decompensation	197 (38.7)	328 (52.9)	< 0.001
Complication			
Hyponatremia	144 (28.3)	249 (40.2)	< 0.001
Ascites	469 (92.1)	496 (80.0)	< 0.001
Bacteria infection	106 (20.8)	75 (12.1)	< 0.001
Gastrointestinal hemorrhage	123 (24.2)	62 (10.0)	< 0.001
Hepatic encephalopathy I-II	100 (19.6)	46 (7.4)	< 0.001
Hepatic encephalopathy III-IV	89 (17.5)	33 (5.3)	< 0.001
Spontaneous bacterial peritonitis	21 (4.1)	19 (3.1)	0.337
Hepatorenal syndrome	44 (8.6)	61 (9.8)	0.492
Organ failures			
Liver	96 (18.9)	152 (24.5)	< 0.001
Kidney	23 (4.5)	64 (10.3)	< 0.001
Cerebral	89 (17.5)	33 (5.3)	< 0.001
Coagulation	56 (11.0)	120 (19.4)	< 0.001
Respiratory	4 (0.8)	19 (3.1)	0.010
Circulation	6 (1.2)	9 (1.5)	0.797
Biochemical parameters			
Alanine aminotransferase (U/L)	130.7 ± 388.4	161.0 ± 428.1	< 0.001
Aspartate aminotransferase (U/L)	125.4 ± 211.3	143.0 ± 322.6	0.005
γ-Glutamyltransferase (U/L)	60.1 ± 80.9	66.5 ± 86.9	0.015
Albumin (g/L)	29.5 ± 16.3	29.7 ± 5.8	0.764
Total bilirubin (mg/dL)	6.8 ± 9.3	9.6 ± 13.7	0.004
Serum creatinine (μmol/L)	80.3 ± 58.1	89.9 ± 84.8	0.016
Serum sodium (mmol/L)	137.0 ± 5.4	134.6 ± 6.8	< 0.001
International normalized ratio	1.7 ± 1.5	2.0 ± 1.3	0.001
White blood cell count ($\times 10^9$/L)	5.5 ± 4.0	6.4 ± 4.8	0.009
Neutrophil count ($\times10^9$/L)	4.1 ± 5.8	–	–
Platelet ($\times10^9$/L)	73.2 ± 55.2	79.1 ± 59.2	0.240
HBV-DNA (log copies/ml)	4.1 ± 1.7	4.4 ± 1.6	< 0.001
Mortality			
7 days	19(3.7)	71(11.5)	< 0.001
14 days	40(7.9)	116(18.7)	< 0.001
28 days	56(11.0)	170(27.4)	< 0.001

Data are the mean ± standard deviation for continuous valiables, and n (%), frequency with percentage for categorical variables

Discussion

In the present study, a novel and easy-to-use nomogram was constructed to evaluate individual prognosis for AD of CHB cirrhosis. This nomogram demonstrated superior predictive capability and clinical usefulness relative to the current prognostic score models, including MELD, CTP, SOFA, and CLIF-C ADs.

In our derivation cohort, 11.0% (56/509) of patients with AD of CHB cirrhosis died within 4 weeks—a result that was similar to that of another study [23]. A total of 13.0% (66/509) of the patients died within 90 days, and 56 of 66 patients died in the first 4 weeks; thus, we set up the 28-day statistical prognostic score model for patients with AD to find out those at the highest risk for death, which

Table 2 Univariate and multivariate Cox regression analyses in patients with acute decompensation of CHB cirrhosis from the derivation cohort (n = 509)

	Univariate analysis		Multivariate analysis	
	HR (95% CI)	*p* value	HR (95% CI)	*p* value
Age (yr)	1.054(1.031–1.079)	< 0.001	1.057(1.032–1.082)	< 0.001
Male sex	2.350(1.391–3.969)	< 0.001		
Mean arterial pressure (mm Hg)	0.979(0.953–1.005)	0.116		
Previous decompensation	2.419(1.420–4.120)	0.001	2.449(1.351–4.438)	0.002
Complication				
Hyponatremia	4.005(2.351–6.823)	< 0.001		
Ascites	0.463(0.113–1.900)	< 0.001		
Bacteria infection	2.479(1.443–4.259)	0.001	5.325(3.015–9.405)	< 0.001
Gastrointestinal hemorrhage	2.301(1.042–5.081)	0.039		
Hepatic encephalopathy I-II	1.426(0.439–4.631)	0.555		
Hepatic encephalopathy III-IV	22.381(10.893–45.983)	< 0.001	4.660(3.115–6.972)	< 0.001
Spontaneous bacterial peritonitis	4.392(1.988–9.703)	< 0.001		
Hepatorenal syndrome	6.345(3.617–11.129)	< 0.001		
Organ failures				
Liver	2.720(1.583–4.672)	< 0.001		
Kidney	4.839(2.370–9.881)	< 0.001		
Cerebral	20.324(10.909–37.863)	< 0.001		
Coagulation	9.389(5.547–16.891)	< 0.001		
Circulation	10.148(3.657–28.166)	< 0.001		
Lung	9.706(3.024–31.154)	< 0.001		
Biochemical parameters				
Alanine aminotransferase (U/L)	1.000(1.000–1.001)	0.298		
Aspartate aminotransferase (U/L)	1.001(1.000–1.002)	0.005		
γ-Glutamyltransferase (U/L)	0.999(0.996–1.003)	0.722		
Albumin (g/L)	0.937(0.890–0.987)	0.015		
Total bilirubin (mg/dL)	1.048(1.029–1.067)	< 0.001	1.053(1.030–1.078)	< 0.001
Serum creatinine (μmol/L)	1.005(1.003–1.007)	< 0.001		
Serum sodium (mmol/L)	0.904(0.872–0.937)	< 0.001		
International normalized ratio	1.963(1.683–2.290)	< 0.001		
White blood cell count (×10^9/L)	1.151(1.108–1.195)	< 0.001		
Neutrophil count (×10^9/L)	1.175(1.128–1.225)	< 0.001		
Platelet (× 10^9/L)	0.998(0.993–1.004)	0.576		
HBV-DNA (log copies/ml)	1.160(0.986–1.366)	0.074		

would enable us to take effective treatment measures as soon as possible. In addition, most of studies on prognosis factors for liver decompensation cirrhosis did not strictly distinguish the etiology, such as viral hepatitis, alcohol, drugs, or other factors [17, 24]. Our study only observed patients with AD of CHB cirrhosis as subjects; both blood biochemical tests and clinical complications were part of our prognosis factors. We also excluded the influence of liver transplantation, considering this has less application in our country. Moreover, to effectively evaluate the predictive ability of our nomogram versus those of established models, we adopted the external validation cohort to reduce the influence of drugs, treatments, and other factors on the results.

The proposed nomogram included age, two liver function indices (previous decompensation, TBil), and two complications (bacterial infection and HE). Many studies have suggested the correlation between age and prognosis in many diseases, and that old age is an important factor in poor prognosis for cirrhosis [25, 26]. Recently, the CANONIC

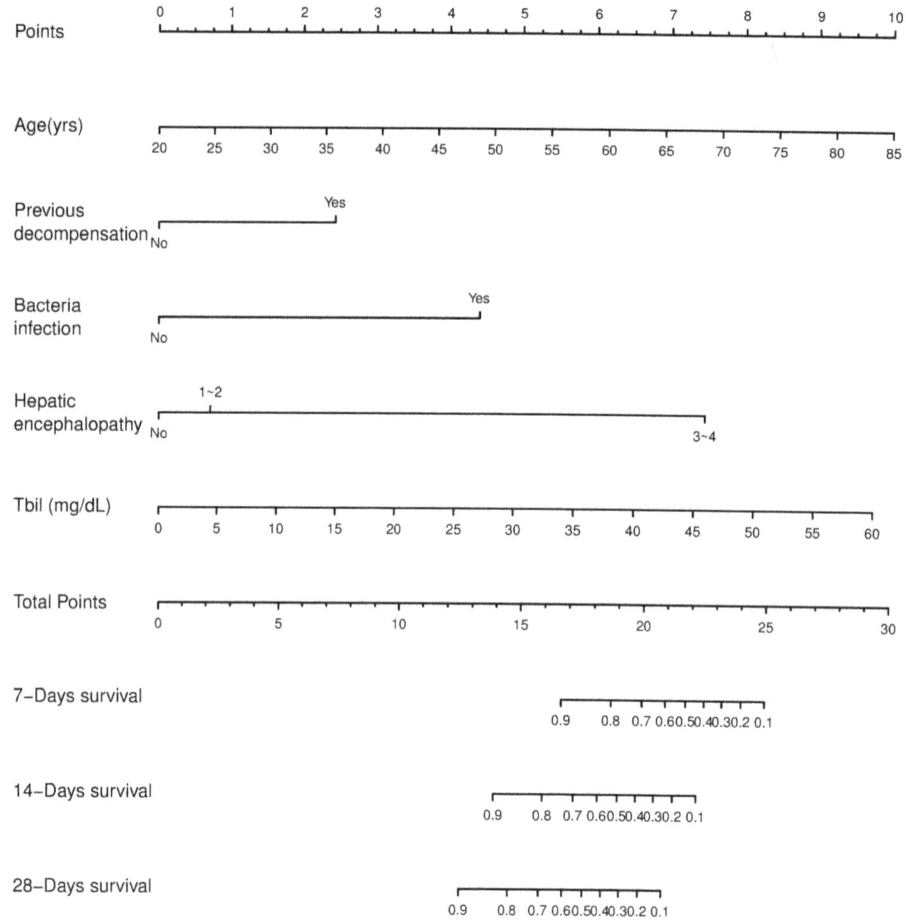

Fig. 1 Acute decompensation of CHB cirrhosis survival nomogram. To use the nomogram, the value of an individual patient is located on each variable axis, and a line is drawn upward to determine the number of points received for the value of each variable. The sum of these numbers is located on the total point axis, and a line is drawn downward to the survival axes to determine the likelihood of 7-, 14-, and 28-day survivals

study team built two models for ACLF (CLIF-C ACLFs) and AD (CLIF-C ADs) patients, where old age was considered an important indicator of poor outcomes [5, 15]. This may be explained by loss of immune function or decline in tissue regeneration and repair [27, 28]. Serum TBil is commonly used as an indicator of the degree of liver damage and reserve function; it is also the main parameter of the CTP and MELD score systems [16, 17]. Previous decompensation could better reflect the underlying disease before the onset of AD. Bacterial infection represent the particularly important cause of liver failure and other complications [29]. The end-organ damaging effect of bacterial infection is more serious in liver cirrhosis and often culminates in newly developed liver and extrahepatic organ failures, which account for significant morbidity and mortality [4, 30]. HE is a frequent and serious complication of cirrhosis [31, 32]. Once HE occurs in patients with cirrhosis, the prognosis is poor, and liver transplant should be performed as soon as possible in order to increase the survival rate [33, 34].

In this study, the nomogram model performed well in predicting survival, as supported by the C-index (0.897 and 0.839 for the primary and validation cohorts respectively) and the calibration curve. Compared with MELD, CTP, SOFA, and CLIF-C ADs, the nomogram showed superior predictive capability for outcomes. Furthermore, the nomogram demonstrated better net benefit and improved performance for 7-, 14-, and 28-day prognostic evaluation in the derivation and validation cohorts compared with MELD, CTP, SOFA, and CLIF-C AD score models.

In current study, some patients didn't received antiviral therapy. One of the reasons is that patients with HE III-IV and gastrointestinal hemorrhage are unable to take drugs. Another reason is that the antiviral therapy was administered not only according to HBV replication levels, but also the willingness of the patient. So, considering the bad financial condition, many patients have to abandon the use of antiviral drugs. Besides, more patients didn't received the antiviral therapy in the validation cohort. The major reason is that the enrollment

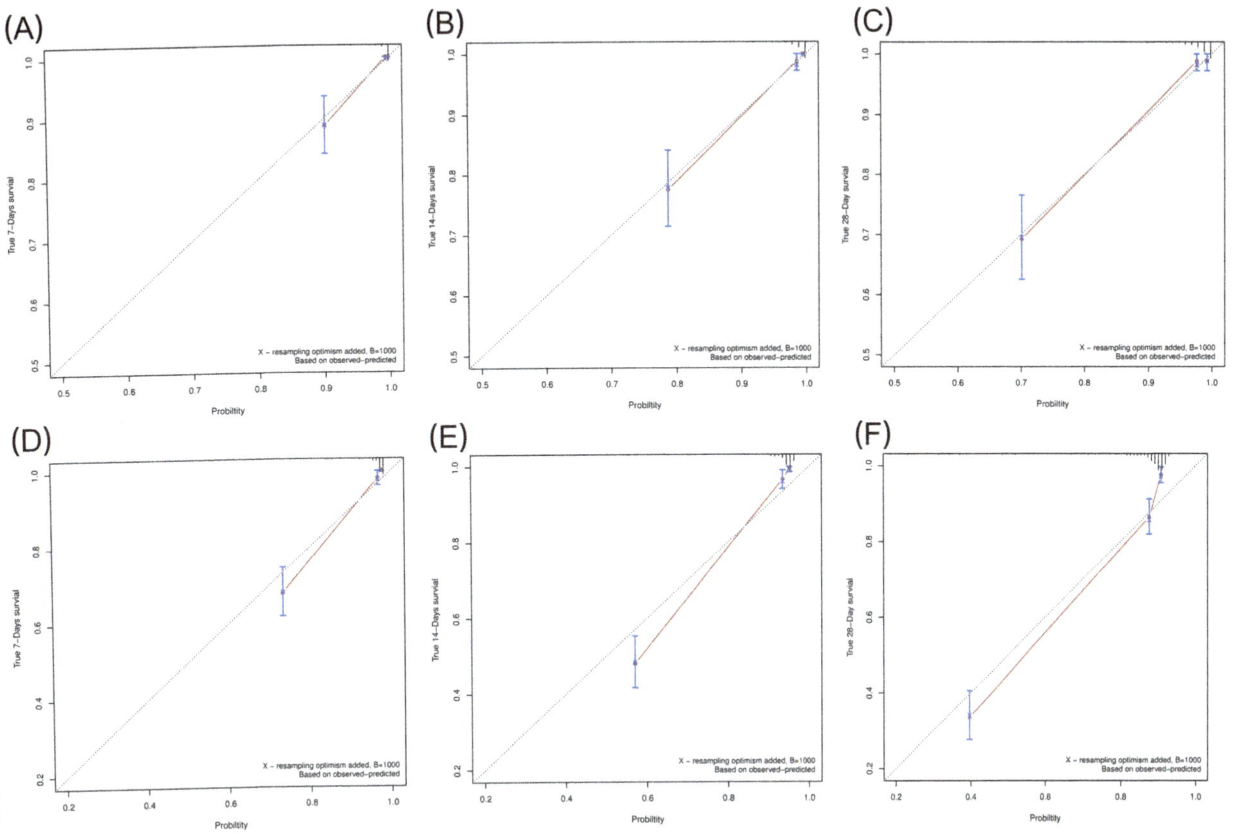

Fig. 2 The calibration curve of overall survival at 7, 14, and 28 days for the derivation cohort (**a-c**) and the external validation cohort (**d-f**). Nomogram-predicted probability of survival is plotted on the x-axis, and the actual survival is plotted on the y-axis. Dashed lines along the 45-degree line through the point of origin represent the perfect calibration models in which the predicted probabilities are identical to the actual probabilities

Table 3 The predictive discrimination ability of the nomogram compared to the MELD, CTP, and SOFA score systems in the primary and validation cohorts

	C-index	95% CI for C-index		Goodness of Fit		Comparison of models			
		Lower	Upper	LR	R^2	Dxy	SD	Z	*P* value
Primary cohort (n = 509)									
MELDs	0.820	0.764	0.878	72.07	0.185	−0.343	0.083	−4.12	< 0.001
CTPs	0.793	0.744	0.842	70.79	0.175	−0.687	0.051	−13.5	< 0.001
SOFAs	0.868	0.829	0.907	119.46	0.282	−0.398	0.075	−5.33	< 0.001
CLIF-C ADs	0.716	0.636	0.796	45.36	0.121	−0.476	0.078	−6.10	< 0.001
Nomogram	0.897	0.850	0.943	165.63	0.374	–	–	–	
Validation cohort (n = 620)									
MELDs	0.826	0.794	0.857	238.69	0.336	0.451	0.045	10.13	< 0.001
CTPs	0.741	0.707	0.776	130.11	0.196	−0.557	0.035	−15.94	< 0.001
SOFAs	0.837	0.807	0.866	255.24	0.349	−0.215	0.049	−4.39	< 0.001
CLIF-C ADs	0.569	0.525	0.615	8.47	0.015	−0.501	0.041	−12.22	< 0.001
Nomogram	0.839	0.811	0.867	268.38	0.363	–	–	–	

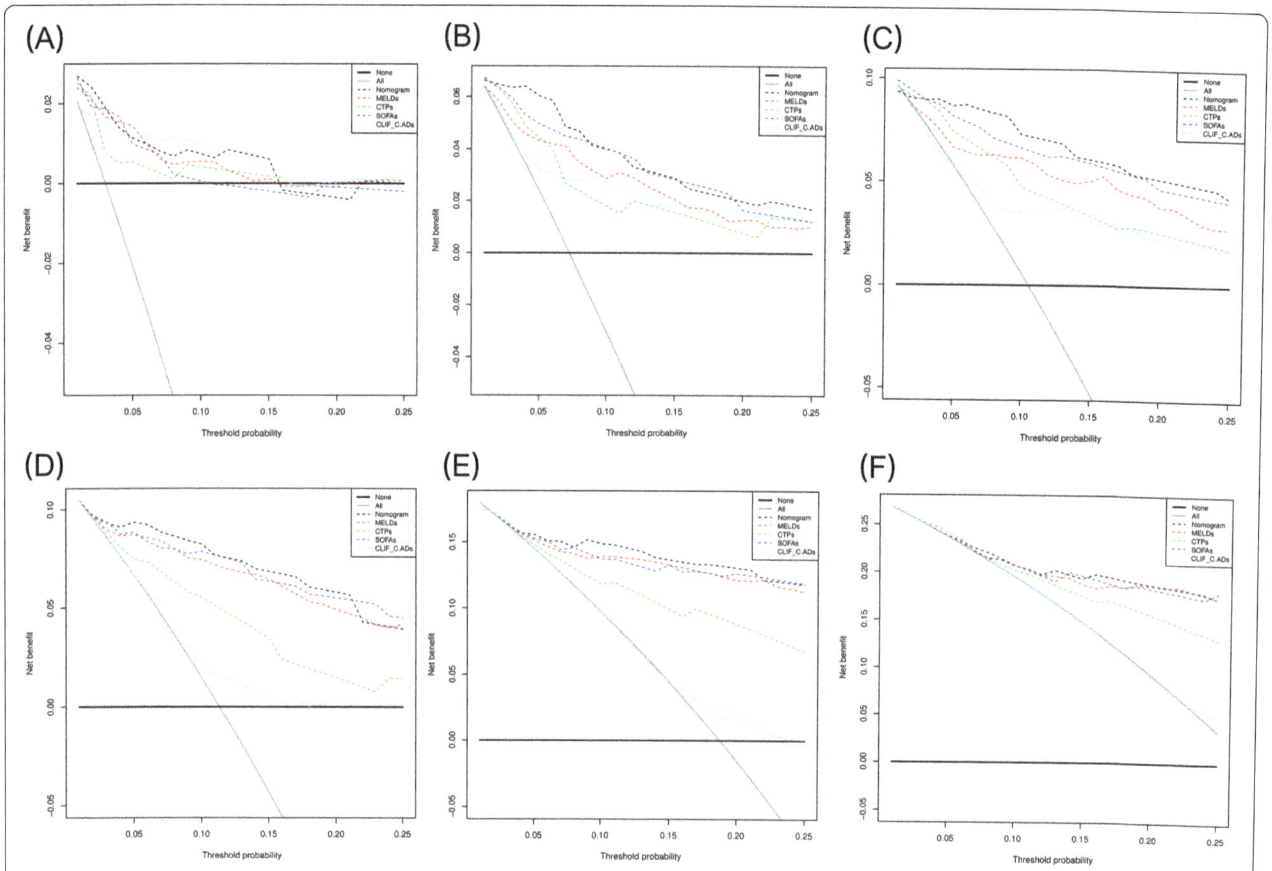

Fig. 3 Decision curve analysis at 7, 14, and 28 days for the derivation cohort (**a-c**) and the external validation cohort (**d-f**). Decision curve analyses depict the clinical net benefit in pairwise comparisons across the different models. The horizontal solid black line represents the assumption that no patients will experience the event, and the solid gray line represents the assumption that all patients will relapse. On decision curve analysis, the nomogram showed superior net benefit compared with other models across a range of threshold probabilities

time of patients in validation cohort is from January 2005 to December 2010, four years ahead of the derivation cohort. Antiviral drugs are more widespread with the development of healthcare in China. This reflects the clinical treatment situation of China objectively.

Our study has several limitations. First, our nomogram only included basic laboratory data. However, this study aimed to construct a reliable prognostic model. To avoid inevitable bias, subjective variables have not been included to construct our nomogram. Second, the nomogram was built on the basis of a retrospective cohort, and selection bias may exist. However, we have validated the model with data from another institution. The results consistently demonstrated the very good performance of our established nomogram.

Conclusions

To our knowledge, the nomogram model here is the first model developed to predict the individual prognosis of AD of cirrhosis in CHB patients to date. This provided better performance than MELD, CTP, SOFA, and CLIF-C AD scores, and it offers a foundation for individualized counseling and clinical treatment.

Abbreviations

AD: acute decompensation; ALB: albumin; ALP: alkaline phosphatase; ALT: alanine aminotransferase; AST: aspartate aminotransferase; CHB: chronic hepatitis B; CIs: confidence intervals; CLIF-C AD: Chronic Liver Failure Consortium Acute Decompensation; CTP: Child-Turcotte-Pugh; DCA: decision curve analysis; GGT: γ-glutamyltranspeptidase; HBV: hepatitis B virus; HE: hepatic encephalopathy; HRs: hazard ratios; INR: international normalized ratio; MELD: Model for End-stage Liver Disease; NC: absolute neutrophil count; PLT: absolute platelet count; SOFA: Sequential Organ Failure Assessment; TBil: total bilirubin; WBC: white blood cell

Acknowledgements

We gratefully recognize the patients who participated in this study. We thank Yan Sang for her help with the data.

Funding

This study was supported by grants from the National Natural Science Foundation of China (No. 81473641) and the Beijing Municipal Administration of Hospitals Clinical Medicine Development of Special Funding Support (ZYLX201707). The funders had no role in study design, data collection and analysis, decision to publish, or preparation of the manuscript.

Authors' contributions

XBW and HL were responsible for the conception and design of the study. FYG, XSL, GW, YXL, QZ, YL and HML were responsible for the acquisition and analysis of data. FYG, XSL and GW drafted the manuscript. All authors participated in interpretation of the findings. XBW revised and commented on the draft, and all authors read and approved the final version of the manuscript. All authors confirm that the content has not been published elsewhere and does not overlap with or duplicate their previously published work. All authors read and approved the final manuscript.

Consent for publication
Not applicable.

Competing interests
The authors declare that they have no conflicts of interest with regard to the publication of this research report.

Author details
[1]Center of Integrative Medicine, Beijing Ditan Hospital, Capital Medical University, Beijing, China. [2]Statistics Room, Beijing Ditan Hospital, Capital Medical University, Beijing, China. [3]Department of Gastroenterology, Ren Ji Hospital, School of Medicine, Shanghai Jiao Tong University, Shanghai, China.

References
1. Dienstag JL, Ghany MG, Morgan TR, Di Bisceglie AM, Bonkovsky HL, Kim HY, et al. A prospective study of the rate of progression in compensated, histologically advanced chronic hepatitis C. Hepatology. 2011;54:396–405.
2. Jepsen P, Ott P, Andersen PK, Sørensen HT, Vilstrup H. Clinical course of alcoholic liver cirrhosis: a Danish population-based cohort study. Hepatology. 2010;51:1675–82.
3. D'Amico G, Garcia-Tsao G, Pagliaro L. Natural history and prognostic indicators of survival in cirrhosis: a systematic review of 118 studies. J Hepatol. 2006;44:217–31.
4. Moreau R, Jalan R, Gines P, Pavesi M, Angeli P, Cordoba J, et al. Acute-on-chronic liver failure is a distinct syndrome that develops in patients with acute decompensation of cirrhosis. Gastroenterology. 2013;144:1426–37 1437.e1–9.
5. Jalan R, Pavesi M, Saliba F, Amorós A, Fernandez J, Holland-Fischer P, et al. The CLIF consortium acute decompensation score (CLIF-C ADs) for prognosis of hospitalised cirrhotic patients without acute-on-chronic liver failure. J Hepatol. 2015;62:831–40.
6. Touijer K, Scardino PT. Nomograms for staging, prognosis, and predicting treatment outcomes. Cancer. 2009;115:3107–11.
7. Kattan MW, Scardino PT. Evidence for the usefulness of nomograms. Nat Clin Pract Urol. 2007;4:638–9.
8. Wan G, Gao F, Chen J, Li Y, Geng M, Sun L, et al. Nomogram prediction of individual prognosis of patients with hepatocellular carcinoma. BMC Cancer. 2017;17:91.
9. Sternberg CN. Are nomograms better than currently available stage groupings for bladder cancer. J Clin Oncol. 2006;24:3819–20.
10. Moore KP, Wong F, Gines P, Bernardi M, Ochs A, Salerno F, et al. The management of ascites in cirrhosis: report on the consensus conference of the international ascites Club. Hepatology. 2003;38:258–66.
11. Blei AT, Córdoba J. Hepatic encephalopathy. Am J Gastroenterol. 2001;96: 1968–76.
12. Garcia-Tsao G, Bosch J. Management of varices and variceal hemorrhage in cirrhosis. N Engl J Med. 2010;362:823–32.
13. Gustot T, Durand F, Lebrec D, Vincent JL, Moreau R. Severe sepsis in cirrhosis. Hepatology. 2009;50:2022–33.
14. Arvaniti V, D'Amico G, Fede G, Manousou P, Tsochatzis E, Pleguezuelo M, et al. Infections in patients with cirrhosis increase mortality four-fold and should be used in determining prognosis. Gastroenterology. 2010;139:1246–56 1256.e1–5.
15. Jalan R, Saliba F, Pavesi M, Amoros A, Moreau R, Ginès P, et al. Development and validation of a prognostic score to predict mortality in patients with acute-on-chronic liver failure. J Hepatol. 2014;61:1038–47.
16. Kamath PS, Kim WR. The model for end-stage liver disease (MELD). Hepatology. 2007;45:797–805.
17. Pugh RN, Murray-Lyon IM, Dawson JL, Pietroni MC, Williams R. Transection of the oesophagus for bleeding oesophageal varices. Br J Surg. 1973;60:646–9.
18. Vincent JL, Moreno R, Takala J, Willatts S, De Mendonça A, Bruining H, et al. The SOFA (Sepsis-related organ failure assessment) score to describe organ dysfunction/failure. On behalf of the working group on Sepsis-related problems of the European Society of Intensive Care Medicine. Intensive Care Med. 1996;22:707–10.
19. Frank E, Harrell J. Rms: Regression Modeling Strategies. R Package version 3. 4–0. https://CRAN.R-project.org/package=Hmisc.
20. Harrell FE Jr, Lee KL, Mark DB. Multivariable prognostic models: issues in developing models, evaluating assumptions and adequacy, and measuring and reducing errors. Stat Med. 1996;15:361–87.
21. Frank E, Harrell Jr. Harrell Miscellaneous. R Package version 3.9–2. https://CRAN.R-project.org/package=Hmisc.
22. Vickers AJ, Elkin EB. Decision curve analysis: a novel method for evaluating prediction models. Med Decis Mak. 2006;26:565–74.
23. McPhail MJ, Shawcross DL, Abeles RD, Chang A, Patel V, Lee GH, et al. Increased survival for patients with cirrhosis and organ failure in liver intensive care and validation of the chronic liver failure-sequential organ failure scoring system. Clin Gastroenterol Hepatol. 2015;13:1353–60 e8.
24. Malinchoc M, Kamath PS, Gordon FD, Peine CJ, Rank J, ter Borg PC. A model to predict poor survival in patients undergoing transjugular intrahepatic portosystemic shunts. Hepatology. 2000;31:864–71.
25. Schiodt FV, Chung RT, Schilsky ML, Hay JE, Christensen E, Lee WM. Outcome of acute liver failure in the elderly. Liver Transpl. 2009;15:1481–7.
26. Faber W, Stockmann M, Schirmer C, Möllerarnd A, Denecke T, Bahra M, et al. Significant impact of patient age on outcome after liver resection for HCC in cirrhosis. Eur J Surg Oncol. 2014;40:208–13.
27. Zeeh J, Platt D. The aging liver: structural and functional changes and their consequences for drug treatment in old age. Gerontology. 2002;48:121–7.
28. Wynne HA, Cope LH, Mutch E, Rawlins MD, Woodhouse KW, James OF. The effect of age upon liver volume and apparent liver blood flow in healthy man. Hepatology. 1989;9:297–301.
29. Jalan R, Fernandez J, Wiest R, Schnabl B, Moreau R, Angeli P, et al. Bacterial infections in cirrhosis: a position statement based on the EASL special conference 2013. J Hepatol. 2014;60:1310–24.
30. Bajaj JS, O'Leary JG, Reddy KR, Wong F, Biggins SW, Patton H, et al. Survival in infection-related acuteon-chronic liver failure is defined by extrahepatic organ failures. Hepatology. 2014;60:250–6.
31. Ferenci P, Lockwood A, Mullen K, Tarter R, Weissenborn K, Blei AT. Hepatic encephalopathy-definition, nomenclature, diagnosis, and quantification: final report of the working party at the 11th world congresses of gastroenterology, Vienna, 1998. Hepatology. 2002;35:716–21.
32. Häussinger D, Schliess F. Pathogenetic mechanisms of hepatic encephalopathy. Gut. 2008;57:1156–65.
33. Orr JG, Morgan CL, Jenkins-Jones S, Hudson M, Conway P, Radwan A, et al. Resource use associated with hepatic encephalopathy in patients with liver disease. J Hepatol. 2014;60:S228–9.
34. Cordoba J, Ventura-Cots M, Simón-Talero M, Amorós À, Pavesi M, Vilstrup H, et al. Characteristics, risk factors, and mortality of cirrhotic patients hospitalized for hepatic encephalopathy with and without acute-on-chronic liver failure (ACLF). J Hepatol. 2014;60:275–81.

23

Distribution and clinical significance of hepatitis B virus genotypes in Pakistan

Majid Mahmood[1,2*], Muhammad Asim Anwar[3], Azra Khanum[4], Nasib Zaman[5] and Abida Raza[6]

Abstract

Background: Hepatitis B virus (HBV) genotype and its role in disease progression and patients' response to antiviral treatment, is not well studied in Pakistan. This comprehensive study was aimed to determine the distribution of HBV genotypes in Pakistan and their possible association with phases of HBV infection.

Methods: A total of 840 HBsAg positive samples was collected and tested for HBV DNA quantity. Samples below 100 IU/ml were excluded from the study. A total of 715 samples representing all the six parts of the country were genotyped by type specific primer PCR method. Clinical data of only 384 patients was compared as the remaining 332 were either receiving antiviral treatment or their infection phase was not confirmed.

Results: Genotype D was found in 509 samples (71.2 %), genotype A in 55 samples (7.7 %) and mixed infection with genotypes A and D in 124 samples (17.3 %). Genotypes B, C and E were identified in less than 1 % of the total samples. Genotype A, D and their mixture (A + D) were compared for severity of HBV infection. Significant differences were not found in distribution of HBV genotypes among different disease stages.

Conclusion: HBV genotype D was the predominant infection in all study areas of Pakistan followed by mixed genotypes infection (A + D) whereas genotype A has 10 times lower prevalence than genotype D. Genotypes B, C, E and F altogether make only 1.5 % of the prevalence. Genotype do not appears to show the severity of liver disease.

Keywords: Hepatitis B virus, HBV genotypes, Liver disease progression, PCR

Abbreviations: AJK, Azad Jammu and Kashmir; ANOVA, Analysis of Variance; bp, Base Pairs; ddH_2O, Double Distilled Water; DNA, Deoxy ribo nucleic acid; FATA, Federally Administered Tribal Areas; FCT, Federal Capital Territory; HBsAg, Hepatitis B Surface Antigen; HBV, Hepatitis B Virus; HCC, Hepatocellular Carcinoma; HEC, Higher Education Commission; IU/ml, International Unit Per Milli Liter; KP, Khyber Pakhtoonkha; NORI, Nuclear Medicine, Oncology and Radiotherapy Institute; PCR, Polymerase Chain Reaction; PMAS, Pir Mehr Ali Shah; SPSS, Statistical Package for Social Sciences; USA, United States of America; °C, Centigrade

Background

Hepatitis B virus (HBV) infection has been a major health problem as about 400 million people carry hepatitis B surface antigen worldwide [1], out of which, nearly 1 million die every year [2]. The infection rate of HBV has decreased significantly in developed countries like United States of America [3], where the acute HBV infection rate has fallen by 78 % during 1990–2005 [4]. Unfortunately, in developing and underdeveloped countries including Pakistan, the infection rate seems to have not decreased, even to any appreciable level. The failure in tackling the infection has been related to the high cost of antiviral drugs, lack of vaccination and public awareness about infection and the mismanagement to address the problem in Pakistan [5].

Eight HBV genotypes have been established on the basis of 8 % or more nucleotide divergence in the genome. These genotypes are named as A, B, C, D [6], E, F [7, 8], G [9] and H [10] which are common [11], while genotype I [12, 13] and J [14] are also introduced as new genotypes but their status is questionable. HBV genotypes have specific pattern of distribution in different geographic regions and ethnic groups of the world. Genotype A is prevalent

* Correspondence: majid1133@gmail.com
[1]Department of Zoology, The University of Poonch, Rawalakot, Azad Jammu and Kashmir 12350, Pakistan
[2]Department of Zoology, Pir Mehr Ali Shah Arid Agriculture University, Rawalpindi 46300, Pakistan

in Brazil, USA, Canada, Northwest Europe, South Asia, Central African countries, Tunisia and Benin [15–17]. Genotype B is common in Japan, Taiwan, Philippines, Hong Kong, China, Vietnam, Thailand, Indonesia and United States of America. Genotype C occurs in Australia, Polynesia, Melanesia, Micronesia, Indonesia, China, Hong Kong, Vietnam, Thailand, Japan, Korea, Taiwan, India, Solomon Islands, Brazil and USA. Genotype D is predominant in Mediterranean region, Spain, Albania, Czech Republic, Russia, Turkey, Middle East, Iran, Afghanistan, South Asia, Solomon Islands, Tunisia, Polynesia, Melanesia, Micronesia, Brazil and USA [17–19]. Genotype E is endemic to Africa where it occurs only in some countries of the Western part of the continent while genotype F is widely distributed in new world. It has been reported from Alaska, Argentina, South America, Central America and Polynesia [17, 20]. Genotypes G has been recorded from North America, France and Germany, genotype H from Central America, South America and Mexico while genotypes I and J were reported only from Vietnam and Japan respectively [17].

HBV genotypes have been reported to have significant association with progression of liver diseases, risk of cirrhosis, development of hepatocellular carcinoma (HCC), viral load, HBsAg sero-clearance, HBeAg sero-conversion and response to antiviral therapy [21]. Co-infection with two different virus genotypes has been reported to be associated with worse prognosis of the disease. Some studies showed that co-infection with HBV/B and HBV/C is associated with high viral load and more severe liver disease as compared to single genotype infection [22, 23]. The patients with HBV/A have been reported to be more sensitive to interferon α treatment as compared to those infected with HBV/D [24] while the patients having infection with HBV/B have a higher response rate to interferon α treatment as compared to the patients infected with HBV/C [25]. Moreover, infection with genotype C alone was also found to be associated with significantly higher risks of liver cirrhosis and hepatocellular carcinoma as compared to genotype B infection [26, 27] while HBV/B shown an earlier HBsAg sero-clearance rate as compared to HBV/C [28]. In another study, HBV/A was found to have significantly higher sero-conversion rate of HBeAg as compared to HBV/B, HBV/C, HBV/D and HBV/F [29]. From all the studies mentioned above it's quite clear that genotypes influence disease condition as well as response to treatment.

The picture regarding distribution of HBV genotypes in Pakistan and its association with disease stage has not been clearly understood yet. In fact, all of the available studies are mostly confined to specific cities/areas like Karachi (Sind) and Lahore (Punjab) and none of them contain data from other parts of the country. A vast range of areas from different regions of Pakistan still remains unexplored for HBV genotypes. Moreover, the existing state of knowledge regarding the distribution and prevalence of HBV genotypes in Pakistan seems to be sketchy and questionable too. For example, four studies [5, 30–32] are in agreement that genotype D infection is most prevalent in the country while three studies [18, 33, 34] reported that genotype C is the most common ones in Pakistan. Yet in an another study, genotype C and D have been cited as most common HBV genotypes in Pakistan [35]. In view of the presence of the inadequate data, it was felt that a comprehensive study is required to determine the current distribution of HBV genotypes in all the six provinces of Pakistan and their possible association with different phases of HBV infection.

Methods

Patients

Eight hundred and forty (840) samples from HBsAg positive patients were collected during October 2010 to March 2013 from different locations of six regions of Pakistan which include Punjab and Federal Capital Territory of Islamabad ($n = 359$); Khyber Pakhtoonkhwa along with Federally Administered Tribal Areas ($n = 115$); Azad Jammu and Kashmir ($n = 81$); Gilgit-Baltistan ($n = 111$); Sind province including Karachi city ($n = 107$); and Baluchistan ($n = 67$). The sampling sites and the details of patients are given in Fig. 1 and Table 1 respectively. All the patients were diagnosed as chronic HBV carriers. Serum samples were acquired from the different hospitals and diagnostic laboratories of the above regions where they were originally collected for routine diagnostic purposes. All the available data of clinical and demographic importance were collected at the time of sample collection by filling out a questionnaire. All the samples were then brought to Nuclear Medicine, Oncology and Radiotherapy Institute (NORI), Islamabad and stored at −25 °C for further analysis. The samples were tested for positivity and quantity of HBV DNA. Only the samples having more than 100 IU/ml of viral load were subjected to HBV genotyping (Table 1). The samples with lower than 100 IU/ml of viral load were excluded because their genotyping was not successful in most of the cases. All the routine tests including HBsAg, ALT, and anti-HBe were performed in Central Laboratories, NORI using commercially available kits (Abott Diagnostics, USA).

The stage of HBV infection was primarily assigned by the local physician and further confirmed by the status of different HBV markers and biochemical tests. Only 384 patients were included in the study of genotypes influence on disease stage. All the patients (331) who had already received antiviral treatment or had co-infection with HIV, HCV or HDV were excluded from this part of study. The liver disease stage was primary assigned by

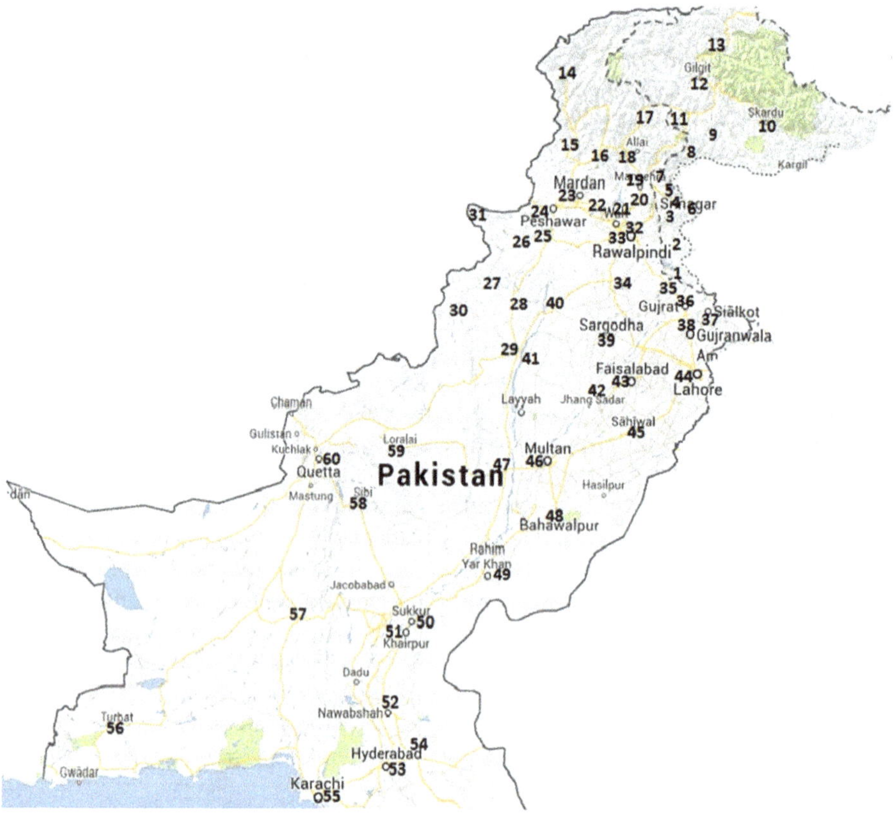

Fig. 1 The map shows the sampling sites in all regions of Pakistan. Sites are indicated with numerals. Sites: 1. Mirpur; 2. Kotli; 3. Palandari; 4. Rawalakot; 5. Bagh; 6. Kahuta; 7. Muzaffarabad; 8. Neelum; 9. Astor; 10. Sikardu; 11. Diamir; 12. Gilgit; 13. Hunza; 14. Chitral; 15. Dir; 16. Swat; 17. Kohistan; 18. Batgram; 19. Mansehra; 20. Abottabad; 21. Haripur; 22. Nowshera; 23. Mardan; 24. Peshawar; 25. Kohat; 26. Hangu; 27. Bannu; 28. LakkiMarwat; 29. D I Khan; 30. Wana; 31. Parachinar; 32. Islamabad; 33. Rawalpindi; 34; Chakwal; 35. Jhelum; 36. Gujrat; 37. Sialkot; 38. Gujranwala; 39. Sargodha; 40. Mianwali; 41. Bhakkar; 42. Jhang; 43. Faisalabad; 44. Lahore; 45. Sahiwal; 46. Multan; 47. D.G. Khan; 48. Bahawalpur; 49. Rahim Yar Khan; 50. Sukhar; 51. Khairpur; 52. Nawabshah; 53. Hyderabad; 54. Mirpur Khas; 55. Karachi; 56. Turbat; 57; Khuzdar; 58. Sibi; 59. Loralai; 60. Quetta. Regions: 1–8, Azad Jammu & Kashmir; 9–13, Gilgit-Baltistan; 14–31, Khyber Pakhtunkhwa; 32, Federal Capital Territory of Islamabad (FCT); 33–49, Punjab; 50–55, Sind; 56–60, Baluchitan

classified gastroenterologists and then the disease phase was further confirmed on the base of patients' HBV viral load, ALT levels, HBeAg status and the presence or absence of anti HBe antibodies (Table 3). The study was approved by institutional ethics committee of PMAS Arid Agriculture University Rawalpindi and each patient gave written consent.

HBV DNA extraction and quantification

HBV DNA was extracted from the plasma according to manufacturer's protocol using "Instant Virus DNA kit" (AJ Roboscreen, Analytikajena Biosolutions, GmbH, Germany) while the DNA was quantified using RoboGene® HBV Quantification kit (AJ Roboscreen, analytikajena Biosolutions, GmbH, Germany) according to manufacturer's instructions.

HBV genotyping

The genotyping was performed using PCR method with genotype specific primers described by Naito et al. [36] with some modifications in cycling profile and PCR constituents. For regular PCR, 10 μl of GoTaq® Green Master mix (Promega, USA), 1 μl each of universal primers P1A

Table 1 Samples collected and selected for HBV genotyping from different regions of the country

Total no of samples (No of male and female samples)							
	Punjab and FCT	KP and FATA	AJK	Gilgit-Baltistan	Sind	Baluchistan	Total
Total collected	359 (243 + 116)	115 (78 + 37)	81 (50 + 31)	111 (83 + 28)	107 (68 + 39)	67 (39 + 28)	840 (561 + 279)
Negative HBV DNA	29 (18 + 11)	7 (5 + 2)	6 (4 + 2)	8 (6 + 2)	13 (7 + 6)	6 (4 + 2)	69 (44 + 25)
<100 IU/ml	19 (11 + 8)	9 (6 + 3)	7 (4 + 3)	10 (6 + 4)	10 (7 + 3)	1 (0 + 1)	56 (34 + 22)
Total Genotyped	311 (214 + 97)	99 (67 + 32)	68 (42 + 26)	93 (71 + 22)	84 (54 + 30)	60 (35 + 25)	715 (483 + 232)

Abbreviations: *FCT* federal capital territory, *KP* Khyber Pkhtoonkhwa, *FATA* federally administered tribal areas, *AJK* Azad Jammu and Kashmir and S1-2, 2 μl of ddH_2O and 6 μl of diluted template (DNA) were used to make 20 μl of reaction volume. The thermal profile was; 10 min at 95 °C, then 30 cycles of; 94 °C for 20 s, 55 °C for 20 s and 72 °C for 1 min, then another 7 min at 72 °C (ABI 9700, USA). Two mixes were used in nested PCR. Mix 1 had the forward primers for genotype A, B and C with a common reverse primer while mix two had reverse primers for genotypes D, E and F with common forward primer. Two μl of product from 1st round of PCR were added to each mix as DNA template with 8 μl of GoTaq® Green Master mix, 8 μl of ddH2O and 1 μl of each primer to make 22 μl of final volume. The cycling profile for nested PCR was; 95 °C for 10 min, then 40 cycles of 94 °C for 45 s, 63 °C for 20 s, and 72 °C for 60 s, and then another 7 min at 72 °C (ABI 9700, USA). Products were run on 2 % agarose gel which was stained in a solution of ethidium bromide, and then observed under ultraviolet fluorescence (BioRad Gel Doc-XR, USA). Amplified products in mix 1 were 68 bp, 281 bp and 122 bp in size for genotypes A, B and C respectively while the product sizes in mix 2 were 119 bp, 167 bp and 97 bp for genotypes D, E and F respectively. The product's size was estimated with reference to a 50-bp DNA ladder (GeneRuler™ Fermentas) and the genotype was determined for each sample according to the sizes of DNA product obtained in both mixes (Fig. 2). The term untypable was assigned to those samples which had higher than 100 IU/ml of viral load but were not successfully genotype or their genotype was not identified by the method.

Statistical analysis

Chi square test was applied to evaluate the relationship HBV genotype and HBV infection phase with each other as well as with patients' gender while one way analysis of variance (ANOVA) was performed to analyze the relationship of HBV genotype and HBV infection phase with the age of patients. A value of p less than 0.05 was considered as statistically significant. SPSS version-16.0 was used for all the analyses.

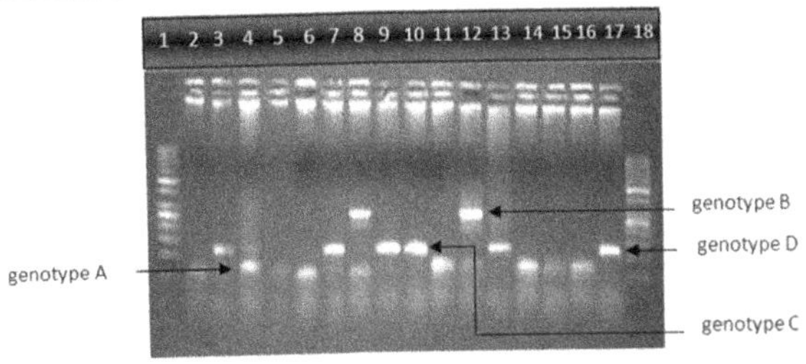

Fig. 2 Amplified PCR products on 2 % gel showing bands for four genotypes. Lanes 2, 4, 6, 8, 10, 12, 14 and 16: the product bands of mix 1. Lanes 3, 5, 7, 9, 11, 13, 15 and 17: the product bands of mix 2. Lanes 1 and 18: 50 bp DNA ladder. lanes 2 + 3: genotype D. lanes 4 + 5: genotype A. lanes 6 + 7: genotype A + D. lanes 8 + 9: genotype A + B + D. lanes 10 + 11: genotype C and a nonspecific band. lanes 12 + 13: genotype B + D. lanes 14 + 15: genotype A. lanes 16 + 17; Genotype A + D

Results

Out of total 840 samples, 125 were excluded from the study as HBV DNA was not detected in them. The remaining 715 samples were further analyzed (Table 1).

Regional distribution of HBV genotypes

Out of the 715 samples taken for genotyping, 699 were successfully genotyped while 16 (2.2 %) remained untypable. HBV genotypes A, B, C, D and E were detected in 55 (7.7 %), 4 (0.6 %), 6 (0.8 %), 509 (71.2 %) and 1 (0.1 %) samples respectively (Table 2). A total of 124 (17.3 %) patients were infected with more than one genotype i.e. mix genotype infection. The mix genotype infection comprised six combinations in different proportions which were - A + B (0.3 %), A + D (13.7 %), B + D (1.9 %), C + D (1.0 %), E + D (0.1 %) and A + B + D (0.3 %).

Concerning the regions included in this study, genotype D was always the predominant one with the prevalence ranging from 63.3 to 88.3 % (Table 2). Genotype A and the mix genotype combination A + D was also present in all regions. The prevalence of genotype A, D and mix genotypes respectively was 10 %, 63.3 % and 23.5 % in Punjab and FCT region; 7 %, 68 % and 18 % in KP and FATA region; 4.4 %, 82.3 % and 11.8 % in AJK region; 3.2 %, 80.6 % and 12.8 % in Gilgilt-Baltistan region; 10.7 %, 72.6 % and 13 % in Sind region; 3.3 %, 88.3 % and 5 % in Baluchistan region (Fig. 3).

Multiple genotype infections presented the second more prevalent group of genotypes with 17.3 % of the total samples infected with 6 different combinations of genotypes (Table 2). Mix infection with A + D genotype was the major combination found among multiple genotype infections which was 98/124 of the samples. Other mix genotype combinations identified were B + D, C + D, A + B, A + B + D and E + D which were 1.9 %, 1.0 %, 0.3 %, 0.3 % and 0.1 % of the samples respectively. None of the combinations except A + D was found in more than 2 % of the samples. This combination was detected from all parts of the Pakistan, though it was highest in Punjab and FCT region (21.8 %) as compared to all other parts (Table 2).

Distribution HBV genotypes in different phases of disease

All statistical comparisons performed for genotypes A, D and A + D as the other genotypes and their combinations in mix infections were rare (Table 2). Out of total 715 patients included in the study, 331 (46.3 %) had either already received antiviral treatment or had co-infection with HIV, HCV or HDV or had genotype other than A and D. Thus the remaining 384 (53.7 %) patients who were not exposed to any treatment till the time of sample

Table 2 Distribution of HBV genotypes and their combinations in the samples taken from different regions of Pakistan. The numbers and proportions (%) are given against each genotype or the genotypic combination

Genotype	KP and FATA	AJK	Gilgit-Baltistan	Sind	Punjab and FCT	Baluchistan	Total
A	7 (7)	3 (4.4)	3 (3.2)	9 (10.7)	31 (10)	2 (3.3)	55 (7.7)
B	2 (2)	0	1 (1.1)	0	1 (0.3)	0	4 (0.6)
C	3 (3)	1 (1.5)	0	0	1 (0.3)	1 (1.7)	6 (0.8)
D	67 (68)	56 (82.3)	75 (80.6)	61 (72.6)	197 (63.3)	53 (88.3)	509 (71.2)
E	0	0	0	1 (1.2)	0	0	1 (0.1)
Mix	18 (18)	8 (11.8)	11 (12.8)	11 (13)	73 (23.5)	3 (5)	124 (17.3)
A + B	2 (2.0)	0	0	0	0	0	2 (0.3)
A + D	9 (9.1)	5 (7.3)	4 (4.3)	9 (10.7)	68 (21.8)	3 (5.0)	98 (13.7)
B + D	2 (2.0)	0	6 (6.4)	2 (2.3)	4 (1.3)	0	14 (1.9)
C + D	4 (2.0)	3 (4.4)	0	0	0	0	7 (1.0)
E + D	0	0	0	0	1 (0.3)	0	1 (0.1)
A + B + D	1 (1.0)	0	1 (1.1)	0	0	0	2 (0.3)
Untypable	2 (2.0)	0	3 (3.2)	2 (2.3)	8 (2.5)	1 (1.7)	16 (2.2)
Total	99	68	93	84	311	60	715

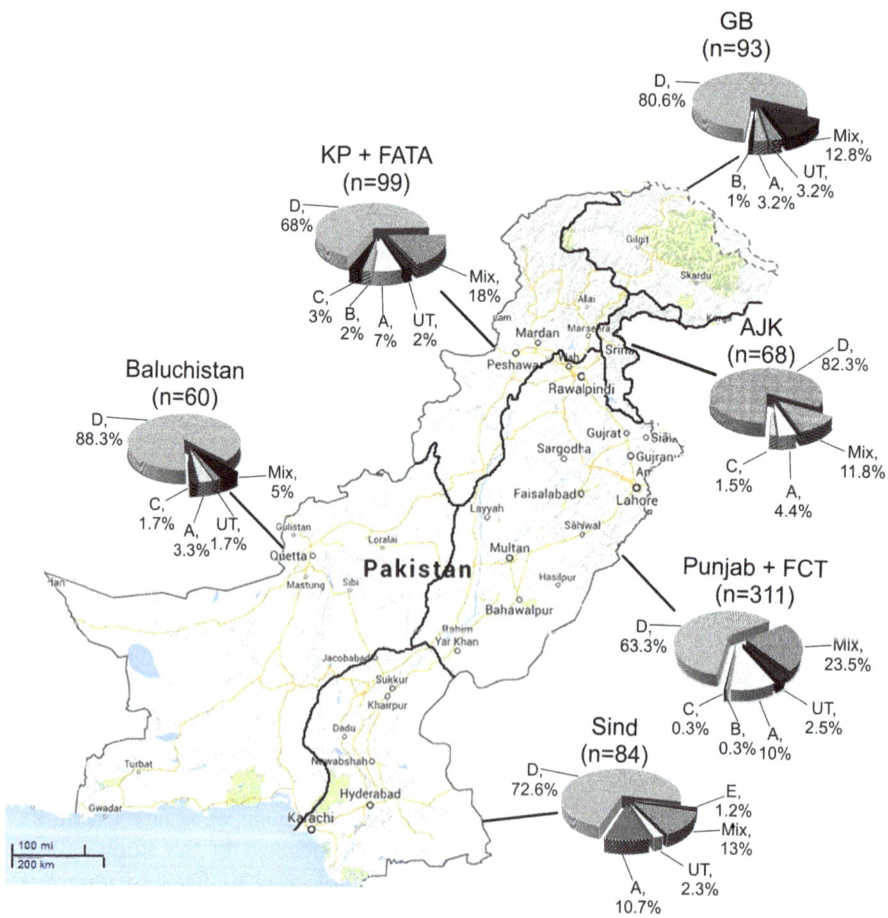

Fig. 3 Genotype prevalence of hepatitis B virus in all regions of the country. UT stands for un-typable and mix means all the infections with more than one genotypes

collection were classified in four different phases of liver disease: 56 (14.6 %) were in immune control phase, 89 (23.2 %) in immune tolerant phase, 153 (39.8 %) in immune clearance phase and 86 (22.4 %) in immune escape phase (Table 3). None of the patients had liver cirrhosis or hepatocellular carcinoma in this study. The mean age of the patients and gender ratio was statistically equal among all the disease phases. Genotype D ($n = 279$) was the most prevalent in all groups of patients with 36 patients in immune control group, 67 in immune tolerant group, 112 in immune clearance and 64 in immune escape group. The second more prevalent was the mix infection A + D ($n = 62$) with 13, 12, 26 and 11 cases in immune control, immune tolerant, immune clearance and immune escape groups respectively. Genotype A ($n = 43$) was the least prevalent with 7, 10, 15 and 11 cases in immune control, immune tolerant, immune clearance and immune escape phases respectively. The differences in distribution of genotypes in disease phases were not statistically significant. Similarly, there were no statistical differences of age and gender among the three genotype groups compared (Table 3).

Discussion

The present study is the first of its kind which included a cohort of 715 patients with chronic HBV infection from all six regions of Pakistan. The study analyzed the patients for HBV genotypes and their possible associations with liver disease severity in 384 consecutive chronic HBV carriers. According to the results, genotypes A, B, C, D, E and mix genotype infections with 6 different genotypic combinations are present in Pakistan, but the majority of patients (92.6 %) were infected with either genotype D, or genotype A or a mixture of both (A + D). The pre-dominant genotype in all regions was D followed by genotype A and mix genotype infection with A + D. Genotypes B, C, E and F were rare and collectively form only 1.5 % of the total prevalence.

HBV genotypes were not studied exclusively from all over the Pakistan so far. Table 4 summarizes some available data on the topic from Pakistan along with the results of present study. Most of the available data are from Karachi and Lahore or Punjab and Sind while none of the study has explored the regions of FATA, Gilgit-Baltistan, AJK, some parts of Khyber Pakhtoonkha province and most of the Baluchistan province. Though three studies carried out by Awan et al. [18], Alam et al. [30] and Idrees et al. [34] investigated the provinces of KP and Baluchistan additionally but the number of samples taken were not satisfactory to conclude the genotype distribution in these provinces (Table 4). None of the studies included the regions of Gilgit-Baltistan, AJK and FATA. Two of these three [18, 34] studies reported genotype C as predominant while one [30] found genotype D as predominant one. Genotype B which was not reported from Pakistan in any other study has also been reported in all three of these studies from 18 to 25 % of the samples. These results are contradictory to these studies.

All the studies confined to the samples from Punjab and Sind reported genotype D as predominant except one [33] which reported prevalence of genotype C and D as 75 and 25 % respectively. The remaining six studies [5, 31, 32, 37–39] reported genotype D as the commonest one in Pakistan with percentage distribution of 59, 84, 70, 98.2, 84 and 93.2 % respectively (Table 4). The results of present study representing all parts of the country with significant number of samples is in agreement with the later group [5, 31, 32, 37–39] that reported genotype D as the most prevalent HBV genotype in Pakistan. Genotype A was found to be the second more prevalent single genotype infection with 7.7 %. Genotype A was also reported in most of the previous studies [5, 18, 30, 32, 34, 39] in different proportions ranging from 0.8 to 21.4 % and a mean prevalence of 11.7 % (Table 4). Genotype B was present only in 0.6 % of present study samples while it was reported in proportions ranging from 18 to 24.5 % by previous studies from Pakistan [18, 30, 34]. None of the other studies reported genotype B infection, however mix infections involving genotype B were reported by some studies [18, 30, 31, 38] as high as 16 % of the samples (Table 4). Genotype C was detected

Table 3 Characteristics of patients infected with different HBV genotypes ($n = 384$)

Characteristics		Genotype A	Genotype D	Genotype A + D	Sig.
Number of patients (%)		43 (11.2)	279 (72.7)	62 (16.1)	
Age (Mean ± SD)		32.4 ± 11.7	34.1 ± 12.1	35.1 ± 12.8	NS[a]
Gender (M/F)		32/11	202/77	40/22	NS[b]
Immune Control ($N = 56$)	normal ALT, HBeAg negative, anti HBe positive, low viral load	7 (16.3 %)	36 (12.9 %)	13 (21.0 %)	NS[b]
Immune Tolerant ($N = 89$)	normal ALT, HBeAg positive, anti HBe negative, high viral load	10 (23.2 %)	67 (24.0 %)	12 (19.3 %)	NS[b]
Immune Clearance ($N = 153$)	elevated ALT, HBeAg positive, high viral load	15 (34.9 %)	112 (40.1 %)	26 (41.9 %)	NS[b]
Immune Escape ($N = 86$)	Normal or elevated ALT, HBeAg negative, anti HBe positive, High HBV DNA,	11 (25.6 %)	64 (22.9 %)	11 (17.7 %)	NS[b]

[a]One way Analysis of Variance, [b]Pearson Chi Square Test, NS for non significant

Table 4 The prevalence of different HBV genotypes in our study compared to previously published studies

Source	Place of sampling	Sample size	Proportion of genotype as percent of total samples								
			A	B	C	D	E	F	Mix	Mixed combinations	UT
Hanif et al., 2013 [5]	Karachi, Islamabad/Rawalpindi	200 (40, 160)	10	-	-	59	-	-	31	A + D	-
Awan et al., 2010 [18]	Punjab, KP, Sind, Baluchistan	300 (222, 36, 26, 15)	14	18	28	13	0.6	1.3	16	A + B + D, A + D + F, A + C, A + D, A + E, A + F, B + C, B + E, C + D	10.3
Ahmed et al., 2009 [39]	Punjab, Sind	236	0.8	-	5.9	93.2	-	-	-	-	-
Baig et al., 2009 [32]	Karachi	315	20	-	-	70	-	-	10	A + D	-
Noorali et al., 2008 [31]	Karachi	180	-	-	-	84	-	-	16	B + D	-
Hakim et al., 2008 [38]	Karachi	180	-	-	-	84	-	-	16	B + D	-
Alam et al., 2007 [30]	Punjab, KP, Sind Baluchistan	110 (30, 28, 25, 18)	4.5	24.5	-	60	-	-	2.7	A + D, B + D	8.2
Abbas et al., 2006 [37]	Karachi	109	-	-	-	98.2	-	-	1.8	A + D	-
Idrees et al., 2004 [34]	Punjab, KP, Sind Baluchistan	112 (Details not available)	21.4	17.9	41.1	8.0	-	-	7.1	Details not available	4.5
Naaz, 2001 [33]	Lahore	12	-	-	75	25	-	-	-	-	-
This study	Punjab, KP, Sind, Baluchistan, AJK, Gilgit-Baltistan	715 (311, 99, 84, 60, 68, 93)	7.7	0.6	0.8	71.2	0.1	-	17.3	A + D, B + D, C + D, A + B, A + B + D, E + D	2.2

UT stands for Un-typable

in only 0.8 % of the samples in our study while three previous studies [18, 33, 34] have reported it as predominant genotype in Pakistan, whereas one study [39] reported it as second more prevalent genotype in the country. Genotype C was not reported by any of the other six studies (Table 4). Genotype E and F were not reported by any previous study except [18] which reported them in the proportions of 0.6 and 1.3 %. As already mentioned, genotypes E and F are endemic to Africa and the New World respectively [17, 20] and the fact that they were found in only 1 case (genotype E) was quite expected. Present study thus supports the conclusion that not only genotypes E and F but also genotypes B and C were rare in Pakistan (Table 4).

The relationship of HBV genotypes with liver disease is still not very clear. Although some studies have reported that HBV genotype influence the severity of liver disease and course of chronic HBV infection [26, 28, 40–44]. Some other studies showed that HBV genotype had no influence on course of HBV infection [43, 45, 46]. Present study is in concordance with the later group [43, 45, 46]. Most of the studies compared genotype B and C in Asia and reported that the latter is more associated to severe liver disease than the former. On the other hand the genotype B is associated with an early HBeAg sero-conversion, more sustained remission after HBeAg sero-conversion, less active hepatic necroinflammation, a slower rate of progression to cirrhosis, and a lower rate of hepatocellular carcinoma (HCC) development as compared to genotype C [26, 28, 41, 43, 44]. A study from Pakistan compared genotype A, D and A + D for their association with complex liver diseases and concluded that genotype A is associated with more complex liver disease [47]. However, present study did not find any association of genotypes with disease stage. The relatively high prevalence of mix infection with genotypes A + D is a confirmation of the data reported by several previous findings about HBV genotyping in Pakistan [5, 18, 30, 32, 34, 37].

Conclusions

In conclusion, it has been observed in the present study that the distribution of HBV genotypes was almost similar in all the regions of Pakistan. Genotype D was the most common one (71.2 %) followed by mix infection with genotypes A and D (17.3 %) and genotype A (7.7 %). Although genotypes B, C, E and F were also detected but their prevalence was very low (1.5 %). Furthermore, genotype was not found to have any significant influence on liver disease progression in Pakistan.

Acknowledgements
The authors are thankful to Professor Ferruccio Bonino and Professor Mirza Azhar Beg for critically reviewing the article and setting its language.

Funding
The study was partially funded by Higher Education Commission of Pakistan (HEC) in the form of indigenous PhD fellowship (PIN: 074-2673-Bm4-145). There was no role of the funding body in design of the study, data collection, analysis and publication.

Authors' contributions
MM, AR and AK conceived and designed the study and experiments. MM, MAA and NZ performed the experiments and collected the data. MM and NZ analyzed the data. MM prepared the initial draft of manuscript. AK, AR, and MAA critically reviewed and revised the manuscript. All authors read and approved the final manuscript.

Competing interests
The authors declare that they have no competing interests. The study is a part of PhD thesis of Majid Mahmood.

Consent for publication
Not applicable.

Author details
[1]Department of Zoology, The University of Poonch, Rawalakot, Azad Jammu and Kashmir 12350, Pakistan. [2]Department of Zoology, Pir Mehr Ali Shah Arid Agriculture University, Rawalpindi 46300, Pakistan. [3]Department of General Medicine, Pakistan Atomic Energy Commission (PAEC) General Hospital, Islamabad 44000, Pakistan. [4]Barani Institute of Management Sciences (BIMS), Rawalpindi 46300, Pakistan. [5]Center for Biotechnology & Microbiology, University of Swat, Swat 19130, Pakistan. [6]Diagnostic Department, Nuclear Medicine, Oncology and Radiotherapy Institute (NORI), Islamabad 44000, Pakistan.

References
1. Bonino F. Introduction to hepatitis B virus heterogeneity – a means to personalized care. Antivir Ther. 2010;15 Suppl 3:1–2.
2. Boesecke C, Wasmuth JC. Hepatitis B. In: Mauss S, Berg T, Rockstroh J, Sarrazin C, Wedemeyer H, editors. Hepatology a clinical text book. 3rd ed. Wuppertal: Flying Publishers; 2012. p. 32–35.
3. Rantala M, Van de Laar MJ. Surveillance and epidemiology of hepatitis B and C in Europe – a review. Eurosurveillance. 2008;13(21):1-8.
4. Wasley A, Grytdal S, Gallagher K. Surveillance for acute viral hepatitis–United States. MMWR Surveill Summ. 2008;57:1–24.
5. Hanif M, Zaidi P, Habib S, Ahmed A, Raza A, et al. Study of genotypes and subgenotypes of Hepatitis B virus prevalent in big cities of Pakistan. Afr J Microbiol Res. 2013;3:152–7.
6. Okamoto H, Tsuda F, Sakugawa H, Sastrosoewignjo RI, Imai M, et al. Typing hepatitis B virus by homology in nucleotide sequence: comparison of surface antigen subtypes. J Gen Virol. 1988;69:2575–83.
7. Naumann H, Schaefer S, Yoshida CFT, Gaspar AMC, Repp R, et al. Identification of a new hepatitis-B-virus (HBV) genotype from Brazil that expresses HBV surface antigen subtype adw4. J Gen Virol. 1993;74:1627–32.
8. Norder H, Courouce AM, Magnius LO. Complete genomes, phylogenetic relatedness, and structural proteins of six strains of the hepatitis B virus, four of which represent two new genotypes. Virol. 1994;198:489–503.
9. Stuyver L, De Gendt S, Van Geyt C, Zoulim F, Fried M, et al. A new genotype of hepatitis B virus: complete genome and phylogenetic relatedness. J Gen Virol. 2000;81:67–74.
10. Arauz-Ruiz P, Norder H, Robertson BH, Magnius LO. Genotype H: a new Amerindian genotype of hepatitis B virus revealed in Central America. J Gen Virol. 2002;83:2059–73.
11. Kay A, Zoulim F. Hepatitis B virus genetic variability and evolution. Virus Res. 2007;127:164–76.
12. Tran TT, Trinh TN, Abe K. New complex recombinant genotype of hepatitis B virus identified in Vietnam. J Virol. 2008;82:5657–63.
13. Olinger CM, Jutavijittum P, Hubschen JM, Yousukh A, Samountry B, et al. Possible new hepatitis B virus genotype, southeast Asia. Emerg Infect Dis. 2008;14:1777–80.

14. Tatematsu K, Tanaka Y, Kurbanov F, Sugauchi F, Mano S, et al. A genetic variant of hepatitis B virus divergent from known human and ape genotypes isolated from a Japanese patient and provisionally assigned to new genotype J. J Virol. 1995;83:10538–47.
15. Kidd-Ljunggren K, Oberg M, Kidd AH. The hepatitis B virus X gene: analysis of functional domain variation and gene phylogeny using multiple sequences. J Gen Virol. 1995;76:2119–30.
16. Bowyer SM, Staden LV, Kew MC, Sim JG. A unique segment of the hepatitis B virus group A genotype identified in isolates from South Africa. J Gen Virol. 1997;78:1719–29.
17. Bonino F, Teerha P, Brunetto MR, Yun-Fan L. Diagnostic markers of chronic hepatitis B infection and disease. Antivir Ther. 2010;15 Suppl 3:35–44.
18. Awan Z, Idrees M, Amin I, Butt S, Afzal S, et al. Pattern and molecular epidemiology of Hepatitis B virus genotypes circulating in Pakistan. Infect Genet Evol. 2010;8:1242–6.
19. Datta S. An overview of molecular epidemiology of hepatitis B virus (HBV) in India. Virol J. 2008;5:156.
20. Nakano T, Lu L, Hu X, Mizokami M, Orito E, et al. Characterization of hepatitis B virus genotypes among Yucpa Indians in Venezuela. J Gen Virol. 2001;82:359–65.
21. Cao GW. Clinical relevance and public health significance of hepatitis B virus genomic variations. World J Gastroenterol. 2009;46:5761–9.
22. Toan NL, le Song H, Kremsner PG, Duy DN, Binh VQ, et al. Impact of the hepatitis B virus genotype and genotype mixtures on the course of liver disease in Vietnam. Hepatology. 2006;43:1375–84.
23. Yin J, Zhang H, Li C, Gao C, He Y, et al. Role of hepatitis B virus genotype mixture, subgenotypes C2 and B2 on hepatocellular carcinoma: compared with chronic hepatitis B and asymptomatic carrier state in the same area. Carcinogenesis. 2008;29:1685–91.
24. Erhardt A, Blondin D, Hauck K, Sagir A, Kohnle T, et al. Response to interferon alfa is hepatitis B virus genotype dependent: genotype A is more sensitive to interferon than genotype D. Gut. 2005;54:1009–13.
25. Wai CT, Chu CJ, Hussain M, Lok AS. HBV genotype B is associated with better response to interferon therapy in HBeAg(+) chronic hepatitis than genotype C. Hepatology. 2002;36:1425–30.
26. Chan HL, Hui AY, Wong ML, Tse AM, Hung LC, et al. Genotype C hepatitis B virus infection is associated with an increased risk of hepatocellular carcinoma. Gut. 2004;53:1494–8.
27. Chan HL, Wong GL, Tse CH, Chim AM, Yiu KK, et al. Hepatitis B Virus Genotype C Is Associated With More Severe Liver Fibrosis Than Genotype B. Clin Gastroenterol Hepatol. 2009;7:1361–6.
28. Chu CJ, Hussain M, Lok AS. Hepatitis B virus genotype B is associated with earlier HBeAg seroconversion compared with hepatitis B virus genotype C. Gastroenterology. 2002;122:1756–62.
29. Livingston SE, Simonetti JP, Bulkow LR, Homan CE, Snowball MM, et al. Clearance of hepatitis B e antigen in patients with chronic hepatitis B and genotypes A, B, C, D, and F. Gastroenterology. 2007;133:1452–7.
30. Alam MM, Zaidi SZ, Malik SA, Shaukat S, Naeem A, et al. Molecular epidemiology of Hepatitis B virus genotypes in Pakistan. BMC Infect Dis. 2007;7:115.
31. Noorali S, Hakim ST, McLean D, Kazmi SU, Bagasra O. Prevalence of Hepatitis B virus genotype D in females in Karachi, Pakistan. J Infect Dev Ctries. 2008; 2:373–8.
32. Baig S, Siddiqui A, Chakravarty R, Moatter T. Hepatitis B virus subgenotypes D1 and D3 are prevalent in Pakistan. BMC Res Notes. 2009;2:1.
33. Naaz A. Variability analysis in immunogenic region of surface gene of Pakistani isolates of Hepatitis B Virus. PhD thesis. University of Punjab 2001, pp. 68-113
34. Idrees M, Khan S, Riazuddin S. Common genotypes of hepatitis B virus. J Coll Physicians Surg Pak. 2004;14:344–7.
35. Ali M, Idrees M, Ali L, Hussain A, Rehman IU, et al. Hepatitis B virus in Pakistan: A systematic review of prevalence, risk factors, awareness status and genotypes. Virol J. 2011;8:102.
36. Naito H, Hayashi S, Abe K. Rapid and Specific Genotyping System for Hepatitis B Virus Corresponding to Six Major Genotypes by PCR Using Type-Specific Primers. J Clin Microbiol. 2001;39:362–4.
37. Abbas Z, Muzaffar R, Siddiqui A, Naqvi SAA, Rizvi SAH. Genetic variability in the precore and core promoter regions of hepatitis B virus strains in Karachi. BMC Gastroenterol. 2006;6:20.
38. Hakim ST, Kazmi SU, Bagasra O. Seroprevalence of Hepatitis B and C Genotypes Among Young Apparently Healthy Females of Karachi-Pakistan. Lib J Med. 2008;3:66–70.
39. Ahmed CS, Wang ZH, Bin Z, Chen JJ, Hou JL. Hepatitis B virus genotypes, subgenotypes, precore, and basal core promoter mutations in the two largest provinces of Pakistan. J Gastroenterol Hepatol. 2009;24:569–73.
40. Lindh M, Hannoun C, Dhillon AP, Norkrans G, Horal P. Core promoter mutations and genotypes in relation to viral replication and liver damage in East Asian hepatitis B virus carriers. J Infect Dis. 1999;179:775–82.
41. Kao JH, Chen PJ, Lai MY, Chen DS. Hepatitis B genotypes correlate with clinical outcomes in patients with chronic hepatitis B. Gastroenterology. 2000;118:554–9.
42. Orito E, Mizokami M, Sakugawa H, Michitaka K, Ishikawa K, et al. A case-control study for clinical and molecular biological differences between hepatitis B viruses of genotypes B and C. Hepatology. 2001;33:218–23.
43. Sumi H, Yokosuka O, Seki N, Arai M, Imazeki F, et al. Influence of hepatitis B virus genotypes on the progression of chronic type B liver disease. Hepatology. 2003;37:19–26.
44. Chu CM, Liaw YF. Genotype C hepatitis B virus infection is associated with a higher risk of reactivation of hepatitis B and progression to cirrhosis than genotype B: a longitudinal study of hepatitis B e antigen-positive patients with normal amino-transferase levels at baseline. J Hepatol. 2005;3:411–7.
45. Gandhe SS, Chadha MS, Arankalle VA. Hepatitis B virus genotypes and serotypes in western India: lack of clinical significance. J Med Virol. 2003;69:324–30.
46. Zeng G, Wang Z, Wen S, Jiang J, Wang L, et al. Geographic distribution, virologic and clinical characteristics of hepatitis B virus genotypes in China. J Vir Hepat. 2005;12:609–17.
47. Baig S, Siddiqui A, Ahmed W, Qureshi H, Arif A. The association of complex liver disorders with HBV genotypes prevalent in Pakistan. Virol J. 2007;4:128.

Economic evaluation of pegylated interferon plus ribavirin for treatment of chronic hepatitis C in Thailand: genotype 1 and 6

Nattiya Kapol[1*], Surasit Lochid-amnuay[1] and Yot Teerawattananon[2]

Abstract

Background: Pegylated interferon alpha 2a, alpha 2b and ribavirin have been included to the National List of Essential Medicines (NLEM) for treatment of only chronic hepatitis C genotypes 2 and 3 in Thailand. This reimbursement policy has not covered for other genotypes of hepatitis C virus infection (HCV) especially for genotypes 1 and 6 that account for 30-50 % of all HCV infection in Thailand. Therefore, this research determined whether pegylated interferon alpha 2a or alpha 2b plus ribavirin is more cost-effective than a palliative care for treatment of HCV genotype 1 and 6 in Thailand.

Methods: A cost-utility analysis using a model-based economic evaluation was conducted based on a societal perspective. A Markov model was developed to estimate costs and quality-adjusted life years (QALYs) comparing between the combination of pegylated interferon alpha 2a or alpha 2b and ribavirin with a usual palliative care for genotype 1 and 6 HCV patients. Health-state transition probabilities, virological responses, and utility values were obtained from published literatures. Direct medical and direct non-medical costs were included and retrieved from published articles and Thai Standard Cost List for Health Technology Assessment. The incremental cost-effectiveness ratio (ICER) was presented as costs in Thai baht per QALY gained.

Results: HCV treatment with pegylated interferon alpha 2a or alpha 2b plus ribavirin was dominant or cost-saving in Thailand compared to a palliative care. The ICER value was negative with lower in total costs (peg 2a- 747,718vs. peg 2b- 819,921 vs. palliative care- 1,169,121 Thai baht) and more in QALYs (peg 2a- 13.44 vs. peg 2b- 13.14 vs. palliative care- 11.63 years) both in HCV genotypes 1 and 6.

Conclusion: As cost-saving results, the Subcommittee for Development of the NLEM decided to include both pegylated interferon alpha 2a and alpha 2b into the NLEM for treatment of HCV genotype 1 and 6 recently. Economic evaluation for these current drugs can be further applied to other novel medications for HCV treatment.

Keywords: Chronic hepatitis C, Economic evaluation, Pegylated interferon, Ribavirin

* Correspondence: kapol_n@su.ac.th; kpnatty@gmail.com
[1]Department of Community Pharmacy, Faculty of Pharmacy, Silpakorn University, Nakhon Pathom, Thailand73000

Background

Chronic hepatitis C virus infection (CHC) is a global important health burden [1]. Untreated infected patients may develop chronic liver problems, including hepatitis, cirrhosis and hepatocellular carcinoma (HCC), and progress to premature death finally [2]. World Health Organization (WHO) reported 150–170 million patients infected with hepatitis C virus and caused 350,000 deaths a year [3]. A global prevalence rate of hepatitis C virus (HCV) infection is 2.5 % [4]. In Thailand, a prevalence of CHC is approximately 2.8 % [5]. Additionally, CHC-related treatment influences an economic burden worldwide [6, 7]. HCV can be transmitted through infected blood include blood transfusions, contaminated needles, body piercing, and hemodialysis. Most of CHC patients are asymptomatic or no specific symptoms then the diseases are silently progressed. A blood screening test by determining anti-HCV antibodies and serum HCV RNA level is recommended for a high risk people [8].

HCV has been classified into six major genotypes, which are distributed differently worldwide. HCV genotype 1, 2, and 3 are broadly distributed in North America, Northern and Western Europe, South America, Asia and Australia. Genotypes 4 and 5 are common in Africa and Middle East, whereas genotype 6 is mainly found in Southeast Asia [9]. The treatment regimen of HCV infection depends on virus genotypes. The American Association for the Study of Liver Diseases (AASLD) [10], the Asian Pacific Association for the Study of the Liver (APASL) [8], the European Association for the Study of the Liver (EASL) [11], and the Thai Association for the Study of the Liver (THASL) [12] recommend pegylated interferon alpha 2a or alpha 2b plus ribavirin as a standard treatment for all genotypes of HCV infection. Treatment of CHC aims to improve quality of life and prevent deaths from cirrhosis and carcinoma. Primary achievement of treatment is undetectable HCV RNA (<50 IU/ml) 24 weeks after the end of treatment or sustained virological response (SVR) [8, 10–12].

Although a combination of pegylated interferon and ribavirin is clinically effective for CHC treatment, some patients cannot afford to pay for drug costs. A palliative care is used for those patients. In 2011, cost-effectiveness of pegylated interferon alpha 2a, alpha 2b and ribavirin have been included to the National List of Essential Medicines (NLEM) in Thailand for treatment of only CHC genotypes 2 and 3 in Thailand since they demonstrates the cost saving comparing to the palliative care [13]. This policy decision, however, has not covered for other genotypes of HCV. Among all genotypes, genotypes 2 and 3 are mainly found in Thailand (40 %). Most of the remaining is genotype 1 and genotype 6, accounting for 20-30 % and 10-20 % of all HCV infection, respectively.

Compared to HCV genotypes 2 and 3, pegylated interferon alpha 2a or alpha 2b plus ribavirin produced a greater SVR than in HCV genotype 6 but less than in HCV genotype 1 [14]. However, most economic evaluation studies of CHC treatment were conducted in Europe [15–17], US [18] and South America [19, 20]. No study of the combination of pegylated interferon alpha 2a or alpha 2b and ribavirin for HCV genotypes 1 and 6 in Southeast Asia including Thailand has been investigated. Therefore, this study aimed to determine and compare costs and health outcomes of pegylated interferon alpha 2a or alpha 2b plus ribavirin and a palliative care for treatment of genotype 1 and 6 HCV infection in Thailand.

Methods

Study design

This study was a model-based economic evaluation. A Markov model was developed from a societal perspective to estimate costs and health outcomes of CHC patients treated with a combination of pegylated interferon alpha 2a or alpha 2b and ribavirin versus a usual palliative care. The study population was a hypothetical cohort of 1000 CHC genotypes 1 or 6 patients. Although, the Thai treatment guidelines (THASL) [12] recommends pegylated interferon and ribavirin combination to an 18-year-old HCV patient, this model cohort assume the patients received treatment at 45 years which is likely to be an average age of current patients in Thailand and other countries [16, 17]. At the beginning of the study, according to THASL guidelines [12], CHC patients genotypes 1 or 6 were 45 years old, a positive RNA test and METAVIR score ≥ 2. The treatment regimens were designed based on THASL guidelines [12] as follows: 1) pegylated interferon alpha-2a 180 μg once a week plus ribavirin 1000 mg/day for 48 weeks, or 2) pegylated interferon alpha-2b 1.5 μg/kg weekly plus ribavirin 800 mg/day for 48 weeks, or 3) a palliative care. SVR rate was assessed 24 weeks after treatment discontinuation, as the achievement. If HCV RNA was undetectable (less than 50 IU/ml) at week 4, defined as a rapid virological responce (RVR), the treatment stopped at 24 weeks. If HCV RNA was undetectable at week 12, defined as an early virological response (EVR), the treatment stopped at 48 weeks. If HCV RNA was reduced by less than 2 log at week 12 compared with the baseline level, defined as a null response (NR), the treatment was stopped at week 12. For the remaining cases, we assumed the treatment results as a partial nonresponse (PR), which the treatment was stopped at week 24. Figure 1 presents the study treatment guidelines. In the base-case analysis, costs and health outcomes were discounted at 3 % annually [21].

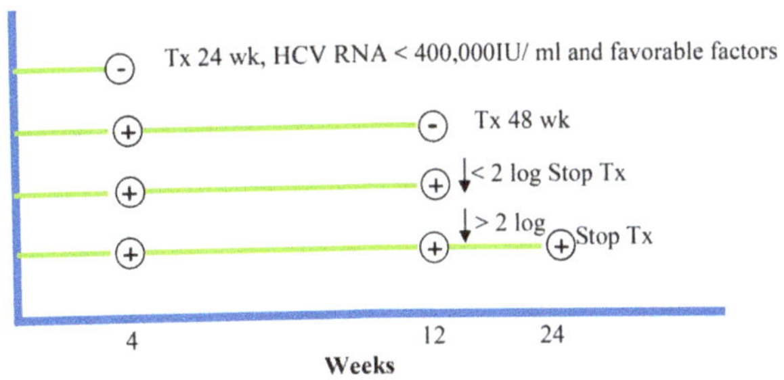

Fig. 1 The study treatment guidelines

Model structure

Figure 2 illustrates the schematic diagram of the Markov model composing of six health states, including CHC, compensated cirrhosis, decompensated cirrhosis, HCC, healthy person, and death. The patients were moved through health states based on transition probabilities. The model started at CHC patients who meet the inclusion criteria for a treatment. If the CHC patients achieved a treatment, they could proceed to the healthy person state, if not, they could continue to the compensated cirrhosis or HCC or death states. The patients in the compensated cirrhosis, decompensated cirrhosis, and HCC could not reverse to CHC or healthy person states. This model assumptions were: 1) the CHC patients weigh sixty kilograms, 2) the patients failure to the treatment are not re-treated, 3) the patients respond to the treatment were not re-infected from HCV, and 4) the patients are 100 % compliant with the treatment. This model was simulated throughout the patients' lifetime with a 1-year cycle length.

Model parameters

The parameters used in the model were health state transition probabilities, efficacy data, utility data, and cost data. Health state transition probabilities and utility data were based on the study by Werayingyong, P. and Teerawattananon, Y [13], which conducted a systematic review from published literatures and a meta-analysis of CHC patients' utility according to their health states (Table 1). Efficacy data of treatment with a combination of pegylated interferon alpha 2a or alpha 2b and ribavirin versus a usual palliative care for CHC genotype 1 were retrieved from a meta-analysis study [22] which included randomized controlled trial studies. According to the expert meeting, the inclusion criteria of RCT studies recruited in the study were publishing after 2008, and reporting SVR and RVR. Finally, the SVR and RVR from three RCT studies, and NR from two RCT studies were pooled to calculated for SVR, RVR and NR. Additionally, Thai general population death rates at each age were used in the analysis [23]. For a 45 year old patient, probability of death from other causes was 0.0044 and varied throughout the patient's lifetime. All input parameters used in the model presented in Table 1.

The costs of CHC treatment composed of direct medical costs and direct non-medical costs. To avoid double

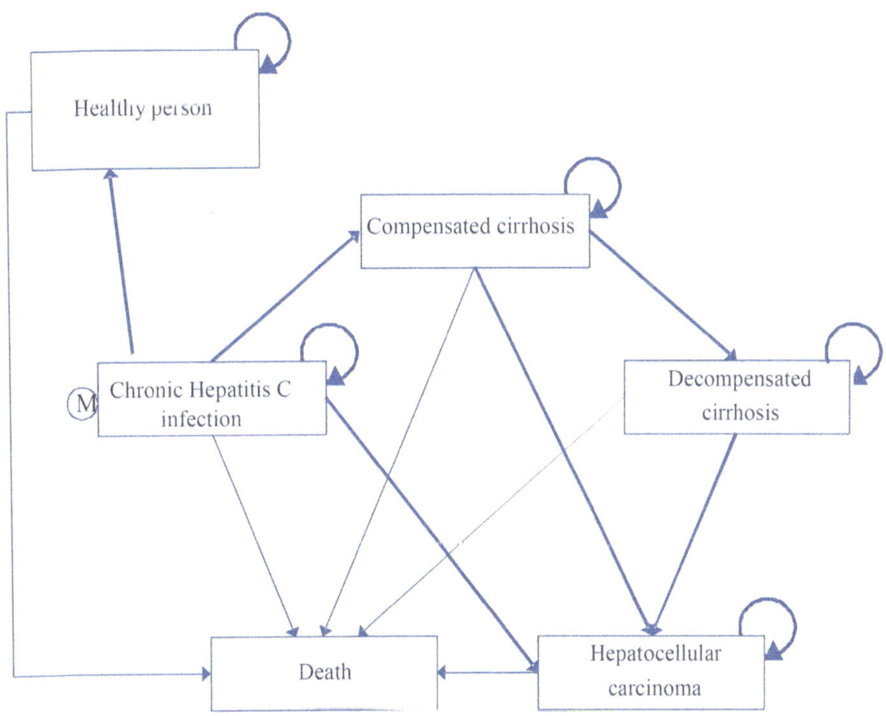

Fig. 2 The schematic diagram of the markov model

Table 1 Input parameters used in the model

Input parameters	Mean	Standard error	Distribution	Ref.
Transition probability parameters				
Genotype 1				
chronic HCV to compensated cirrhosis year 1-10	0.0057	0.0057	Beta	[24]
chronic HCV to compensated cirrhosis year 11-20	0.0143	0.0141	Beta	[24]
chronic HCV to compensated cirrhosis year 21-30	0.0207	0.0203	Beta	[24]
chronic HCV to HCC year 1-10	0.0007	0.0007	Beta	[24]
chronic HCV to HCC year 11-20	0.0032	0.0032	Beta	[24]
chronic HCV to HCC year 21-30	0.0063	0.0062	Beta	[24]
chronic HCV to death	0.0070	0.0070	Beta	[25]
compensated cirrhosis to decompensated cirrhosis year1-3	0.0417	0.0400	Beta	[26]
compensated cirrhosis to decompensated cirrhosis year 4-5	0.0945	0.0855	Beta	[26]
compensated cirrhosis to decompensated cirrhosis year 6-10	0.0662	0.0618	Beta	[26]
compensated cirrhosis to HCC year 1-3	0.0135	0.0133	Beta	[26]
compensated cirrhosis to HCC year 4-5	0.0356	0.0344	Beta	[26]
compensated cirrhosis to HCC year 6-10	0.0297	0.0288	Beta	[26]
compensated cirrhosis to death year 1-3	0.0135	0.0133	Beta	[26]
compensated cirrhosis to death year 4-5	0.0461	0.0439	Beta	[26]
compensated cirrhosis to death year 6-10	0.0461	0.0439	Beta	[26]
decompensated cirrhosis to HCC	0.0681	0.0635	Beta	[27]
decompensated cirrhosis to death year 1	0.2600	0.1924	Beta	[24]
decompensated cirrhosis to death year 2	0.3900	0.2379	Beta	[24]
decompensated cirrhosis to death year 3-5	0.2394	0.1821	Beta	[24]
HCC to death year 1	0.8482	0.0011	Beta	[28]
HCC to death year 2	0.9201	0.0009	Beta	[28]
Genotype 6				
chronic HCV to compensated cirrhosis year 1-10	0.0057	0.0057	Beta	[24]
chronic HCV to compensated cirrhosis year 11-20	0.0143	0.0141	Beta	[24]
chronic HCV to compensated cirrhosis year 21-30	0.0207	0.0203	Beta	[24]
chronic HCV to HCC year 1-10	0.0007	0.0007	Beta	[24]
chronic HCV to HCC year 11-20	0.0032	0.0032	Beta	[24]
chronic HCV to HCC year 21-30	0.0063	0.0062	Beta	[24]
chronic HCV to death	0.0070	0.0070	Beta	[25]
compensated cirrhosis to decompensated cirrhosis year 1-3	0.0417	0.0400	Beta	[26]
compensated cirrhosis to decompensated cirrhosis year 4-5	0.0945	0.0855	Beta	[26]
compensated cirrhosis to decompensated cirrhosis year 6-10	0.0662	0.0618	Beta	[26]
compensated cirrhosis to HCC year 1-3	0.0135	0.0133	Beta	[26]
compensated cirrhosis to HCC year 4-5	0.0356	0.0344	Beta	[26]
compensated cirrhosis to HCC year 6-10	0.0297	0.0288	Beta	[26]
compensated cirrhosis to death year 1-3	0.0135	0.0133	Beta	[26]
compensated cirrhosis to death year 4-5	0.0461	0.0439	Beta	[26]
compensated cirrhosis to death year 6-10	0.0461	0.0439	Beta	[26]
decompensated cirrhosis to HCC	0.0681	0.0635	Beta	[27]
decompensated cirrhosis to death year 1	0.2600	0.1924	Beta	[24]
decompensated cirrhosis to death year 2	0.3900	0.2379	Beta	[24]

Table 1 Input parameters used in the model *(Continued)*

decompensated cirrhosis to death year 3-5	0.2394	0.1821	Beta	[24]
HCC to death year 1	0.8482	0.0011	Beta	[28]
HCC to death year 2	0.9201	0.0009	Beta	[28]
Virological responses				
Genotype 1				
Pegylated interferon alpha 2b and Ribavirin				
Probability of SVR	0.2720	0.0057	Beta	[29–31]
Probability of RVR	0.1302	0.0033	Beta	[29–31]
Probability to change from RVR to SVR	0.8620	0.1190	Beta	[29]
Probability of NR	0.2449	0.0055	Beta	[29, 31]
Pegylated interferon alpha 2a and Ribavirin				
RR of SVR (peg 2a vs peg 2b)	1.1950	0.0492	Log normal	calculated
RR of RVR (peg 2a vs peg 2b)	1.1300	0.0353	Log normal	calculated
RR of NR (peg 2a vs peg 2b)	0.6960	0.1134	Log normal	calculated
Genotype 6				
RR of SVR (gen 6 vs gen 1)	1.2200		Log normal	[32]
RR of RVR (gen 6 vs gen 1)	1.6800		Log normal	[32]
Health utility				
Chronic hepatitis C infection	0.7284	0.0011	Beta	[13]
Compensated cirrhosis	0.7023	0.0020	Beta	[13]
Decompensated cirrhosis	0.5774	0.0020	Beta	[13]
Hepatocellular carcinoma	0.5778	0.0023	Beta	[13]
SVR (Healthy)	0.7955	0.0018	Beta	[13]

counting for utility outcomes, indirect costs were excluded. Direct medical costs included drugs (pegylated interferon and ribavirin), laboratory tests (investigation and monitoring) and complication treatment. The prices of pegylated interferon and ribavirin were obtained from the prices that the drug companies presented to the NLEM committee. The types and the number of laboratory tests used in the model were estimated by the expert panel. The tests for investigation included complete blood count (CBC), liver function test, prothrombin time, genotype, viral load, HIV, creatinin, thyroid-stimulating hormone, antinuclear antibodies, abdominal ultrasound, pregnancy test, alanine aminotransferase (ALT), and aspartate aminotransferase (AST). For monitoring, CBC, creatinin, ALT and viral load were included.

Direct non-medical costs included transportation and food expenditure of patients. The number of OPD visits, IPD admissions and length of stay were retrieved from the existing study conducted in Thailand [33]. The unit costs of transportation and food expenditure were derived from Thai Standard Cost List for Health Technology Assessment [34]. All costs were converted in 2013 values by using consumer price index (CPI) and discounted at a rate of 3 %. The average exchange rate of Thai baht (THB) to 1 $US was 35 Baht (Table 2).

Model structure and all parameters were approved by the experts during the expert consultation meeting.

Sensitivity analysis

A one-way sensitivity analysis and a probabilistic sensitivity analysis (PSA) were performed to determine the uncertainty of model parameters. For one-way sensitivity analysis, each parameter was varied at a time across the plausible range and shown graphically as a tornado diagram. In addition, PSA were carried out by varying all parameters randomly within the plausible range. The Monte Carlo Simulation was generated in order to randomly select a value of each parameter for 1000 times and calculated for expected cost and outcome. The results of PSA were presented by a cost-effectiveness plans and acceptability curves.

Results

The total costs and QALYs gained of all treatments in patients with HCV genotypes 1 and 6 infection were presented in Table 3. Comparing to palliative care treatment, HCV treatment with pegylated interferon alpha 2a or alpha 2b plus ribavirin both in HCV genotypes 1 and 6 provided the negative ICER value that mean higher in outcomes and lower in costs. The results showed a

Table 2 Costs of CHC treatment

Cost parameters	Mean	Standard error	Distribution	Ref.
Medication, laboratory and diagnostic tests costs				
Pegylated interferon alfa-2a + Ribavirin (per week)	3,150	630	Gamma	[35]
Pegylated interferon alfa-2b + Ribavirin (per week)	3,150	630	Gamma	[35]
Investigation and monitoring	16,277	3,255	Gamma	[34]
Direct medical cost for complication treatment				
Costs of chronic HCV infection (per year)	65,640	19,723	Gamma	[33]
Costs of compensated cirrhosis (per year)	73,532	18,605	Gamma	[33]
Costs of decompensated cirrhosis (per year)	138,141	18,996	Gamma	[33]
Costs of hepatocellular carcinoma (per year)	168,899	11,601	Gamma	[33]
Direct non-medical cost for complication treatment				
Costs of chronic HCV infection (per year)	4,303	430.3	Gamma	[33, 34]
Costs of compensated cirrhosis (per year)	4,216	421.6	Gamma	[33, 34]
Costs of decompensated cirrhosis (per year)	5,823	582.3	Gamma	[33, 34]
Costs of hepatocellular carcinoma (per year)	9,516	951.6	Gamma	[33, 34]

superior of pegylated interferon alpha 2a plus ribavirin over pegylated interferon alpha 2b plus ribavirin in both genotype 1 and 6. In addition, pegylated interferon plus ribavirin provided less cost and higher outcome in HCV genotype 6 than genotype 1.

The one-way sensitivity analysis of the most cost-saving intervention was presented by a tornado diagram (Fig. 3). Only fifteen parameters most influencing on the model's results of each HCV genotype was shown from the greatest to the least. For genotype 1, they were as follows: cost of HCV treatment, rate of SVR, transitional probability from HCV state to death, and transitional probability from HCV state to compensated cirrhosis state.

The PSA results of both HCV genotypes 1 and 6 treatment were illustrated by cost-effectiveness plane (Fig. 4) and acceptability curves (Fig. 5). The cost-effectiveness acceptability curves showed the superior of pegylated interferon alpha 2a or alpha 2b plus ribavirin over palliative care for all willingness to pay values. In addition, the combination of pegylated interferon alpha 2a and ribavirin was presented a higher probability to cost-effectiveness than that of pegylated interferon alpha 2b and ribavirin.

Discussion

The findings have shown that the treatment with pegylated interferon alpha 2a or alpha 2b plus ribavirin had lower costs and higher outcomes since early HCV infection treatment will decrease complications and death from decompensated cirrhosis, compensated cirrhosis and HCC. These results were relevant with the study of Gerkens [16] that showed cost-effectiveness of pegylated interferon alpha 2a plus ribavirin in the treatment of CHC genotypes 1 and 6 comparing to the palliative care in Belgium and the study of Gheorghe [17] that showed cost-effectiveness of pegylated interferon alpha 2a plus ribavirin over pegylated interferon alpha 2b, and standard interferon and ribavirin combination in Romania.

For the treatment of CHC genotype 6 with pegylated interferon alpha 2a or alpha 2b plus ribavirin, the results revealed the superior of outcome to HCV infection and inferior of total treatment costs than CHC genotype 1. Despite the fact, the treatment in CHC genotype 6 had more cost-effectiveness than that of CHC genotype 1, the ICER results of both genotypes indicated pegylated interferon alpha 2a or alpha 2b plus ribavirin were dominant comparing to palliative care.

Table 3 Total costs and QALYs gained

Alternative treatment	Genotype 1			Genotype 6		
	Total costs (Baht)	QALYs (Year)	ICER (compare to palliative care)	Total costs (Baht)	QALYs (Year)	ICER (compare to palliative care)
Palliative care	1,169,121	11.63	-	1,150,417	11.67	-
Peg 2a + RBV	747,718	13.44	Dominant	558,868	14.07	Dominant
Peg 2b + RBV	819,921	13.14	Dominant	655,697	13.69	Dominant

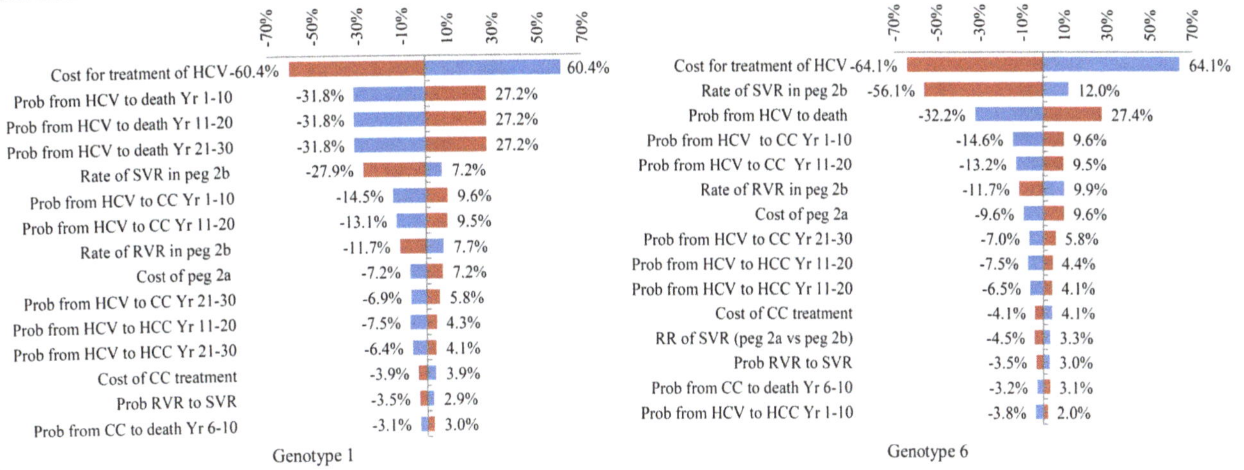

Fig. 3 Tornado diagram

There were limitations for this study need to be reported. First, due to a lack of randomized controlled trial to compare pegylated interferon alpha 2a plus ribavirin and alpha 2b plus ribavirin in CHC genotype 6 patients, the SVR and RVR rate were calculated using the relative risk (RR) in HCV genotype 1 versus HCV genotype 6 patients from a prospective study in Thailand. Although, these rates may not indicate the exact values for genotype 6 patients, they were accepted from the expert consultation meeting and the Subcommittee for Development of the NLEM. Second, the patients who were not achieved SVR and RVR were assumed as treatment failure. We applied the number of patients who were discontinued the treatment because of virological response for null response patients and the rest of treatment failure were partial response. This may not be the exact number of those groups of patients but the number was assumed to estimate cost of treatment. Thirdly, this study assumed that the patients are 100 % complied with the treatment throughout 24 or 48 weeks. In the actual circumstances, the patients may not abide by 100 % with treatment [36], which may affect the lower effectiveness. Last, the utility score of patients in each health state was obtained from studies in other countries that may be different from Thai patients. It is noted that Thai patients' utility score is needed for further study.

Given that this modeling study was performed before the current era of direct-acting antiviral (DAA) therapies, and DAAs are not currently available in Thailand, our study examined the available standard of care for HCV treatment in Thailand. Recently, sofosbuvir, a new antiviral drug has been approved in the US and Europe for treating CHC patients. AASLD and EASL guidelines have changed the standard treatment of HCV infection into DAAs. Although DAA showed the superior effects than pegylated interferon [37], this study did not include any DAAs in the model since the study was conducted before the drug approval. However, the study is certainly valuable to support an evidence for other developing countries who are considering the combination of

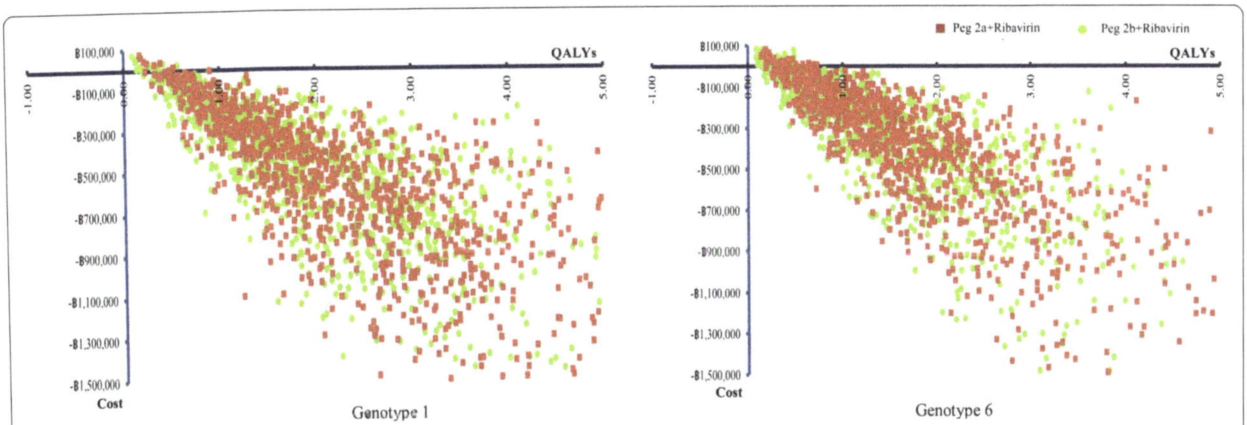

Fig. 4 Incremental cost-effectiveness plane

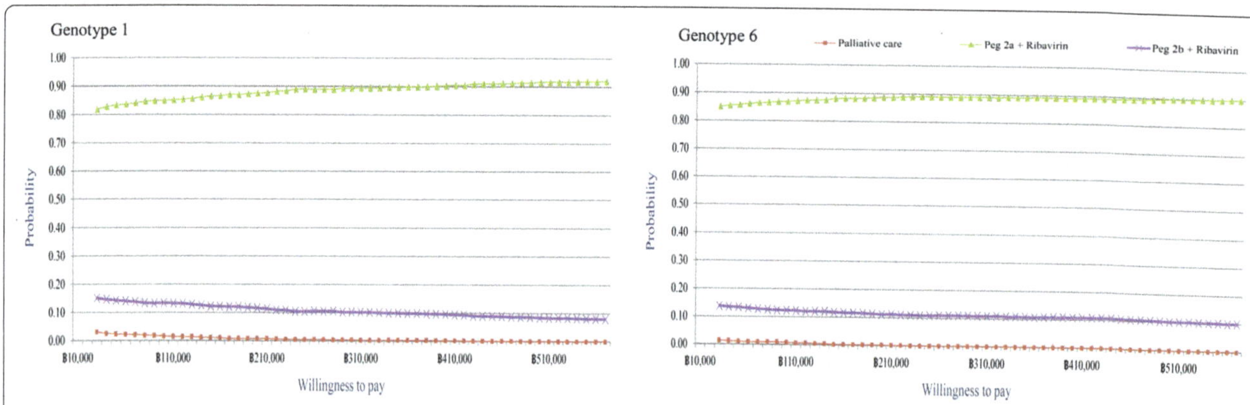

Fig. 5 Acceptability curve

pegylated interferon and ribavirin into their national drug lists. In addition, this Markov model is the first approval model for HCV treatment in Thailand. The model was validated for CHC patients along with the THASL guidelines [12], which are comparable to other guidelines [8, 10, 11]. Therefore, the model can be applied to other countries and other novel medications of HCV infection treatment. Not only is the application of the model utilized, but also the acceptance of Health Technology Assessment (HTA) for national policy making is a crucial model for other countries.

Conclusions

The treatment of CHC infection genotypes 1 and 6 with pegylated interferon alpha 2a or alpha 2b plus ribavirin comparing to the palliative care showed cost-saving in Thailand. As cost-saving results, our study proposed the Subcommittee for Development of the NLEM to include both pegylated interferon alpha 2a and alpha 2b into the NLEM. Successively, the Subcommittee for Development of the NLEM approved to include both pegylated interferon alpha 2a and alpha 2b into the NLEM in 2014.

Abbreviations

CHC, chronic hepatitis C virus infection; CPI, consumer price index; EVR, early virological response; HCC, hepatocellular carcinoma; HCV, hepatitis C virus infection; ICER, incremental cost-effectiveness ratio; NLEM, national list of essential medicines; NR, null response; PR, partial nonresponse; PSA, probabilistic sensitivity analysis; QALY, quality-adjusted life year; RVR, rapid virological response; SVR, sustained virological response; THB, Thai baht

Acknowledgements

We gratefully acknowledge all experts involved in the study for their comments on model and parameters validation. In addition, we would like to thank Professor Pornsak Sriamornsak for helping us editing the manuscript.

Funding

The Health Intervention and Technology Assessment Program (HITAP) is funded by the Thailand Research Fund under the senior research scholar on Health Technology Assessment. HITAP's international unit was established with support from the International Decision Support Initiative (funded by the Bill & Melinda Gates Foundation and the Department for International Development, UK), and the Rockefeller Foundation to provide technical assistance on health intervention and technology assessment for governments of low- and middle-income countries. The findings, interpretations, and conclusions expressed in this article do not necessarily reflect the views of the previous funding agencies.

Authors' contributions

NK reviewed literature, developed protocol, conducted study analysis and drafted manuscript, SL reviewed literature, conducted study analysis and involved in protocol development. YT involved in protocol development and provided critical comments. All authors read and approved the final manuscript.

Competing interests

The authors declare that they have no competing interests.

Consent for publication

Not Applicable.

Author details

[1]Department of Community Pharmacy, Faculty of Pharmacy, Silpakorn University, Nakhon Pathom, Thailand73000. [2]Health Intervention and Technology Assessment Program (HITAP), Ministry of Public Health, Nonthaburi, Thailand.

References

1. World Health Organization. Hepatitis. 2014. http://apps.who.int/gb/ebwha/pdf_files/WHA67/A67_R6-en.pdf. Accessed 15 Oct 2014.
2. Centers for Disease Control and Prevention. Hepatitis C: General information. 2010. http://www.cdc.gov/hepatitis/hcv/pdfs/hepcgeneralfactsheet.pdf. Accessed 20 Apr 2014.
3. World Health Organization. Hepatitis C. 2013. http://www.who.int/mediacentre/factsheets/fs164/en/. Accessed 12 Apr 2013.
4. Mohd Hanafiah K, Groeger J, Flaxman AD, Wiersma ST. Global epidemiology of hepatitis C virus infection: new estimates of age-specific antibody to HCV seroprevalence. Hepatology. 2013;57(4):1333–42.
5. Sievert W, Altraif I, Razavi HA, Abdo A, Ahmed EA, AlOmair A, et al. A systematic review of hepatitis C virus epidemiology in Asia, Australia and Egypt. Liver International. 2011;31(s2):61–80.
6. El Khoury AC, Klimack WK, Wallace C, Razavi H. Economic burden of hepatitis C-associated diseases in the United States. J Viral Hepat. 2012;19(3):153–60.
7. El Khoury AC, Wallace C, Klimack WK, Razavi H. Economic burden of hepatitis C-associated diseases: Europe, Asia Pacific, and the Americas. J Med Econ. 2012;15(5):87–96.
8. Omata M, Kanda T, Yu ML, Yokosuka O, Lim SG, Jafri W, et al. APASL consensus statements and management algorithms for hepatitis C virus infection. Hepatol Int. 2012;6(2):409–35.

9. Bunchorntavakul C, Chavalitdhamrong D, Tanwandee T. Hepatitis C genotype 6: A concise review and response-guided therapy proposal. World J Hepatol. 2013;5(9):496–504.
10. Ghany MG, Strader DB, Thomas DL, Seeff LB. Diagnosis, management, and treatment of hepatitis C: an update. Hepatology. 2009;49(4):1335–74.
11. Europaean Association for the Study of the Liver. EASL Clinical Practice Guidelines: management of hepatitis C virus infection. J Hepatol. 2014; 60(2):392–420.
12. Thai Association for the Study of the Liver. Thailand practice guideline for management of chronic hepatitis B and C 2012. 2nd ed. Bangkok: Thai Association for the Study of the Liver; 2012. p. 52.
13. Werayingyong P, Teerawattananon Y. Cost-utility and budget impact of the chronic hepatitis C treatment. In: International Health Policy Program (IHPP) and Health Intervention and Technology Assessment Program (HITAP), editor. Research for development of health benefit package under universal health care coverage scheme: Issue 1. Nontaburi: The Graphico System Co. Ltd; 2011. p. 147–72.
14. Nguyen NH, VuTien P, Garcia RT, Trinh H, Nguyen H, Nguyen K, et al. Response to pegylated interferon and ribavirin in Asian American patients with chronic hepatitis C genotypes 1 vs 2/3 vs 6. J Viral Hepat. 2010;17(10):691–7.
15. Siebert U, Sroczynski G, Rossol S, Wasem J, Ravens-Sieberer U, et al. Cost effectiveness of peginterferon alpha-2b plus ribavirin versus interferon alpha-2b plus ribavirin for initial treatment of chronic hepatitis C. Gut. 2003; 52(3):425–32.
16. Gerkens S, Nechelput M, Annemans L, Peraux B, Mouchart M, Beguin C, et al. A health economic model to assess the cost-effectiveness of PEG IFN alpha-2a and ribavirin in patients with mild chronic hepatitis C. J Viral Hepat. 2007;14(8):523–36.
17. Gheorghe L, Baculea S. Cost-effectiveness of peginterferon alpha-2a and peginterferon alpha-2b combination regimens in genotype-1 naive patients with chronic hepatitis C. Hepatogastroenterology. 2010;57(101):939–44.
18. Sullivan SD, Jensen DM, Bernstein DE, Hassanein TI, Foster GR, Lee SS, et al. Cost-effectiveness of combination peginterferon alpha-2a and ribavirin compared with interferon alpha-2b and ribavirin in patients with chronic hepatitis C. Am J Gastroenterol. 2004;99(8):1490–6.
19. Fonseca MC, Araujo GT, Araujo DV. Cost effectiveness of peginterferon alfa-2B combined with ribavirin for the treatment of chronic hepatitis C in Brazil. Braz J Infect Dis. 2009;13(3):191–9.
20. Barros FMR, Cheinquer H, Tsuchiya CT, Santos EAV. Cost-effectiveness analysis of treatment with peginterferon-alfa-2a versus peginterferon-alfa-2b for patients with chronic hepatitis C under the public payer perspective in Brazil. Cost Eff Resour Alloc. 2013;11(25):1–9.
21. Permsuwan U, Guntawongwan K, Buddhawongsa P. Handling time in economic evaluation studies. J Med Assoc Thai. 2008;91 Suppl 2:S53–58.
22. Flori N, Funakoshi N, Duny Y, Valats JC, Bismuth M, Christophorou D, et al. Pegylated interferon-alpha2a and ribavirin versus pegylated interferon-alpha2b and ribavirin in chronic hepatitis C: a meta-analysis. Drugs. 2013;73(3):263–77.
23. Bureau of Policy and Strategy, Ministry of Public Health. Public health statistics 2011. Bangkok: The War Veterans Organization of Thailand Printing House. 2012. p. 58–61.
24. Krahn M, Wong JB, Heathcote J, Scully L, Seeff L. Estimating the prognosis of hepatitis C patients infected by transfusion in Canada between 1986 and 1990. Med Decis Making. 2004;24(1):20–9.
25. Omland LH, Krarup H, Jepsen P, Georgsen J, Harritshoj LH, Riison K, et al. Mortality in patients with chronic and cleared hepatitis C viral infection: a nationwide cohort study. J Hepatol. 2010;53(1):36–42.
26. Fattovich G, Giustina G, Degos F, Tremolada F, Diodati G, Almasio P, et al. Morbidity and mortality in compensated cirrhosis type C: a retrospective follow-up study of 384 patients. Gastroenterology. 1997;112(2):463–72.
27. Planas R, Balleste B, Alvarez MA, Rivera M, Montoliu S, Galeras JA, et al. Natural history of decompensated hepatitis C virus-related cirrhosis. A study of 200 patients. J Hepatol. 2004;40(5):823–30.
28. Sithinamsuwan P, Piratvisuth T, Tanomkiat W, Apakupakul N, Tongyoo S. Review of 336 patients with hepatocellular carcinoma at Songklanagarind Hospital. World J Gastroenterol. 2000;6(3):339–43.
29. McHutchison JG, Lawitz EJ, Shiffman ML, Muir AJ, Galler GW, McCone J, et al. Peginterferon alfa-2b or alfa 2a with ribavirin for treatment of hepatitis C infection. N Engl J Med. 2009;361(6):580 93.
30. Rumi MG, Aghemo A, Prati GM, D'Ambrosio R, Donato MF, Soffredini R, et al. Randomized study of peginterferon-alpha2a plus ribavirin vs peginterferon-alpha2b plus ribavirin in chronic hepatitis C. Gastroenterology. 2010;138(1):108–15.
31. Miyase S, Haraoka K, Ouchida Y, Morishita Y, Fujiyama S. Randomized trial of peginterferon alpha-2a plus ribavirin versus peginterferon alpha-2b plus ribavirin for chronic hepatitis C in Japanese patients. J Gastroenterol. 2012;47(9):1014–21.
32. Tangkijvanich P, Komolmit P, Mahachai V, Poovorawan K, Akkarathamrongsin S, Poovorawan Y. Response-guided therapy for patients with hepatitis C virus genotype 6 infection: a pilot study. J Viral Hepat. 2012;19(6):423–30.
33. Thongsawat S, Piratvisuth T, Pramoolsinsap C, Chutaputti A, Tanwandee T, Thongsuk D. Resource Utilization and Direct Medical Costs of Chronic Hepatitis C in Thailand: A Heavy but Manageable Economic Burden. Value Health Reg Issues. 2014;3:12–8.
34. Riewpaiboon A. Standard Cost List for Health Technology Assessment. 2010. http://costingmenu.hitap.net/. Accessed 10 Nov 2013.
35. Ministry of Public Health. Drug and medical supply information center. 2013. http://dmsic.moph.go.th/dmsic/index.php?p=1&id=1. Accessed 10 Nov 2013.
36. Piratvisuth T, Tanwandee T, Mahachai V, Chutaputti A, Thongsawat S, Khow-Ean U, et al. The efficacy of peginterferon alfa-2b plus ribavirin combination in Thai patients with chronic hepatitis c. Thai J Gastroenterol. 2004;5(1):2–7.
37. Yang HJ, Ryoo JY, Yoo BK. Meta-analysis of the efficacy and safety of sofosbuvir for the treatment of hepatitis C virus infection. Int J Clin Pharm. 2015;37(5):698–708.

25

Off-treatment durability of antiviral response to nucleoside analogues in patients with chronic hepatitis B

Naruhiko Nagata, Tatehiro Kagawa*, Shunji Hirose, Yoshitaka Arase, Kota Tsuruya, Kazuya Anzai, Koichi Shiraishi and Tetsuya Mine

Abstract

Background: Off-treatment durability of nucleoside analogue (NA) therapy in patients with chronic hepatitis B has not been well investigated. In this study we monitored antiviral effect of NA therapy and evaluated off-treatment durability after NA cessation in patients with chronic hepatitis B.

Patients and methods: A total of 94 consecutive patients (39 HBeAg-negative and 55 HBeAg-positive patients) who received NA therapy were followed up for approximately 9 years. We discontinued NA according to the following criteria; undetectable serum HBV-DNA by polymerase chain reaction (PCR) on three separate occasions at least 6 months apart in HBeAg-negative patients (APASL stopping recommendation), and seroconversion from HBeAg-positive to HBeAb-positive and undetectable serum HBV-DNA by PCR for at least 12 months in HBeAg-positive patients.

Results: The cumulative rate of relapse after NA cessation was 48 % and 40 % in HBeAg-negative and -positive patients, respectively. Higher baseline serum alanine aminotransferase level was the only significant predictor for maintaining remission. No patients experienced decompensation after relapse. HBsAg loss occurred at an annual rate of 1.4 % and 0.4 % in HBeAg-negative and -positive patients, respectively. Hepatocellular carcinoma developed at an annual rate of 0.6 % in both HBeAg-negative and -positive patients.

Conclusions: Almost half of the patients did not relapse after cessation of NA therapy in both HBeAg-negative and -positive patients. Therefore, NA therapy could be discontinued with close monitoring if the APASL stopping recommendation is satisfied even in HBeAg-negative patients.

Keywords: Chronic hepatitis B, Nucleoside analogue, Durability, Hepatocellular carcinoma, HBs antigen

Background

Nucleoside analogues (NAs) are shown to improve prognosis of patients with chronic hepatitis B. Continuous treatment with lamivudine (LMV) delayed clinical progression defined by hepatic decompensation, hepatocellular carcinoma (HCC), spontaneous bacterial peritonitis, bleeding gastroesophageal varices, or liver disease-related death in patients with chronic hepatitis B and advanced fibrosis or cirrhosis [1]. NAs can suppress hepatic inflammation by inhibiting viral proliferation in most cases, however, this effect is transient. Relapse after NA cessation is frequently observed [2–9]. Alanine aminotransferase (ALT) flare with 10 times higher than normal upper limit was reported in up to 20 % [2, 3] of patients who discontinued NA treatment. These results suggest that NA discontinuation should be decided with caution. On the other hand, considerable number of patients are receiving NA treatment even if they actually no longer need NA. Therefore, making a discrimination of patients who can discontinue NA treatment is important from the viewpoint of health care economics.

Currently there is no clear consensus on when to stop NA treatment. For HBeAg-negative patients, the guidelines from the American Association for the Study of Liver Diseases (AASLD) [10] and the European Association for the Study of the Liver (EASL) [11] recommend

* Correspondence: kagawa@tokai.ac.jp
Division of Gastroenterology and Hepatology, Department of Internal Medicine, Tokai University School of Medicine, Shimokasuya 143, Isehara 259-1193, Japan

long-term NA treatment until HBsAg seroclearance has been achieved. Although HBsAg seroclearance is an ideal goal of NA treatment, it takes place in only a minority of patients (<1 % per year [10]). On the other hand, the Asian-Pacific Association for the Study of the Liver (APASL) guideline [12] suggests that treatment discontinuation can be considered if patients have been treated for at least 2 years with undetectable HBV-DNA documented on three separate occasions 6 months apart, even if HBsAg seroclearance is not achieved. For HBeAg-positive patients, the AASLD, EASL and APASL guidelines recommend that NA treatment can be discontinued when HBeAg seroconversion with undetectable HBV-DNA has been maintained for 6-12 months.

There have been several studies on off-treatment durability of NA's antiviral effect (see review [13]), however, the results considerably vary by study. Therefore, the accumulation of further data is required.

In this study we monitored antiviral effect of NA therapy and evaluated off-treatment durability after NA cessation according to the APASL stopping recommendation in patients with chronic hepatitis B.

Methods

We consecutively enrolled the patients who started treatment with LMV or entecavir (ETV) from December 1999 through June 2010. Most patients started with ETV since ETV was approved in Japan (July 2006). These patients were positive for serum HBsAg and HBV-DNA, and had elevated ALT at least twice before initiating treatment. We excluded patients who were co-infected with HCV or HIV, and those with liver cirrhosis or HCC. We discontinued NA treatment after obtaining verbal informed consent when patients satisfied the APASL stopping recommendation [12]; undetectable serum HBV-DNA by polymerase chain reaction (PCR) on three separate occasions at least 6 months apart in HBeAg-negative patients, and seroconversion from HBeAg-positive to HBeAb-positive and undetectable serum HBV-DNA by PCR for at least 12 months in HBeAg-positive patients. Treatment for at least 2 years was not a prerequisite for NA discontinuation in this study. Patients were followed up every one to three months to monitor blood chemistry and HBV markers. They received ultrasonography for the surveillance of HCC every 6 months. Relapse after NA discontinuation was defined as serum ALT elevation more than twice the upper limit of normal or serum HBV-DNA elevation higher than 5 log copy/mL at 2 consecutive examinations. Serum HBV-DNA levels were measured by COBAS TaqMan HBV test (Roche Molecular Systems, Inc., Pleasanton, CA). Serum HBsAg was quantitated by Architect assay (Abbott Japan, Co., Ltd., Tokyo, Japan). A part of serum samples were stored at −80°C until measurement. This study had been approved by Institutional Review Board for Clinical Research, Tokai University Hospital, and was performed in accordance with the Declaration of Helsinki.

Statistical analysis

Pearson chi-square and Fisher exact probability tests were performed to compare the frequency distributions of categorical variables between groups. One-way analysis of variance was used to test the differences in means between groups for continuous variables. The probabilities of satisfying NA discontinuation criteria, relapse, disappearance of serum HBsAg, and progression to HCC were estimated using the Kaplan-Meier method, and differences between groups were compared using the log-rank test. Analyzed baseline factors included age, gender, HBV genotype, serum ALT, HBV-DNA, HBsAg, and liver histology assessed by METAVIR classification [14]. The factors with P value < .1 by univariate analysis were evaluated with a Cox proportional hazards regression model. All statistical analyses were performed using SPSS version 22 (SPSS Japan, Tokyo, Japan). All reported P values are 2-sided, with $P < .05$ considered statistically significant.

Results

Patient characteristics

The cohort consisted of 94 patients; 39 and 55 patients were negative and positive for HBeAg, respectively (Table 1). The HBeAg-negative patients were significantly older than the HBeAg-positive patients. Most patients were infected with genotype C HBV (84 % and 97 % in HBeAg-negative and -positive patients, respectively). The serum HBV-DNA levels were significantly higher in the HBeAg-positive patients. The mean ± SD of the follow-up period was 108 ± 42 (min-max: 18-182) and 111 ± 42 (min-max: 16-178) months in HBeAg-negative and -positive patients, respectively.

Outcome of the patients

HBeAg-negative patients

Twenty-five (64 %) patients received LMV, while the remaining 14 (36 %) received ETV (Fig. 1). Most of the patients (23/25, 92 %) receiving LMV met the APASL stopping recommendation. Of 23 patients 17 agreed to stop LMV treatment, and 10 of these 17 patients (59 %) maintained remission. In 7 patients who relapsed, 3 achieved remission afterwards and 4 started ETV treatment. All of 14 patients (100 %) receiving ETV met the stopping criteria. Six of 14 patients agreed to stop ETV treatment, and 2 of 6 (33 %) maintained remission. In 4 relapsers, 2 achieved remission afterwards, and 2 restarted ETV. The mean ± SD of NA treatment duration until discontinuation was 40 ± 41 (min-max: 8–141) and 26 ± 17 (min-max: 9–50) months in patients who received LMV and

Table 1 Patient characteristics

Variables	HBeAg (-) (n=39)		HBeAg (+) (n=55)		*P* value
	no.	%	no.	%	
Age, <40/40-59/60≤	7/22/10	18/56/26	22/23/10	40/42/18	0.07
Age (y/o)	50.0 ± 11.8		44.3 ± 14.5		0.03
Gender, female/male	11/28	28/72	18/37	33/67	0.7
Drug, LAM/ETV	25/14	64/36	38/17	69/31	0.7
ALT (IU/L), <100/100-199/200≤	12/16/11	31/41/28	20/13/22	36/24/40	0.19
HBV-DNA (Log copy/mL), <6/6-7.6/7.6<	11/22/6	28/56/15	4/20/31	7/36/56	0.001
Genotype*, B/C	5/26	16/84	1/37	3/97	0.07
HBsAg (IU/mL)*, <1000/1000-10000/10000≤	7/11/5	30/48/22	3/9/8	15/45/40	0.09
Histology (METAVIR Staging)*, 1/2/3	13/8/6	48/30/22	11/13/7	35/42/23	0.6
Histology (METAVIR Grading)*, 1/2/3	7/17/3	26/63/11	8/15/8	26/48/26	0.3

*Data were not available in some patients

ETV, respectively. The difference between LMV and ETV was not statistically significant. A total of 11 patients (48 %) experienced relapse. Most relapses occurred within 1 year after NA cessation. The cumulative relapse rate at 1 year, 2 years, and 5 years were 30 %, 35 %, and 39 %, respectively. In contrast, 44 % of patients were under control without NA administration.

HBeAg-positive patients

Thirty-eight (69 %) patients received LMV and the remaining 17 (31 %) received ETV (Fig. 2). In patients who received LMV, 13 patients (34 %) met the stopping criteria. Six (60 %) of 10 patients who consented to stop LMV maintained remission. The mean ± SD of treatment duration until discontinuation was 44 ± 23 (min-max: 15–86) months. In 4 relapsers, 2 achieved remission afterwards, while 2 restarted ETV. Only 2 of 17 who received ETV met stopping criteria, and both continued ETV treatment. Finally, 4 patients (40 %) relapsed. The 1-year, 2-year, and 5-year cumulative relapse rates were 20 %, 30 %, and 30 %, respectively, whereas 15 % of patients were under control without NA administration.

Predictive factors for meeting the stopping criteria

HBeAg-negative patients were more likely to meet the stopping criteria than HBeAg-positive patients (95 % vs. 27 %, $P < 0.001$, Fig. 3). We analyzed the predictive factors for meeting the stopping criteria in HBeAg-positive patients. Multivariate analysis revealed lower serum HBV-DNA level as the only predictive factor ($P = 0.02$). The proportion of patients who met the stopping criteria was 42 % (10/24) in those with serum HBV-DNA of 7.6

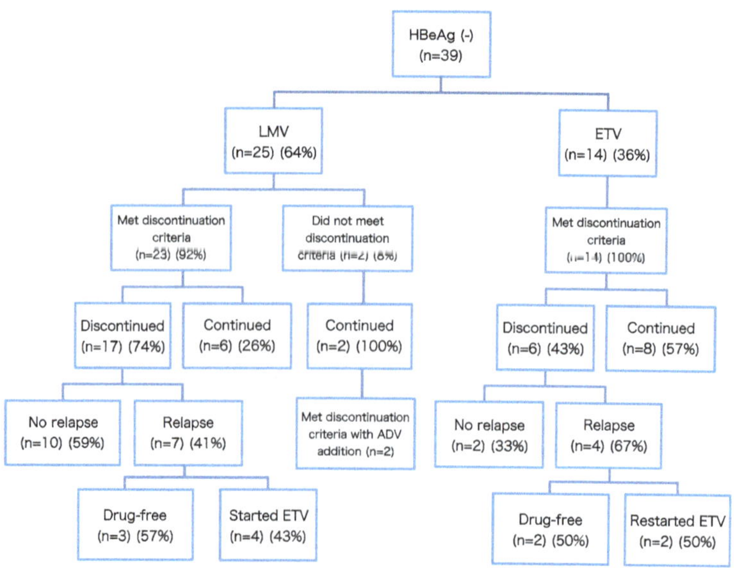

Fig. 1 Flow chart of HBeAg-negative patients. LMV: lamivudine, ETV: entecavir, ADV: adefovir

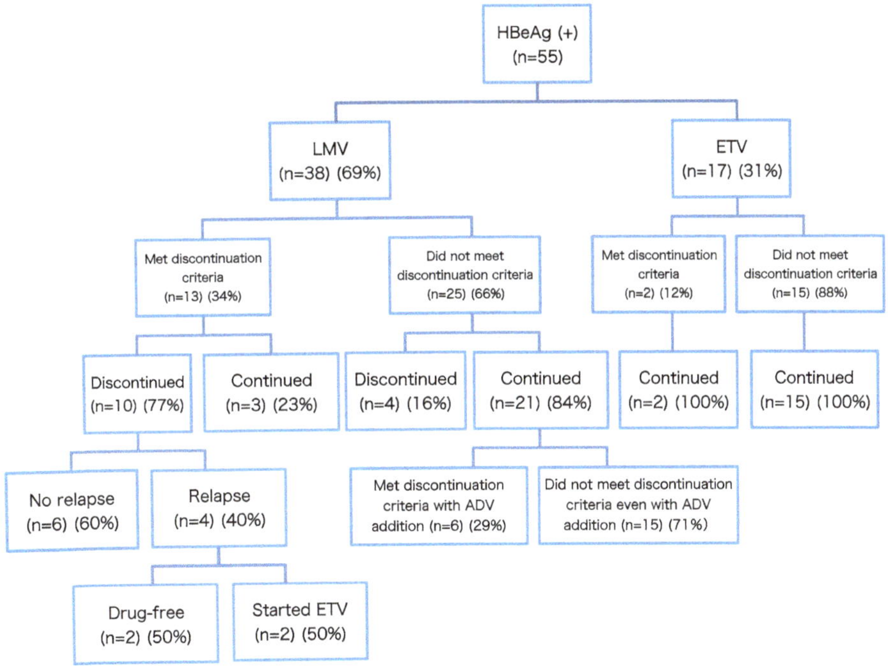

Fig. 2 Flow chart of HBeAg-positive patients. LMV: lamivudine, ETV: entecavir, ADV: adefovir

log copy/mL or less, whereas it was 15 % (5/31) in those with serum HBV-DNA higher than 7.6 log copy/mL.

Predictive factors for relapse

A total of 15 (45 %) among 33 patients who discontinued NA treatment relapsed, while the remaining 18 (55 %) maintained remission. We analyzed the baseline variables associated with relapse. Multivariate analysis demonstrated that serum ALT was the only predictive factor for relapse. Relapse rate was 50 % (2/4), 71 % (10/14), and 20 % (3/15) in patients with ALT < 100, 100–199, and ≥ 200 IU/mL, respectively. The patients with ALT ≥ 200 IU mL were more likely to maintain remission (Fig. 4, $P = 0.02$).

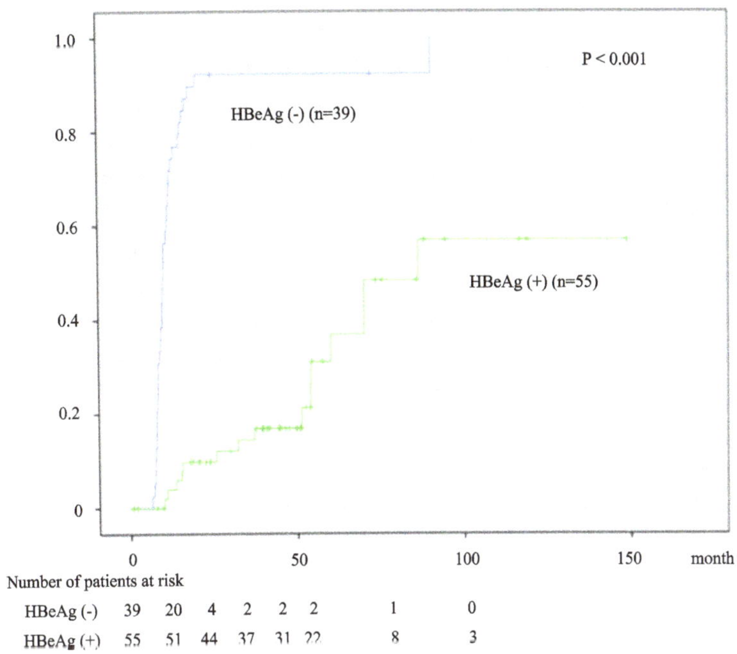

Fig. 3 Cumulative rate of satisfying NA stopping criteria according to the HBeAg status

Serum ALT elevated up to more than 500 IU/mL in 4 of 15 relapsers (27 %), however, none experienced decompensation.

HBsAg disappearance

Serum HBsAg disappeared in 7 patients (7.4 %), resulting in an annual HBsAg disappearance rate of 0.8 %; 1.4 % and 0.4 % for HBeAg-negative and -positive patients, respectively. We analyzed the baseline factors associated with HBsAg loss. Serum HBV-DNA was the only predictive variable by multivariate analysis; HBsAg loss was observed in 5 of 15 patients (33 %) with serum HBV-DNA less than 6 log copy/mL, while 2 of 79 patients (3 %) with serum HBV-DNA of 6 log copy/mL or higher ($P = 0.001$). The accumulated HBsAg loss was observed more frequently in those with lower HBV-DNA (Fig. 5, $P = 0.02$).

HCC progression

Five of 94 (5.3 %) patients progressed to HCC, resulting in an annual HCC progression rate of 0.6 % in both HBeAg-negative and -positive patients. Age was the only predictive variable for HCC progression by multivariate analysis ($P = 0.01$). Only one of 74 (1.4 %) patients younger than 60 years progressed to HCC, whereas did 4 of 20 (20 %) patients aged 60 or older ($P = 0.01$, Fig. 6). Four patients died, all of whom were HBeAg-positive. One died of HCC and the remaining 3 died of the diseases unrelated to the liver (pancreatic cancer, gastric cancer, and unknown).

Discussion

In approximately 9 years after initiating NA administration, 44 % (17/39) of HBeAg-negative patients and 15 % (8/55) of HBeAg-positive patients were under control without NA. In other words, more than half of HBeAg-negative and most of HBeAg-positive patients still need NA therapy, suggesting difficulty in stopping NA therapy.

In this study we adopted the APASL stopping recommendation [12]. Most of the HBeAg-negative patients (95 %) satisfied this stopping criteria, whereas only one forth of the HBeAg-positive patients (27 %) did. These results are in agreement with a study [15] reporting that seroconversion from HBeAg-positive to HBeAb-positive occurred only in 38 % of HBeAg-positive patients through 4 year-treatment of ETV. Multivariate analysis revealed that patients with lower serum HBV-DNA levels were more likely to meet the stopping criteria in concordance with the previous study [15]. Thus, patients with higher serum HBV-DNA will have difficulty to cease NA treatment once it started.

In HBeAg-negative patients, the cumulative relapse rate after discontinuation of NA therapy was 48 % (11/23), which was comparable with the previous studies [9, 16-19]. Jeng et al. [19] evaluated off-therapy durability in 95 patients who discontinued ETV treatment according to the APASL stopping recommendation as we adopted. The cumulative 1-year relapse rate was 45.3 %. On the other hand, another prospectively study [20] enrolling 184 patients in which ETV was stopped according to the APASL stopping recommendation demonstrated an

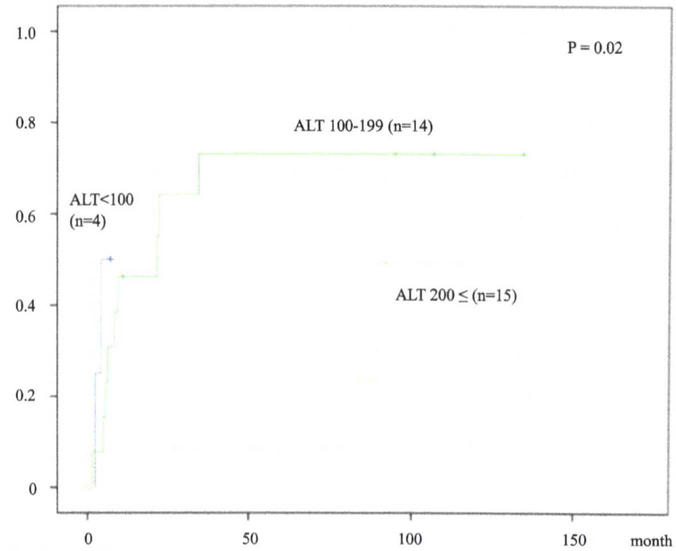

Number of patients at risk

ALT<100	4	0				
ALT 100-199	13	4	3	3	2	1
ALT 200 ≤	15	11	9	6	1	

Fig. 4 Cumulative rate of relapse after NA discontinuation according to the serum ALT levels

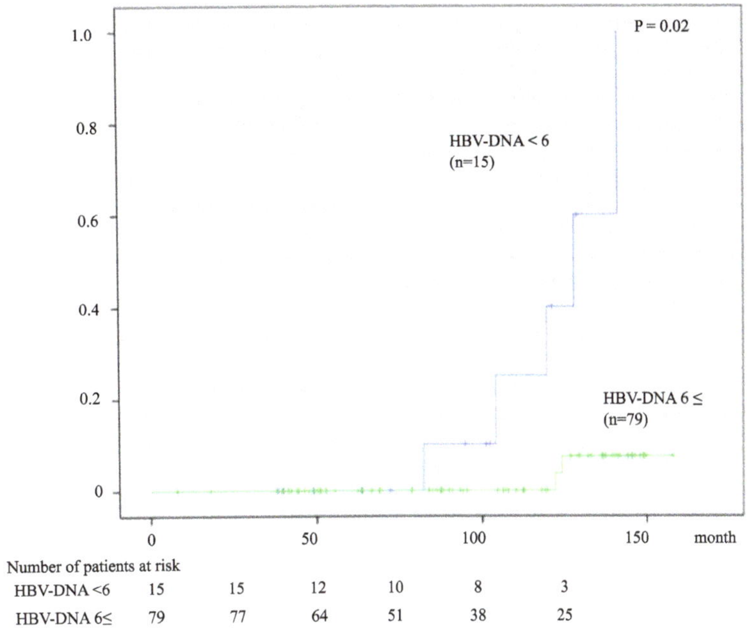

Fig. 5 Cumulative rate of HBsAg loss according to the viral load

exceptionally high cumulative 1-year relapse rate of 91.4 %. Although reason for the discrepancy in the reported relapse rates is unclear, the differences in patients background and study design may be involved. The AASLD and EASL recommend long-term NA therapy until HBsAg seroclearance is achieved, however, this goal is unrealistic considering very low HBsAg seroclearance rate (<1 % per year [10]). The others and we showed that approximately half of the HBeAg-negative patients remained remission after cessation of NA therapy according to the APASL stopping recommendation. Thus, NA therapy can be stopped with proper monitoring.

In the HBeAg-positive patients, cumulative relapse rate after discontinuation of NA therapy was 40 % (4/10), which is in concordance with other studies ranging 29–77 %

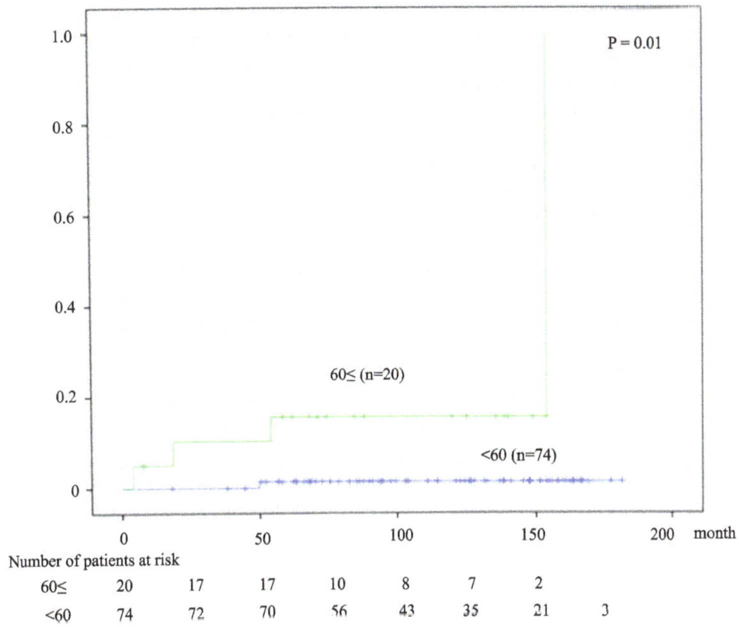

Fig. 6 Cumulative rate of HCC occurrence according to the age

[5, 6, 8, 20-24]. According to a retrospective study of Song et al. analyzing 98 HBeAg-positive patients who stopped LMV therapy after HBeAg seroconversion, the cumulative relapse rates at 1 year and 2 years were 37.5 % and 49.2 %, respectively [5].

Our study demonstrated that relapse was less frequently observed in patients with higher ALT levels in agreement with a previous study [6]. Patients with high ALT indicating strong immunological reaction against HBV may be on the transition state from immune clearance phase to low replicative phase in which relapse is relatively rare. Although lower baseline serum HBV-DNA [5, 6, 19] and younger age [9, 25–27], and longer treatment duration [5, 27] were associated with lower relapse rate in other studies, we could not find these associations.

Four of 15 relapsers (27 %) underwent serum ALT flare above 500 IU/L, however, they did not progress to liver failure. ALT flare with 10 times higher than normal upper limit was reported in up to 20 % [2, 3] of patients who discontinued NA treatment. We similarly observed ALT flare, but did not experience decompensation as previous studies [9, 19, 20, 22].

HBsAg disappeared at an annual rate of 0.8 %; 1.4 % in HBeAg-negative and 0.4 % in HBeAg-positive patients. These results are compatible with other studies [28-32]. Low baseline serum HBV-DNA was the only predictor for HBsAg disappearance in our study, in agreement with a previous study [33]. Kim et al. [33] revealed 0.33 % annual HBsAg seroclearance rate by 6-year-follow-up of 5409 patients (two-thirds were HBeAg positive) receiving LMV or ETV therapy, and demonstrated baseline low HBV-DNA, high ALT, HBeAg negativity, and absence of cirrhosis as predictors for HBsAg loss.

The progression to HCC was observed at an annual rate of 0.6 % in both HBeAg-negative and -positive patients, which results are in agreement with previous studies [33-36]. The decrease of HCC occurrence by long-term NA treatment is confirmed by a randomized study [1] and a meta-analysis [37]. The only predictive factor for HCC progression was age of 60 years or older, which is also reported in a previous study [36].

This study has limitations; the study was conducted in a retrospective manner in a single institution, and number of patients was small. Our patients predominantly consisted of genotype C. However, the data on off-treatment durability of NA's antiviral effect are still insufficient, and we believe our results provide important information.

Conclusions

Approximately half of the patients did not relapse after cessation of NA therapy in both HBeAg-negative and -positive patients. The relapsers did not experience decompensation. Therefore, NA therapy could be discontinued with close monitoring if the APASL stopping recommendation is satisfied even in HBeAg-negative patients.

Competing interests

The authors declare that they have no competing interests.

Authors' contributions

NN collected patients' data, performed statistical analysis, and drafted the manuscript. TK participated in the design of the study, performed statistical analysis, and helped to draft the manuscript. SH, YA, KT, KA, KS, and TM participated in the collection of patients' data. All authors read and approved the final manuscript.

Acknowledgments

This study was supported in part by a research grant from the Ministry of Health, Labor and Welfare of Japan.

References

1. Liaw YF, Sung JJ, Chow WC, Farrell G, Lee CZ, Yuen H, Tanwandee T, Tao QM, Shue K, Keene ON, Dixon JS, Gray DF, Sabbat J. Lamivudine for patients with chronic hepatitis B and advanced liver disease. N Engl J Med. 2004;351:1521–31.
2. Honkoop P, de Man RA, Niesters HG, Zondervan PE, Schalm SW. Acute exacerbation of chronic hepatitis B virus infection after withdrawal of lamivudine therapy. Hepatology. 2000;32:635–9.
3. Honkoop P, de Man RA, Niesters HG, Zondervan PE, Schalm SW. Acute exacerbation of chronic hepatitis B virus infection after withdrawal of lamivudine therapy. Hepatology. 2000;32:635–9.
4. Santantonio T, Mazzola M, Iacovazzi T, Miglietta A, Guastadisegni A, Pastore G. Long-term follow-up of patients with anti-HBe/HBV DNA-positive chronic hepatitis B treated for 12 months with lamivudine. J Hepatol. 2000;32:300–6.
5. Song BC, Suh DJ, Lee HC, Chung YH, Lee YS. Hepatitis B e antigen seroconversion after lamivudine therapy is not durable in patients with chronic hepatitis B in Korea. Hepatology. 2000;32:803–6.
6. van Nunen AB, Hansen BE, Suh DJ, Lohr HF, Chemello L, Fontaine H, Heathcote J, Song BC, Janssen HL, de Man RA, Schalm SW. Durability of HBeAg seroconversion following antiviral therapy for chronic hepatitis B: relation to type of therapy and pretreatment serum hepatitis B virus DNA and alanine aminotransferase. Gut. 2003;52:420–4.
7. Ito K, Tanaka Y, Orito E, Hirashima N, Ide T, Hino T, Kumashiro R, Kato A, Nukaya H, Sakakibara K, Mukaide M, Ito H, Sata M, Ueda R, Mizokami M. Predicting relapse after cessation of Lamivudine monotherapy for chronic hepatitis B virus infection. Clin Infect Dis. 2004;38:490–5.
8. Reijnders JG, Perquin MJ, Zhang N, Hansen BE, Janssen HL. Nucleos(t)ide analogues only induce temporary hepatitis B e antigen seroconversion in most patients with chronic hepatitis B. Gastroenterology. 2010;139:491–8.
9. Liu F, Wang L, Li XY, Liu YD, Wang JB, Zhang ZH, et al. Poor durability of lamivudine effectiveness despite stringent cessation criteria: a prospective clinical study in hepatitis B e antigen-negative chronic hepatitis B patients. J Gastroenterol Hepatol. 2011;26:456–60.
10. Lok AS, McMahon BJ. Chronic hepatitis B: update 2009. Hepatology. 2009;50:661–2.
11. European Association For The Study Of The Liver. EASL clinical practice guidelines: Management of chronic hepatitis B virus infection. J Hepatol. 2012;57:167–85.
12. Liaw Y-F, Kao J-H, Piratvisuth T, Chan H, Chien R-N, Liu C-J, Gane E, Locarnini S, Lim S-G, K-H. H, Amarapurkar D, Cooksley G, Jafri W, Mohamed R, Hou J-L, Chuang W-L, Lesmana L, JD. S, Suh D-J, Omata M. Asian-Pacific consensus statement on the management of chronic hepatitis B: a 2012 update. Hepatology International. 2012;6:531–61.
13. Kang W, Park JY. When to stop nucleos(t)ide analogues treatment for chronic hepatitis B? Durability of antiviral response. World J Gastroenterol. 2014;20:7207–12.
14. Bedossa P, Poynard T. An algorithm for the grading of activity in chronic hepatitis C. The METAVIR Cooperative Study Group. Hepatology. 1996;24:289–93.
15. Ono A, Suzuki F, Kawamura Y, Sezaki H, Hosaka T, Akuta N, Kobayashi M, Suzuki Y, Saitou S, Arase Y, Ikeda K, Kobayashi M, Watahiki S, Mineta R,

Kumada H. Long-term continuous entecavir therapy in nucleos(t)ide-naive chronic hepatitis B patients. J Hepatol. 2012;57:508–14.
16. Fung SK, Wong F, Hussain M, Lok AS. Sustained response after a 2-year course of lamivudine treatment of hepatitis B e antigen-negative chronic hepatitis B. J Viral Hepat. 2004;11:432–8.
17. Paik YH, Kim JK, Kim do Y, Park JY, Ahn SH, Han KH, Chon CY, Lee KS. Clinical efficacy of a 24-months course of lamivudine therapy in patients with HBeAg negative chronic hepatitis B: a long-term prospective study. J Korean Med Sci. 2010;25:882–7.
18. Hadziyannis SJ, Sevastianos V, Rapti I, Vassilopoulos D, Hadziyannis E. Sustained responses and loss of HBsAg in HBeAg-negative patients with chronic hepatitis B who stop long-term treatment with adefovir. Gastroenterology. 2012;143:629–36.
19. Jeng WJ, Sheen IS, Chen YC, Hsu CW, Chien RN, Chu CM, Liaw YF. Off-therapy durability of response to entecavir therapy in hepatitis B e antigen-negative chronic hepatitis B patients. Hepatology. 2013;58:1888–96.
20. Seto WK, Hui AJ, Wong VW, Wong GL, Liu KS, Lai CL, Yuen MF, Chan HL. Treatment cessation of entecavir in Asian patients with hepatitis B e antigen negative chronic hepatitis B: a multicentre prospective study. Gut. 2015;64:667–72.
21. Chien RN, Yeh CT, Tsai SL, Chu CM, Liaw YF. Determinants for sustained HBeAg response to lamivudine therapy. Hepatology. 2003;38:1267–73.
22. Dienstag JL, Cianciara J, Karayalcin S, Kowdley KV, Willems B, Plisek S, Woessner M, Gardner S, Schiff E. Durability of serologic response after lamivudine treatment of chronic hepatitis B. Hepatology. 2003;37:748–55.
23. Fung J, Lai CL, Tanaka Y, Mizokami M, Yuen J, Wong DK, Yuen MF. The duration of lamivudine therapy for chronic hepatitis B: cessation vs. continuation of treatment after HBeAg seroconversion. Am J Gastroenterol. 2009;104:1940–6.
24. Lee HW, Lee HJ, Hwang JS, Sohn JH, Jang JY, Han KJ, Park JY, Kim do Y, Ahn SH, Paik YH, Lee CK, Lee KS, Chon CY, Han KH. Lamivudine maintenance beyond one year after HBeAg seroconversion is a major factor for sustained virologic response in HBeAg-positive chronic hepatitis B. Hepatology. 2010;51:415–21.
25. Wang L, Liu F, Liu YD, Li XY, Wang JB, Zhang ZH, Park JY, Kim do Y, Ahn SH, Paik YH, Lee CK, Lee KS, Chon CY, Han KH. Stringent cessation criterion results in better durability of lamivudine treatment: a prospective clinical study in hepatitis B e antigen-positive chronic hepatitis B patients. J Viral Hepat. 2010;17:298–304.
26. Ha M, Zhang G, Diao S, Lin M, Sun L, She H, Kuan C, Shen L, Huang C, Shen W, Huang Z. A prospective clinical study in hepatitis B e antigen-negative chronic hepatitis B patients with stringent cessation criteria for adefovir. Arch Virol. 2012;157:285–90.
27. Song MJ, Song do S, Kim HY, Yoo SH, Bae SH, Choi JY, Yoon SK, Paik YH, Lee JS, Lee HW, Kim HJ. Durability of viral response after off treatment in HBeAg positive chronic hepatitis B. World J Gastroenterol. 2012;18:6277–83.
28. Chang TT, Lai CL, Kew Yoon S, Lee SS, Coelho HS, Carrilho FJ, Poordad F, Halota W, Horsmans Y, Tsai N, Zhang H, Tenney DJ, Tamez R, Iloeje U. Entecavir treatment for up to 5 years in patients with hepatitis B e antigen-positive chronic hepatitis B. Hepatology. 2010;51:422–30.
29. Gish RG, Chang TT, Lai CL, de Man R, Gadano A, Poordad F, Yang J, Brett-Smith H, Tamez R. Loss of HBsAg antigen during treatment with entecavir or lamivudine in nucleoside-naive HBeAg-positive patients with chronic hepatitis B. J Viral Hepat. 2010;17:16–22.
30. Zoutendijk R, Reijnders JG, Brown A, Zoulim F, Mutimer D, Deterding K, Petersen J, Hofmann WP, Buti M, Santantonio T, van Bommel F, Pradat P, Oo Y, Luetgehetmann M, Berg T, Hansen BE, Wedemeyer H, Janssen HL, Group VSS. Entecavir treatment for chronic hepatitis B: adaptation is not needed for the majority of naive patients with a partial virological response. Hepatology. 2011;54:443–51.
31. Hosaka T, Suzuki F, Kobayashi M, Seko Y, Kawamura Y, Sezaki H, Petersen J, Hofmann WP, Buti M, Santantonio T, van Bommel F, Pradat P, Oo Y, Luetgehetmann M, Berg T, Hansen BE, Wedemeyer H, Janssen HL, Group VSS: Entecavir treatment for chronic hepatitis B: adaptation is not needed for the majority of naive patients with a partial virological response. Hepatology 2011, 54:443-45131. Hosaka T, Suzuki F, Kobayashi M, Seko Y, Kawamura Y, Sezaki H, Akuta N, Suzuki Y, Saitoh S, Arase Y, Ikeda K, Kobayashi M, Kumada H. Clearance of hepatitis B surface antigen during long-term nucleot(s)ide analog treatment in chronic hepatitis B: results from a nine-year longitudinal study. J Gastroenterol. 2013;48:930–41.
32. Kobayashi M, Hosaka T, Suzuki F, Akuta N, Sezaki H, Suzuki Y, Kawamura Y, Kobayashi M, Saitoh S, Arase Y, Ikeda K, Miyakawa Y, Kumada H. Seroclearance rate of hepatitis B surface antigen in 2,112 patients with chronic hepatitis in Japan during long-term follow-up. J Gastroenterol. 2014;49:538–46.
33. Kim GA, Lim YS, An J, Lee D, Shim JH, Kim KM, Lee HC, Chung YH, Lee YS, Suh DJ. HBsAg seroclearance after nucleoside analogue therapy in patients with chronic hepatitis B: clinical outcomes and durability. Gut. 2014;63:1325–32.
34. Matsumoto A, Tanaka E, Rokuhara A, Kiyosawa K, Kumada H, Omata M, Okita K, Hayashi N, Okanoue T, Iino S, Tanikawa K. Efficacy of lamivudine for preventing hepatocellular carcinoma in chronic hepatitis B: A multicenter retrospective study of 2795 patients. Hepatol Res. 2005;32:173–84.
35. Yuen MF, Seto WK, Chow DH, Tsui K, Wong DK, Ngai VW, Wong BC, Fung J, Yuen JC, Lai CL. Long-term lamivudine therapy reduces the risk of long-term complications of chronic hepatitis B infection even in patients without advanced disease. Antivir Ther. 2007;12:1295–303.
36. Hosaka T, Suzuki F, Kobayashi M, Seko Y, Kawamura Y, Sezaki H, Akuta N, Suzuki Y, Saitoh S, Arase Y, Ikeda K, Kobayashi M, Kumada H. Long-term entecavir treatment reduces hepatocellular carcinoma incidence in patients with hepatitis B virus infection. Hepatology. 2013;58:98–107.
37. Sung JJ, Tsoi KK, Wong VW, Li KC, Chan HL. Meta-analysis: Treatment of hepatitis B infection reduces risk of hepatocellular carcinoma. Aliment Pharmacol Ther. 2008;28:1067–77.

Integrative role of vitamin D related and Interleukin-28B genes polymorphism in predicting treatment outcomes of Chronic Hepatitis C

M. O. El-Derany[1], N. M. Hamdy[1], N. L. Al-Ansari[2] and H. O. El-Mesallamy[1*]

Abstract

Background: Improving prediction of treatment outcomes in chronic hepatitis C (CHC) genotype 4 (G4) is necessary to increase sustained viral response (SVR) rates. Vitamin D related and interferon stimulated genes are good candidates as they are recently crosstalk altering interferon response. Thus single nucleotide polymorphisms (SNPs) within some of these genes and multiple stepwise regression analysis including other independent predictors (IL28B(rs12979860), serum 25OH-vitamin D, serum alfa-fetoprotein (AFP)) were performed on a cohort of 200 Egyptian CHC patients treated with Pegylated interferon-alpha (Peg-IFN) plus ribavirin.

Methods: SNPs in cytochrome P-450 (CYP2R1)(rs10741657AG), vitamin D receptor (VDR)(rs2228570AG, rs1544410CT), oligoadenylate synthetases-like (OASL)(rs1169279CT) and adenosine deaminases acting on RNA (ADAR)(rs1127309TC) genes were analyzed by real-time PCR.

Results: The carrier state of A allele in VDR rs2228570 and CYP2R1 rs10741657 genes were independently associated with SVR [OR 6.453 & 3.536, $p < 0.01$ respectively]. Combining carriers of A allele in CYP2R1 and VDR genes with IL28B C/C genotype increased the probability of SVR from 80 % to reach 87.8 %, 93 % and 100 %. No relation was found between VDR rs1544410CT, ADAR rs1127309TC, OASL rs1169279CT polymorphisms and treatment outcome. Combining VDR rs2228570 A/A genotype with IL28B C/C genotype increased the probability of SVR from 82 % to reach 100 % and from 29 % to reach 80 % in C/T+ T/T IL28B genotype in none F4 liver disease patients.

Conclusion: Vitamin D related (VDR rs2228570 and CYP2R1 rs10741657) and IL28B rs12979860 genes polymorphisms accurately assure SVR in naïve CHC G4 patients treated with low cost standard therapy.

Keywords: CHC, VDR, CYP2R1, Vitamin D, G4

Background

Hepatitis C virus (HCV) is a hepatotropic non-cytopathic positive strand RNA virus, which represents a major cause of chronic hepatitis, cirrhosis, and hepatocellular carcinoma, affecting over 150 million people worldwide. In Egypt the condition is even worse just about every family is touched by hepatitis C it kills an estimated 40,000 Egyptian per year where at least 1 in every 10 of the population aged 15 to 59 is infected [1].

Pegylated interferon-alpha (Peg-IFN) plus ribavirin (RBV) constitutes the standard cornerstone therapy for chronic hepatitis C (CHC). Even though less than half of the patients are able to achieve sustained viral response (SVR) while the rest don't show response or experience sever complications [2]. By the introduction of the novel direct acting antivirals (DAAs), CHC treatment modalities dramatically evolve increasing rates of SVR, treatment efficacy and tolerability especially in patients with advanced liver

* Correspondence: hala.elmesallamy@hotmail.com
[1]Biochemistry Department, Faculty of Pharmacy, Ain Shams University, Cairo, Egypt

disease (fibrosis METAVIR score F3 or F4) [3, 4]. Yet, they are much more expensive if compared to the standard dual therapy [5] and a more questionable issue emerged about its availability in treating all CHC patients especially in low income developing countries [6]. Recently, according to the latest guidelines of the European Association for the Study of the Liver (EASL) six treatment options are available for patients infected with HCV genotype 4 (G4), including two interferon-containing regimens which are sofosbuvir and simeprevir and four interferon-free regimens which are combinations of sofosbuvir and simeprevir or sofosbuvir and ledipasvir or ombitasvir, paritaprevir and ritonavir or sofosbuvir and daily daclatasvir [4]. But EASL declared that the combination of PegIFN and RBV remains acceptable in settings where none of these options are available [4].

Thus, despite progress in DAAs there is still room for optimizing the efficacy of the lower cost standard dual therapy in naïve CHC patients. This aim could be obtained by further refining the treatment factors associated with maximal outcome benefits from dual therapy [7].

Several predictors of successful treatment response of CHC are identified [8]. Some of these depend on the virus itself others are host-related, either genetic (interleukin 28B (IL28B) rs12979860 gene polymorphism, gender and race) or acquired (insulin resistance, obesity, liver steatosis and liver fibrosis stage) [9, 10]. To refine the predictive capacity of these biomarkers for the response to Peg-IFN and RBV, additional baseline predictors of clinical response would be welcomed [10].

Vitamin D appears to possess an important immune-modulator effect beside its classical action on calcium metabolism [11]. Deficiency of vitamin D is very common in CHC patients [12]. Though, conflicting results were found by relating these deficiencies with the success of Peg-IFN and RBV therapy [13, 14]. Vitamin D undergoes two activation processes before its interaction with vitamin D receptor (VDR) [15]. The first activation is performed in the liver by cytochrome P-450 family 2, subfamily R, polypeptide 1 (CYP2R1) and produces 25-hydroxylated form of vitamin D [13]. This step produces the main circulating vitamin D form in serum. By means of CYP27B1, vitamin D is subjected to its second hydroxylation which leads to the production of 1,25(OH) active vitamin D form which interacts with its specific transmembrane receptor VDR to exert its physiological functions [16]. CYP2R1 and VDR genes have different polymorphic forms which are recently suggested to influence the efficacy of antiviral therapy. On the other hand single functional nucleotide polymorphism (SNP) of CYP27B1 gene fails to predict antiviral response in CHC patients mainly genotype 1 [7, 10].

A more recent study found that VDR crosstalk the Jak–STAT pathway through altered expression of interferon stimulated genes (ISGs) which results in calcitriol-mediated increase of hepatocellular response to interferon-alpha (IFN-α) [17]. Where, signaling the expression of ISGs by the administration of exogenous interferon provides antiviral action against HCV through interferon receptors and through Jak–STAT pathway [18]. Of these ISGs functional SNPs at oligoadenylate synthetases-like (OASL) gene and adenosine deaminases acting on RNA (ADAR) gene were found to affect the response to antiviral therapy of HCV genotype 1 [19, 20].

Knowing that different HCV genotypes respond differently to interferon antiviral therapy [21] and based on the aformetioned information we aimed to investigate for the first time the influence of SNPs in CYP2R1 gene, VDR gene, OASL gene and ADAR gene as well as IL28B gene, serum 25-OH vitamin D levels, serum levels of AFP and insulin resistance in treatment outcomes of Egyptian CHC G4 patients treated with Peg-IFN and RBV.

Methods

Study population

Two hundred Egyptian patient infected with HCV G4 were enrolled in this study. Baseline and clinical characteristics are summarized in Table 1. The population study included all patients with CHC G4 attended to Dr. Yassin Abdel Ghaffar center for liver diseases and researches, Cairo, Egypt who were scheduled to receive Peg-IFN and RBV therapy in accordance with the current guidelines [22]. They received Peg-IFN (Pegasys, Roche Corporation, Kenilworth, NJ or Pegintron, Roche, Basel, Switzerland) at a dosage of 180 μg per week and RBV (Copegus, Roche or Rebetol, Schering-Plough, Puerto Rico, U.S.A.) which was administered according to body weight (1000 mg/d for patients weighing <75 kg, 1200 mg/d for those weighting ≥75 kg). Patients were selected according to the following criteria: (1) older than 18 years, (2) lack of co-infection with HBV, HIV, EBV, and CMV, (3) no history of alcohol consumption, (4) no bilharzias or diabetes mellitus, (5) not suffering from other autoimmune or hematological diseases and (6) adherence to treatment. Patients were asked to stick to the follow-up visits scheduled at week 4, 12, 24, 36, 48, 72 and 6 months after end of the treatment date. Patients were defined as having a SVR if they had undetectable serum HCV-RNA (Roche Amplicor™ Assay) levels 6 months after the discontinuation of treatment. All other patients were defined as non-responders (NRs). The study was approved by the Committee on

Table 1 Baseline clinical characteristics of HCV-infected patients included in the present study

Characteristics	SVR ($n = 91$	NR ($n = 109$)	P value	Statistics (univariate) OR(95%CI)
Age mean ± SD (years)	49.7 ± 7.5	51.5 ± 8.5	-	
Gender distribution[n(%)]			-	
Male	61(67)	68(62.4)		
Female	30(33)	41(37.6)		
BMI, median (range), kg/m^2	23 ± 12	24 ± 13.5	-	
No of injections, median (range)	48(24)	48(67)	0.001	1.035(1.013-1.058)
Tolerability, [n(%)]	91(100)	88(80.7)	-	
*Adjusted No of injections ,mean ± SEM	39.23 ± 1.179	38.218 ± 1.072	-	
Viral load median, IU/mL	460,000	760,580	0.025	0.637(0.429-0.945)
400,000 IU/mL[n(%)] > Viral load	41(45.1)	38(34.9)	-	
Viral load ≥400,000 IU/mL[n(%)]	50(54.9)	71(65.1)	-	
[a]AST median (range), μkat/L	1.66(4.65)	1.44(4.22)	-	
[b]ALT median (range), μkat/L	2.04(6.22)	1.7(5.63)	-	
Albumin median (range), g/L	39 ± 20	39 ± 22	-	
Bilirubin median (range), μmol/L	13.68 ± 50.45	15.39 ± 44.46	-	
Hemoglobin median (range), g/dL	13 ± 6.1	13.5 ± 7	-	
Platelets median (range), 10^9/L	190(241)	160(320)	0.012	3.299(1.306-8.334)
[c]TLC median (range), 10^9/μL	6(10)	6.4(6)	-	
Cholesterol mean ± SD, mmol/L	4.41 ± 0.78	4.69 ± 0.66	-	
Glucose median (range), mmol/L	5.27 ± 3.38	5.5 ± 3.1	-	
Insulin median (range), pmol/L	79.8 ± 127	62.5 ± 147.2	-	
[d]HOMA-IR median (range)	2.4 ± 5.71	2.2 ± 6.8	-	
[e]AFP median (range), ng/mL	3.3(29.5)	7(29)	<0.001	0.165(0.071-0.383)
25-OH Vitamin D median (range),ng/mL	28 ± 38	19 ± 38	<0.001	4.877(2.512-9.468)
Cirrhosis, [n(%)]	5(5.5)	15(13.7)	-	
Fibrosis stage, [n(%)]				
F1	21(42)	12(18.4)	0.006	3.198(1.378-7.419)
F2	16(32)	29(44.6)	-	
F3	12(24)	16(24.6)	-	
F4	1(2)	8(12.3)	-	
Necroinflammatory grade, [n(%)]				
A1	26(52)	27(41.5)	-	
A2	22(44)	27(41.5)	-	
A3	2(4)	11(17)	0.04	0.204(0.043-0.97)
IL28B rs12979860 [n(%)]			Chi^2 = 55.2 $p < 0.001$	
C/C	56(61.5)	14(12.8)	<0.001	10.857(5.379-21.913)
C/T	31(34.1)	67(61.5)	<0.001	0.324(0.181-0.579)
T/T	4(4.4)	28(25.7)	<0.001	0.133(0.045-0.395)
T allele carriers/ T allele non carriers	35/56	94/14	<0.001	0.092(0.046-0.186)

[a] AST, aspartate aminotransferase; [b] ALT, alanine aminotransferase; [c] TLC, total leukocyte count; [d] HOMA-IR, homeostatic model of insulin resistance; [e] AFP, alfa feto protein; NR, non-responders; SVR, sustained virological responders; N, number of samples; OR, odds ratio; 95%CI Confidence Interval.; Chi-square test for genotype distribution; IL28B: interleukin 28 B

*Calculated by general linear model with adjustment for tolerability

Medical Ethics of ASUH, and informed consent was obtained from each patient for participation and publishing results obtained. The study was carried out in accordance with the regulations and recommendations of the Declaration of Helsinki. Blood samples for biochemical, virologic and genetic studies were obtained during the month previous to the onset of therapy. Histopathological data were collected when a liver biopsy performed within the previous six months was available. Liver biopsy specimens were scored using the METAVIR system [23]. All biopsies were evaluated and scored by the same pathologist.

Laboratory analyses

Routine hematological and biochemical tests were performed after an overnight fast with the standard methods at the center's laboratory. It includes complete blood count (CBC), serum transaminases (ALT, AST), total and conjugated bilirubin, serum albumin, alpha-feto protein (AFP), blood sugar and serum cholesterol.

Virological testing

For all 200 patient, a baseline serum sample, collected before starting antiviral therapy, was separated and stored at _80 °C until used. The presence or absence of HCV antibodies was detemined by third generation ELISA (Dia Sorin). Serum HCV RNA was detected by using the real time polymerase chain reaction (RT-PCR) (TaqMan Roche Amplicor™ Assay) [24]. Viral load was classified as low (<400.000 IU/ml) or high (≥400.000 IU/ml), according to Wittho¨ft et al. [25].

Genotyping

Genomic DNA was extracted with QIAamp DNA Mini Kit protocol (QIAGEN, Santa Clarita, CA) according to the manufacturer's instructions. DNA samples were subjected to DNA quantitation and purity assessment using the NanoDrop® (ND)-1000 spectrophotometer (NanoDrop Technologies, Inc. Wilmington, USA).

Analyses of interleukin 28B gene

Genotyping was carried out by the use of TaqMan® QRT-PCR Reagents constitutes a ready-to-use system for the detection of IL-28B rs12979860 polymorphism using (Assays-by-Design supplied by Applied Biosystems International ABI; Applied Biosystems, Foster City, CA) according to the manufacturer's instructions.

Analyses of Vitamin D-related genes

Genotyping was carried out by the use of TaqMan probes designed to detect the following SNPs: CYP2R1, rs10741657; VDR, rs2228570; VDR, rs1544410 (custom TaqMan SNP assay C___2958430_10; C___12060045_20 and C___8716062_10 respectively using Assays-by-Design supplied by Applied Biosystems International ABI; Applied Biosystems, Foster City, CA). The SNPs were selected on the basis of allele frequencies and functional clinical implications [7, 10]. The only nonsynonymous SNP confirmed for the VDR gene was included in the study. No other nonsynonymous SNPs have been described to occur in Caucasian individuals with minor allele frequencies over 0.001.

Analysis of interferon stimulated genes

Genotyping was carried out by the use of TaqMan probes designed to detect the following SNPs: OASL rs1169279 and ADAR, rs1127309 (custom TaqMan SNP assay C___1263582_10 and C____131814_1_; using Assays-by-Design supplied by Applied Biosystems International ABI; Applied Biosystems, Foster City, CA). The SNPs were also selected on the basis of allele frequencies and functional of clinical implications [19, 20] (see the website http://www.ncbi.nlm.nih.gov/projects/SNP/).

Putative departures of Hardy-Weinberg Equilibrium was calculated by using the software Haploview 4.1. [26].

Serum 25-OH vitamin D and serum insulin

Serum human 25-OH vitamin D levels were determined by enzyme linked immunosorbent assay (ELISA) using commercially available kits (DRG International, Inc., USA). The data are expressed as nanograms per milliliter. Serum insulin was also quantified using ELISA technique using commercial available kit (Nova Tec Immundiagnostica GmbH, Germany). The homeostasis model assessment of insulin resistance (HOMA-IR) was calculated from fasting insulin and FBG by the following equation: HOMA-IR = fasting insulin (μU/mL) × FBG (mg/dL)/405 [27]. All ELISA procedures were done by Hyprep Automated ELISA system (Hyperion Inc, Miami, FL) according to the manufacturer's instructions.

Statistical analysis

IBM SPSS statistics (V. 22.0, IBM Corp., USA, 2013) was used for data analysis. Shapiro-Wilk test was used to test the normal distribution of data. Continuous variables were expressed as mean ± SD for parametric data while median (range) was used for non- parametric data. Additionally, categorical variables were presented as frequencies (percentage). Comparison between two independent mean groups for parametric data were performed using Student's *t*-test and Wilcoxon rank-sum test was carried out for comparison between two independent groups for non-parametric. The associations between categorical variables were evaluated using a Pearson chi-squared test and, when appropriate, a chi-squared test for linear trend. Hardy–Weinberg equilibrium was assessed in the study population. General linear model was used to control for potential confounders.

Significant covariates at binary logistic regression analysis were included in a multivariate stepwise logistic regression model with a forward approach to identify independent predictors of SVR. In addition, any skewed data were logarithmically transformed before performing simple and multiple binary stepwise regression analyses. The AUROC indicated the prediction capacity of this analysis. The results were reported as odds ratio (OR) and their 95 % confidence intervals (CIs). A difference of $p < 0.05$ was considered significant.

Results

The clinical and demographic characteristics of the 200 patient are shown in Table 1. 54.5 % of the patients (n = 109) were classified as NR and 45.5 % (n = 91) were classified as SVR. The univariate analysis expressed in Table 1 revealed the following variables were significantly linked with SVR rates: lower viral load (OR = 0.637–95 % CI =0.429–0.945- $p = 0.025$), higher platelets count (OR = 3.299–95 % CI =1.306–8.334- $p = 0.012$), lower serum AFP levels (OR = 0.165–95 % CI =0.071–0.383- $p < 0.001$), higher serum 25-OH vitamin D levels (OR = 4.877–95 % CI =2.512–9.468- $p < 0.001$), the absence of higher fibrosis grade (OR = 3.198–95 % CI =1.378–7.419- $p = 0.006$), and the absence of A3 necroinflammatory grade (OR = 0.204–95 % CI =0.043–0.97- $p = 0.04$). Additionally, number of injections was found to be related to SVR with (OR = 1.035–95 % CI =1.013–1.058- $p = 0.001$). General linear model was performed to control confounding variables as (age, gender, BMI and interferon tolerability) and found that all adjusted values for variables were still significantly related to treatment response except for the adjusted number of injections which loses its significance to SVR due to the effect of interferon tolerability where number of injections were found to be heavily dependent on tolerability with $p < 0.001$ rather than on treatment response with $p = 0.204$.

Exploring the association of IL28B rs12979870, CYP2R1 rs10741657, VDR (rs2228570, rs1544410), OASL rs1169279 and ADAR rs1127309 genes polymorphism with response to antiviral treatment were shown in Tables 1 and 2, it was found that the absence of IL28B rs12979870T allele carrier state ($chi^2 = 51.69$- $p < 0.001$), the prescence of CYP2R1 rs10741657 and VDR rs2228570 A allele carrier states ($chi^2 = 4.888$- $p = 0.027$, $chi^2 = 4.138$- $p = 0.042$ respectively), and OASL rs1169279T allele carrier state ($chi^2 = 6.23$- $p = 0.013$), were significantly predicting SVR in CHC G4 patients.

These significant variables were included in the multivariate binary logistics regression analysis after controlling for the confounders. Where, IL28B gene polymorphism showed the highest significance as C/T + T/T genotypes were inversely associated with SVR (OR = 0.064–95 % CI =0.022–0.184- $p < 0.001$). Beside serum AFP levels and basic viral load were found to be inversely related to SVR (OR = 0.241–95 % CI =0.071–0.816- $p = 0.022$) and (OR = 0.523–95 % CI =0.228–0.951- $p = 0.033$), respectively. On the other hand, serum 25-OH vitamin D levels were confirmed by this study to predict SVR (OR = 7.361–95 % CI =2.828–19.162- $p < 0.001$). A negative cut-off value for serum 25-OH vitamin D levels was calculated to be up to 12 ng/ml with a negative predictive value of 87.5 % and sensitivity of 95.6 %. While a positive predictive value of 69.6 % and specificity of 93.6 % was calculated for the positive cut-off value to be up to 38 ng/ml.

Additionally, the carrier state of allele A at CYP2R1 rs10741657 was found to be inversely related to the probability of therapeutic failure (OR = 3.536–95 % CI = 1.444–8.659- $p = 0.006$). Besides, the carrier state of the minor A allele at VDR rs2228570 was significantly related to the probability of obtaining SVR (OR = 6.453–95 % CI =2.348–17.739- $p < 0.001$).

The ROC was plotted in accordance with the same model as expressed in Fig. 1. The predictive capacity of the final model was quite good as indicated by the AUROC 0.887(95 % CI = 0.842–0.993). Multiple stepwise logistic regression analysis was made to establish the increase in the predictive value of the well-known and recognized IL28B rs12979870 C/T polymorphism. It showed that our model presented significantly increase the sensitivity of IL28B rs12979870 from 61.5 % to reach 75.8 % as well as increasing the accuracy of IL28B rs12979870 from 75.5 % to reach 81 % without significantly affecting IL28B rs12979870 specificity to be 85.3 %.

For confirming the integrative role of VDR rs2228570, CYP2R1 rs10741657 polymorphisms with IL28B rs12979870 polymorphism we further classified our SVR data into four groups depending on IL28B genotype regarding the carrier state of both CYP2R1 rs10741657 and VDR rs2228570 gene. Based on our results the rate of SVR was predicted by 80 % of IL28B C/C genotype patients. We confirmed for the first time that the combination of A allele carrier of VDR rs2228570 gene with IL28B C/C genotype increases SVR rate to reach 93 % and 87.8 % for A allele carrier of CYP2R1 rs10741657 gene with IL28B C/C ($P < 0.001$). Additionally, for each examined variable it was found that there is a highly significant linear trend in the decrease of the SVR rate as shown in Table 3. Formulating a model combining A allele carrier of VDR rs2228570 and CYP2R1 rs10741657 gene and IL28B C/C genotype increased the SVR rate reaching 100 % and 17 % in non A allele carrier of VDR rs2228570 and CYP2R1 rs10741657 gene with IL28B C/T + T/T genotype ($P < 0.001$).

Interestingly we investigate the role of our predictors in different fibrosis grade models. Actually liver

Table 2 Association analysis of genes polymorphisms with the response to antiviral treatment

Genotype/ Allele	SVR $N = 91$	NR $N = 109$	P value	OR(95%CI)
CYP2R1 rs10741657 [n(%)]			$Chi^2 = 5.38$ $p = 0.06$	
A/A	7(7.7)	4(3.7)		
A/G	44(48.4)	40(36.7)		
G/G	40(44)	59.6))65	0.028	0.531(0.302-0.933)
A allele carriers/A allele non carriers	51/40	44/65	0.027	1.884(1.072-3.310)
VDR rs2228570 [n(%)]			$Chi^2 = 8.66$ $p = 0.013$	
A/A	13(14.3)	4(3.7)	0.013	4.375(1.374-13.932)
A/G	36(39.6)	39(35.8)		
G/G	42(46.2)	66(60.6)		
A allele carriers/A allele non carriers	49/42	43/66	0.042	1.791(1.019-3.146)
VDR rs1544410 [n(%)]			n.s.	
C/C	30(33)	38(34.9)		
C/T	39(42.9)	47(43.1)		
T/T	22(24.9)	24(22)		
T allele carriers/ T allele non carriers	61/30	71/38		
OASL rs1169279 [n(%)]			$Chi^2 = 5.4$ $p = 0.06$	
C/C	19(20.9)	39(55.8)	0.022	0.474(0.250-0.898)
C/T	52(57.1)	49(45)		
T/T	20(22)	21(19.3)		
T allele carriers/ T allele non carriers	72/19	70/39	0.013	2.26(1.182-4.318)
ADAR rs1127309 [n(%)]			n.s.	
C/C	30(33)	38(34.9)		
C/T	39(42.9)	47(43.1)		
T/T	22(24.2)	24(22)		
T allele carriers/ T allele non carriers	61/30	71/109		

OR, odds ratio; 95%CI Confidence Interval; n.s., non-significant; SVR: sustained viral response; NR: non response; CYP2R1: cytochrome P-450 family 2, subfamily R; VDR: vitamin D receptor; OASL: oligoadenylate synthetases-like; ADAR: adenosine deaminases acting on RNA
Chi-square test for genotype distribution

biopsies were available for 115 patient. So 106 patient remained after excluding advanced fibrosis F4 and cirrhotic patient at which 53.4 % ($n = 57$) were NR and 46.2 % ($n = 49$) were SVR as shown in Table 4. Univariate analysis showed that some variables significantly predict SVR as: higher serum 25-OH vitamin D levels (OR = 1.068–95 % CI =1.024–1.115- $p = 0.002$), the absence of IL28B rs12979870T allele carrier state ($chi^2 = 26.281$- $p < 0.001$) and the presence of VDR rs2228570 A/A genotype state ($chi^2 = 8.511$- $p = 0.018$). CYP2R1 rs10741657 A allele carrier state showed insignificant relation to SVR (chi2 = 2.834- $p = 0.12$). Number of injections was found to be related to SVR (OR = 1.042–95 % CI =1.013–1.072 - $p = 0.004$) and lower serum AFP levels (OR = 0.563–95 % CI =0.342–0.928- $p = 0.024$) yet the adjusted number of injections for interferon tolerability and the adjusted serum AFP levels also lost their significance to SVR with $p = 0.386$ and $p = 0.205$ respectively.

Multivariate binary logistic regression analysis were made after controlling for the confounders and found that IL28B gene polymorphism showed highest significance as C/T + T/T genotypes were inversely associated with SVR (OR = 0.138–95 % CI =0.045–0.423- $p = 0.001$). While, serum 25-OH vitamin D levels (OR = 1.076–95 % CI =1.013–1.144- $p = 0.018$) and also the presence of A/A genotype state of VDR rs2228570 (OR = 10.3–95 % CI =1.118–94.887- $p = 0.04$) were directly associated with SVR. The ROC was plotted in accordance with the same model showed that the AUROC was 0.837 (95 % CI = 0.76–0.951). Multiple stepwise logistic regression analysis showed that our model significantly increase the sensitivity of IL28B rs12979870 from 57.1 % to reach 67.3 % as well as increasing the accuracy of IL28B rs12979870 from

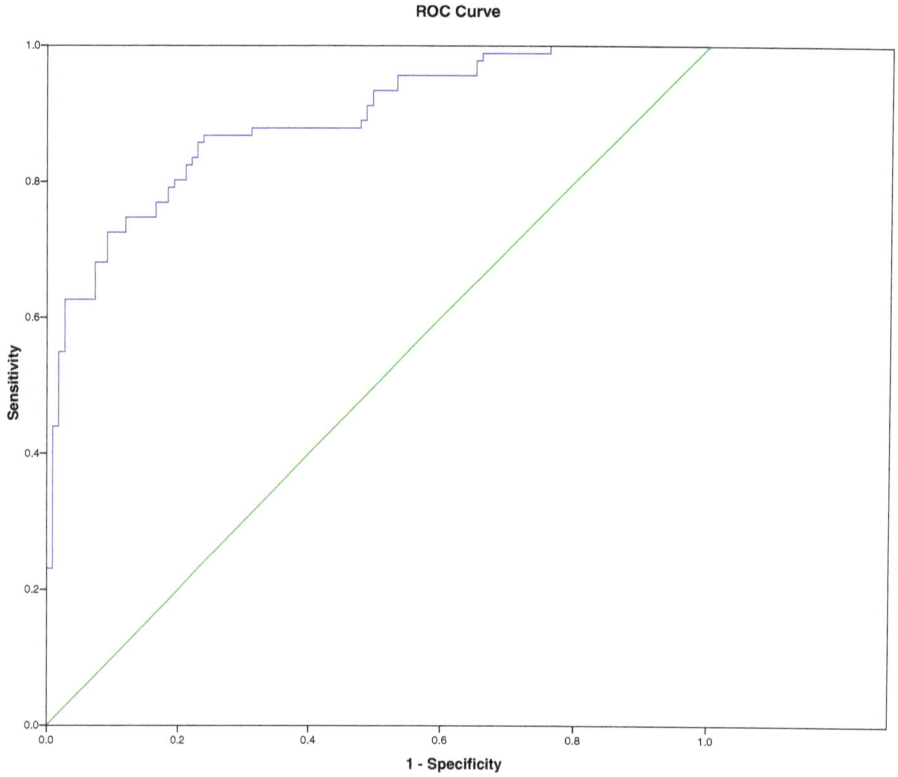

Fig. 1 ROC curve of the multivariate analysis. Area under the curve (AUC) was 0.887 (95 % CI = 0.842–0.993)

74.5 % to reach 77.4 % without significantly affecting IL28B rs12979870 specificity to be 89.5 %.

Classifying our SVR data into four groups depending on IL28B genotype found that combining IL28B C/C genotype with VDR rs2228570 A/A genotype increased the predictive capacity of IL28B C/C genotype from 82.2 % to reach 100 %. More importantly combining VDR rs2228570 A/A genotype with IL28B C/T + T/T increased the SVR from 29 % to reach 80 %.

By formulating a second model excluding F3, F4 and cirrhotic patients 78 patient remained at which 52.5 % ($n = 41$) were NR and 47.4 % ($n = 37$) were SVR. It was found that IL28B C/C genotype is the only predictor of SVR (OR = 20.81–95 % CI =5.394–80.286 - $p < 0.001$). The AUROC equals 0.774 (95 % CI = 0.665–0.883) the calculated specificity, sensitivity and accuracy were 92.7 %, 62.2 % and 78.2 % respectively.

Discussion

The need for optimizing the standard dual anti-HCV therapy is mandatory owing to the high socioeconomic burden associated with recently introduced DAAs [6, 28]. Although DAAs showed strong anti-HCV effects, DAA monotherapy induced drug-resistant and virus mutations. Concluding that the main role of DAAs has been to increase the treatment efficacy of Peg-IFN-α and RBV [29].

Table 3 Rates of SVR in relationship to IL28B rs12979860 and vitamin D related genes polymorphisms

	SVR				*P* value
IL28B rs12979860	C/C	C/C	C/T + T/T	C/T + T/T	
CYP2R1 rs10741657	A allele carrier	Non A carrier	A allele carrier	Non A carrier	
N(%)	29/33 (87.8 %)	27/37(72.9 %)	22/62(35.4 %)	13/68(19.1 %)	<0.001
VDR rs2228570	A allele carrier	Non A carrier	A allele carrier	Non A carrier	
N(%)	27/29(93 %)	29/41(70.7 %)	23/66(34.8 %)	12/64(18.7)	<0.001
CYP2R1 & VDR	A allele carrier	Non A carrier	A allele carrier	Non A carrier	
N(%)	17(100 %)	15/23(65.2 %)	15/30(50 %)	6/35(17 %)	<0.001

The statistical analysis was performed using a chi-squared test for linear trend
IL28B: Interleukin 28 B; SVR: sustained viral response; CYP2R1: cytochrome P-450 family 2, subfamily R; VDR: vitamin D receptor

Table 4 Baseline clinical characteristics of HCV-infected F1, F2 and F3 patients

Characteristics	SVR (*n* = 49)	NR (*n* = 57)	*P* value	Statistics (univariate) OR(95%CI)
Age mean ± SD (years)	50.2 ± 8.5	49.3 ± 7.9	-	
Gender distribution[n(%)]			-	
Male	34(69.3)	34(59.6)		
Female	15(30.6)	23(40.3)		
BMI, median (range), kg/m^2	23 ± 12	23 ± 12	-	
No of injection,s median (range)	48(24)	24(62)	0.004	1.042 (1.013- 1.072)
Tolerability, [n(%)]	49(100)	43(75.4)		
*Adjusted No of injections ,mean ± SEM	37.28 ± 1.74	35.14 ± 1.63	-	
Viral load median, IU/mL	432,210	738,902	-	
[a]AST median (range), µkat/L	1.66(4.23)	1.28(4.2)	-	
[b]ALT median (range), µkat/L	1.78(5.47)	2.091(5.62)	-	
Albumin median (range), g/L	39 ± 20	39 ± 10	-	
Bilirubin median (range), µmol/L	15.39 ± 50.44	13.6 ± 25.6	-	
Hemoglobin median (range), g/dL	13 ± 5.6	13.8 ± 4.6	-	
Platelets median (range), 10^9/L	163(236)	170(207)	-	
[c]TLC mean ± SD, 10^9/µL	6.5(1.7)	6.5(1.3)	-	
Cholesterol mean ± SD, mmol/L	4.1 ± 0.86	4.2 ± 0.6	-	
Glucose median (range), mmol/L	5.27 ± 3.277	5.5 ± 3.1	-	
Insulin median (range), pmol/L	79.6 ± 113.2	63.5 ± 133.3	-	
[d]HOMA-IR median (range)	2.5 ± 5.71	2.16 ± 6.04	-	
[e]AFP median (range), ng/mL	3.5(29.5)	8(26.3)	0.024	0.563 (0.342- 0.928)
*Adjusted AFP, mean ± SE	3.5 ± 0.049	3.448 ± 0.045		
25-OH Vitamin D mean ± SD, ng/mL	27.3 ± 9.2	21.07 ± 10.1	0.002	1.068(1.024-1.115)
IL28B rs12979860 [n(%)]			Chi^2 = 31.35 $p < 0.001$	
C/C	28(57.1)	6(10.5)	<0.001	11.33(4.09-39.35)
C/T	20(40.8)	35(62.4)		
T/T	1(2)	16(28.07)		
T allele carriers/ T allele non carriers	21/28	51/6	<0.001	0.088(0.032-0.244)
VDR rs2228570 [n(%)]			Chi^2 = 8.554 $p = 0.014$	
A/A	9(18.3)	1(1.7)	0.018	12.6(1.53-103.4)
A/G	18(36.7)	24(42.1)		
G/G	22(44.8)	32(56.1)		

[a] AST, aspartate aminotransferase; [b] ALT, alanine aminotransferase; [c] TLC, total leukocyte count; [d] HOMA-IR, homeostatic model of insulin resistance; [e] AFP, alfa feto protein; NR, non-responders; SVR, sustained virological responders; N, number of samples; OR, odds ratio; 95%CI Confidence Interval.; Chi-square test for genotype distribution; IL28B: interleukin 28 B
*Calculated by general linear model with adjustment for tolerability

This paves the way for elucidating new markers that would improve the prediction of Peg-IFN and RBV treatment outcomes. Although several studies have identified specific viral and host genetic factors that predict treatment outcomes, studies regarding G4 are few and the pursuit of further surrogate factors able to optimize therapeutic regimes remains challenging [30]. Due to these facts, we have a great research interest in examining for the first time the relationship between previously described polymorphisms of vitamin D related genes and ISGs with the treatment of HCV G4 patients.

In this study we found a predictive potential of baseline 25-OH vitamin D levels on treatment outcomes. Recent findings from various studies investigating the predictive role of vitamin D levels offered conflicting evidences. On one hand low pretreatment vitamin D concentrations correlated with poor responsiveness to antiviral therapy [31] and on the other hand Kitson et al., showed that vitamin D levels seemed unable to predict treatment response in patients infected with HCV genotype 1 [14]. Yet all these hitherto existing analyses were made on genotype 1 with incomplete consideration of genetic factors affecting vitamin D levels. In this present study only G4 was included and the effect of SNP's within major regulatory enzyme and in vitamin D receptor, which were previously shown to affect vitamin D concentrations, activity and were associated with outcomes of antiviral therapy, were considered [7, 10, 32].

Our results revealed that high serum 25-OH vitamin D levels in the multivariate analysis that included the most potent predictors of viral response at baseline increase the SVR of Peg-IFN and RBV treatment. Also our study concluded that the negative predictive value was 12 ng/ml for 87.5 % of CHC G4 patients who fails to reach SVR and the positive predictive value of 69.6 % was found to be 38 ng/ml which weren't calculated for the Egyptian G4 patients before yet found in agreement to other studies [33]. Interestingly high serum 25-OH vitamin D levels predicted SVR in noneF4 fibrosis grade patients which was recently emphasized by previous studies showing that vitamin D deficiency is associated with advanced liver disease and is an indicator for a poor outcome [34, 35]. This highlights the importance of vitamin D in disease worsening via fibrosis progression and thus it reflects indirectly the importance of fibrosis resolution in CHC treatment [36].

Additionally, the analysis of an already identified SNP (rs10741657) within the CYP2R1 gene on chromosome 11p15, which is one of the main polymorphisms found to be associated with 25(OH) vitamin D circulating levels [37], showed that the carrier state of allele A at CYP2R1 gene predicts SVR. This comes in accordance with a recent study that focused on the association of the absence of A allele with vitamin D insufficiency [38]. Where, our study confirmed that the presence of A allele is associated with higher vitamin D serum levels and is independently predicting SVR in multivariate logistic regression analysis yet it failed to predict response in noneF4 liver disease patients this might be attributed to small sample size.

Moreover, studying the common nonsynonymous SNP in the VDR gene (rs2228570) which cause a threonine-metionine change in the VDR, found that those patients carrying the minor A allele in homo- or heterozygosis obtained SVR at a higher rate than patients with the rs2228570 G/G genotype. This agrees with a recent study made on genotype 1 [10]. Our study additionally showed for the first time that VDR rs2228570 A/A genotype is an independent predictor of SVR in noneF4 fibrosis grade CHC G4 patients which adds to the importance of this rs2228570 in predicting treatment success. In contrast we found no association between SNP in VDR gene (rs1544410) and treatment outcome in our population. This can be explained as our study include only single rs1544410 alone unlike others [10, 39] who categorize the patients as non-carriers/carriers of the rs1544410C- rs7975232C - rs731236A three allelic combination. Thereby, we concluded that we can't account on VDR gene rs1544410 SNP alone in predicting therapeutic failure.

Moreover, a recent study highlighting the possible interaction between VDR and ISGs suggested a role for vitamin D in the response to IFN-α–based therapy [17]. Importantly, and in line with these observations, our study assayed two functional SNPs at two important ISGs which were proven by previous studies to predict antiviral response of CHC genotype 1 [19, 20]. First one was OASL being recognized as a significant molecule in antiviral response with the 2′-5′ oligoadenylate catalytic activity in innate viral clearance. The SNP (rs1169279) is located in the 5′ upstream region of the gene and found to be a promoter polymorphism which may regulate gene expression. Our findings identified that OASL gene polymorphism is not the main player in HCV G4 treatment response as T allele carriers lost their significance in multivariate regression analysis. This can be attributed to the difference in viral genotypes as the previous study was made on genotype 1 [19]. Additionally, it also showed no relation in none-advanced liver disease patients though, larger sample size is recommended to assure our findings.

Regarding the second ISG examined SNP (rs1127309) is a synonymous variant in ADAR gene, our study on the whole populatin and after excluding advanced fibrosis grades patients found no association between ADAR gene polymorphism and Peg-IFN and RBV treatment outcomes. This disagrees with the previous study made by Welzel, et al. [20]. And could be explained by the difference in the percent of genetic variation (presence of T allele) accounted by the selected ADAR SNP. Where in European American the presence of T allele is about (50 %) and our Caucasian population is (66 %). Additionally, the previous study was a Hepatitis C Antiviral Long-term Treatment against Cirrhosis (HALT-C) trial unlike our study which includes insignificant number of cirrhotic patients.

In agreement with other studies suggested adding AFP to the list of predictive factors for treatment response in CHC G4 [40, 41]. Our results showed that increased AFP serum levels are an independent factor of therapeutic failure. This may be explained by intense hepatic progenitor cells expression in NR compared to SVR. Hepatic progenitor cells arise in the periportal region of the liver and may be responsible for liver regeneration and they express high levels of AFP. Quite interestingly, hepatic progenitor cells expression is associated with response to treatment, being higher in NR compared with responders. This may postulate the factor explaining the association of AFP with therapeutic failure [42, 43]. Our results showed that serum AFP levels is not a predictor of SVR in none-advanced liver disease and this also agreed with a study made on G4 [41].

In alignment with other published studies [30, 44] our research didn't find association between cholesterol levels, insulin levels and HOMA-IR with antiviral response this may be probably explained by the absence of diabetes among our patients. On the other hand it was found that baseline lower viral load is a direct predictor to SVR rates as proved previously [45].

Finally we confirmed for the first time that vitamin D related genes (VDR rs2228570 and CYP2R1 rs10741657) polymorphism are completely independent of each other, may be usefully combined to enhance the predictive ability for treatment response. Where combing these two genes with IL28B rs12979860 C/C genotype increase the probability of SVR from 80 % to reach 100 %. Compared with patients carrying the IL28B rs12979860 C/C genotype and who carry at least one A allele of VDR rs2228570 and CYP2R1 rs10741657, the none A allele carriers identified patients showed a lower probability of SVR attainment. Furthermore, carrying at least one T allele of IL28B along with none A allele carrier of VDR rs2228570 and CYP2R1 rs10741657 gene showed the lowest probability of attaining the same viral endpoint. Yet increased the probability of SVR in IL28B C/T + T/T from 27 % to reach 50 %. Advanced fibrosis was proven previously to be a main factor for Peg-IFN and RBV treatment failure [45]. Thus more practically our study interestingly found that only serum levels of 25-OH vitamin D, VDR rs2228570 A/A genotype together with IL28B rs12979860 C/C genotype were the only predictors of SVR in none-F4 CHC patients. Moreover, we proved that the presence of VDR rs2228570 A/A genotype and IL28B rs12979860 C/C genotype increased SVR rates from 82 % reaching 100 % and more importantly combining VDR rs2228570 A/A genotype and IL28B C/T + T/T genotypes dramatically increase SVR from 29 % to reach 80 % which impressively increase treatment success prediction. Although promising yet larger sample size is required to assure our findings.

However in accordance with these data presented vitamin D related genes play an integrative role with IL2B gene in achieving SVR rates in CHC G4 patients.

Conclusions

In conclusion two polymorphic sites in VDR gene and CYP2R1 gene were found to increase the sensitivity and accuracy of IL28B gene in predicting SVR rates for Peg-IFN and RBV therapy in CHC patients G4. The association of these polymorphisms with the response rate is independent from other well-known predictors of response at baseline that were included in the multivariate analysis as potentially confounding factors. The use of these new genes could facilitate the treatment decision and individualize the therapeutic regimens by totally assuring patient's cure under low cost standard basic dual therapy.

Abbreviations

ADAR: adenosine deaminases acting on RNA; AFP: alfa-fetoprotein; ALT: alanine aminotransferase ; AUROC: area under the operating curve; CBC: complete blood count; CHC: chronic hepatitis C; CYP2R1: cytochrome P-450 family 2, subfamily R; DAAs: direct acting antivirals; EASL: European Association for the Study of the Liver; ELISA: enzyme linked immunosorbent assay; G4: genotype 4; HALT-C: Hepatitis C Antiviral Long-term Treatment against Cirrhosis; HCV: hepatitis C virus; HOMA-IR: homeostasis model assessment of insulin resistance; IL28B: interleukin 28B; NR: non-responders; OASL: oligoadenylate synthetases-like; Peg-IFN: Pegylated interferon-alpha; ROC: receiving operating curve; RT-PCR: real time polymerase chain reaction; SNPs: single nucleotide polymorphisms; SVR: sustained viral response; VDR: vitamin D receptor.

Competing interests

The authors declare that there is no conflict of interest that could be perceived as prejudicing the impartiality of the research reported.

Authors' contributions

MO, NH, NA and HO shared in the study design and concept, MO carried out the acquisition of data, MO and HO participated in the analysis and interpretation of data, MO and HO shared the drafting of the manuscript and the critical revision of the manuscript for important intellectual content. MO carried out the statistical analysis, MO, NH, NA and HO all shared the administrative, technical, and material support, HO, NH and NA shared the whole study supervision. All authors read and approved the final manuscript.

Acknowledgements

This research did not receive any specific grant from any funding agency in the public, commercial, or not-for-profit sector.
Authors would like to thank all laboratory team members at Dr. Yassin Abdel Ghaffar center for liver diseases and Dr. Nadia Al-Ansari's private clinic for their aid in technical laboratory analyses. Moreover, the authors would like to thank Prof. Dr Inas Elattar, professor of biostatistics, department of biostatistics and cancer epidemiology, National Cancer Institue, Cairo University for her great impact in revising the whole study statistics.

Author details

[1]Biochemistry Department, Faculty of Pharmacy, Ain Shams University, Cairo, Egypt. [2]Endemic Medicine Department & Hepatology Unit, Faculty of Medicine, Ain Shams University, Cairo, Egypt.

References

1. Wedemeyer H, Dore GJ, Ward JW. Estimates on HCV disease burden worldwide - filling the gaps. J Viral Hepat. 2015;22 Suppl 1:1–5. Epub 2015/01/07. eng.
2. Ghany MG, Strader DB, Thomas DL, Seeff LB. Diagnosis, management, and treatment of hepatitis C: an update. Hepatology (Baltimore, Md). 2009;49(4):1335–74. Epub 2009/03/31. eng.
3. Zimmermann HW, Tacke F. Sofosbuvir for hepatitis C - is brevity the soul of wit? Zeitschrift fur Gastroenterologie. 2013;51(9):1110–2. Epub 2013/09/12. Sofosbuvir fur Hepatitis C - Liegt die Wurze in der Kurze? ger.
4. EASL. Recommendations on Treatment of Hepatitis C 2015. J Hepatol. 2015;63(1):199–236. Epub 2015/04/26. eng.
5. Kim DD, Hutton DW, Raouf AA, et al. Cost-effectiveness model for hepatitis C screening and treatment: Implications for Egypt and other countries with

high prevalence. Glob Public Health. 2015;10(3):296–317. Pubmed Central PMCID: PMC4320005, Epub 2014/12/04. eng.

6. Camma C, Petta S, Enea M, et al. Cost-effectiveness of boceprevir or telaprevir for untreated patients with genotype 1 chronic hepatitis C. Hepatology (Baltimore, Md). 2012;56(3):850–60. Epub 2012/03/29. eng.
7. Falleti E, Cmet S, Fabris C, et al. Genetic polymorphisms of vitamin D pathway predict antiviral treatment outcome in slow responder naive patients with chronic hepatitis C. PLoS One. 2013;8(11):e80764. Pubmed Central PMCID: PMC3828272, Epub 2013/11/19. eng.
8. Asselah T, Estrabaud E, Bieche I, et al. Hepatitis C: viral and host factors associated with non-response to pegylated interferon plus ribavirin. Liver Int. 2010;30(9):1259–69. Pubmed Central PMCID: PMC3071938, Epub 2010/07/17. eng.
9. Maekawa S, Sakamoto M, Miura M, et al. Comprehensive analysis for viral elements and interleukin-28B polymorphisms in response to pegylated interferon plus ribavirin therapy in hepatitis C virus 1B infection. Hepatology (Baltimore, Md). 2012;56(5):1611–21. Epub 2012/05/12. eng.
10. Garcia-Martin E, Agundez JA, Maestro ML, et al. Influence of vitamin D-related gene polymorphisms (CYP27B and VDR) on the response to interferon/ribavirin therapy in chronic hepatitis C. PLoS One. 2013;8(9):e74764. Pubmed Central PMCID: PMC3779247, Epub 2013/09/28. eng.
11. White JH. Vitamin D, metabolism and signaling in the immune system. Rev Endocr Metab Disord. 2012;13(1):21–9. Epub 2011/08/17. eng.
12. Miroliaee A, Nasiri-Toosi M, Khalilzadeh O, Esteghamati A, Abdollahi A, Mazloumi M. Disturbances of parathyroid hormone-vitamin D axis in non-cholestatic chronic liver disease: a cross-sectional study. Hepatol Int. 2010;4(3):634–40. Pubmed Central PMCID: PMC2940008, Epub 2010/11/11. eng.
13. Bitetto D, Fattovich G, Fabris C, et al. Complementary role of vitamin D deficiency and the interleukin-28B rs12979860 C/T polymorphism in predicting antiviral response in chronic hepatitis C. Hepatology (Baltimore, Md). 2011;53(4):1118–26. Epub 2011/04/12. eng.
14. Kitson MT, Dore GJ, George J, et al. Vitamin D status does not predict sustained virologic response or fibrosis stage in chronic hepatitis C genotype 1 infection. J Hepatol. 2013;58(3):467–72. Epub 2012/11/28. eng.
15. Holick MF. Vitamin D: evolutionary, physiological and health perspectives. Curr Drug Targets. 2011;12(1):4–18. Epub 2010/08/28. eng.
16. Rosen CJ, Adams JS, Bikle DD, et al. The nonskeletal effects of vitamin D: an Endocrine Society scientific statement. Endocr Rev. 2012;33(3):456–92. Pubmed Central PMCID: PMC3365859, Epub 2012/05/19. eng.
17. Lange CM, Gouttenoire J, Duong FH, Morikawa K, Heim MH, Moradpour D. Vitamin D receptor and Jak-STAT signaling crosstalk results in calcitriol-mediated increase of hepatocellular response to IFN-alpha. J Immunol (Baltimore, Md : 1950). 2014;192(12):6037–44. Epub 2014/05/14. eng.
18. Feld JJ, Hoofnagle JH. Mechanism of action of interferon and ribavirin in treatment of hepatitis C. Nature. 2005;436(7053):967–72. Epub 2005/08/19. eng.
19. Su X, Yee LJ, Im K, et al. Association of single nucleotide polymorphisms in interferon signaling pathway genes and interferon-stimulated genes with the response to interferon therapy for chronic hepatitis C. J Hepatol. 2008;49(2):184–91. Pubmed Central PMCID: PMC2609954, Epub 2008/06/24. eng.
20. Welzel TM, Morgan TR, Bonkovsky HL, et al. Variants in interferon-alpha pathway genes and response to pegylated interferon-Alpha2a plus ribavirin for treatment of chronic hepatitis C virus infection in the hepatitis C antiviral long-term treatment against cirrhosis trial. Hepatology (Baltimore, Md). 2009;49(6):1847–58. Pubmed Central PMCID: PMC2692559. Epub 2009/05/13. eng.
21. Holmes JA, Congiu M, Bonanzinga S, et al. The relationships between IFNL4 genotype, intrahepatic interferon-stimulated gene expression and interferon treatment response differs in HCV-1 compared with HCV-3. Aliment Pharmacol Ther. 2015;42:296–306.
22. EASL. Clinical Practice Guidelines: management of hepatitis C virus infection. J Hepatol. 2011;55(2):245–64. Epub 2011/03/05. eng.
23. Intraobserver and interobserver variations in liver biopsy interpretation in patients with chronic hepatitis C. The French METAVIR Cooperative Study Group. Hepatology (Baltimore, Md). 1994; 20(1 Pt 1):15–20. Epub 1994/07/01. eng.
24. Heid CA, Stevens J, Livak KJ, Williams PM. Real time quantitative PCR. Genome Res. 1996;6(10):986–94. Epub 1996/10/01. eng.
25. Witthoft T, Moller B, Wiedmann KH, et al. Safety, tolerability and efficacy of peginterferon alpha-2a and ribavirin in chronic hepatitis C in clinical practice: The German Open Safety Trial. J Viral Hepat. 2007;14(11):788–96. Pubmed Central PMCID: PMC2156112, Epub 2007/10/12. eng.
26. Ladero JM, Martin EG, Fernandez C, et al. Predicting response to therapy in chronic hepatitis C: an approach combining interleukin-28B gene polymorphisms and clinical data. J Gastroenterol Hepatol. 2012;27(2):279–85. Epub 2011/07/05. eng.
27. Matthews DR, Hosker JP, Rudenski AS, Naylor BA, Treacher DF, Turner RC. Homeostasis model assessment: insulin resistance and beta-cell function from fasting plasma glucose and insulin concentrations in man. Diabetologia. 1985;28(7):412–9. Epub 1985/07/01. eng.
28. Hezode C. Boceprevir and telaprevir for the treatment of chronic hepatitis C: safety management in clinical practice. Liver Int. 2012;32 Suppl 1:32–8. Epub 2012/01/11. eng.
29. Poveda E, Wyles DL, Mena A, Pedreira JD, Castro-Iglesias A, Cachay E. Update on hepatitis C virus resistance to direct-acting antiviral agents. Antiviral Res. 2014;108:181–91. Epub 2014/06/10. eng.
30. Vidal-Castineira JR, Lopez-Vazquez A, Alonso-Arias R, et al. A predictive model of treatment outcome in patients with chronic HCV infection using IL28B and PD-1 genotyping. J Hepatol. 2012;56(6):1230–8. Epub 2012/02/11. eng.
31. Nimer A, Mouch A. Vitamin D improves viral response in hepatitis C genotype 2-3 naive patients. World J Gastroenterol. 2012;18(8):800–5. Pubmed Central PMCID: PMC3286143, Epub 2012/03/01. eng.
32. Wang TJ, Zhang F, Richards JB, et al. Common genetic determinants of vitamin D insufficiency: a genome-wide association study. Lancet. 2010; 376(9736):180–8. Pubmed Central PMCID: PMC3086761, Epub 2010/06/15. eng.
33. Villar LM, Del Campo JA, Ranchal I, Lampe E, Romero-Gomez M. Association between vitamin D and hepatitis C virus infection: a meta-analysis. World J Gastroenterol. 2013;19(35):5917–24. Pubmed Central PMCID: PMC3793147, Epub 2013/10/15. eng.
34. Fernandez Fernandez N, Linares Torres P, Joao Matias D, Jorquera Plaza F, Olcoz Goni JL. [Vitamin D deficiency in chronic liver disease, clinical-epidemiological analysis and report after vitamin d supplementation]. Gastroenterologia y hepatologia. 2015 Nov 16. Epub 2015/11/26. Deficit de vitamina D en la enfermedad hepatica cronica, analisis clinico epidemiologico y tras aporte vitaminico. Spa.
35. Finkelmeier F, Kronenberger B, Zeuzem S, Piiper A, Waidmann O. Low 25-Hydroxyvitamin D Levels Are Associated with Infections and Mortality in Patients with Cirrhosis. PLoS One. 2015;10(6):e0132119. Pubmed Central PMCID: PMC4487892, Epub 2015/06/30. eng.
36. Tacke F, Trautwein C. Mechanisms of liver fibrosis resolution. J Hepatol. 2015;63(4):1038–9. Epub 2015/08/02. eng.
37. Cheng JB, Levine MA, Bell NH, Mangelsdorf DJ, Russell DW. Genetic evidence that the human CYP2R1 enzyme is a key vitamin D 25-hydroxylase. Proc Natl Acad Sci U S A. 2004;101(20):7711–5. Pubmed Central PMCID: PMC419671, Epub 2004/05/07. eng.
38. Nissen J, Rasmussen LB, Ravn-Haren G, et al. Common variants in CYP2R1 and GC genes predict vitamin D concentrations in healthy Danish children and adults. PLoS One. 2014;9(2):e89907. Pubmed Central PMCID: PMC3937412, Epub 2014/03/04. eng.
39. Baur K, Mertens JC, Schmitt J, et al. The vitamin D receptor gene bAt (CCA) haplotype impairs the response to pegylated-interferon/ribavirin-based therapy in chronic hepatitis C patients. Antivir Ther. 2012;17(3):541–7. Epub 2012/02/04. eng.
40. Khairy M, Fouad R, Mabrouk M, et al. The impact of interleukin 28b gene polymorphism on the virological response to combined pegylated interferon and ribavirin therapy in chronic HCV genotype 4 infected egyptian patients using data mining analysis. Hepat Mon. 2013;13(7):e10509. Pubmed Central PMCID: PMC3776149, Epub 2013/09/26. eng.
41. Youssef SS, Abbas EA, Abd-el-Aal AM, Omran MH, Barakat A, Seif SM. IL28B rs 12979860 predicts response to treatment in Egyptian hepatitis C virus genotype 4 patients and alpha fetoprotein increases its predictive strength. J Interferon Cytokine Res. 2014;34(7):505–9. Epub 2014/03/26. eng.
42. Tsamandas AC, Syrokosta I, Thomopoulos K, et al. Potential role of hepatic progenitor cells expression in cases of chronic hepatitis C and their relation to response to therapy: a clinicopathologic study. Liver Int. 2006;26(7):817–26. Epub 2006/08/17. eng.

43. Abdoul H, Mallet V, Pol S, Fontanet A. Serum alpha-fetoprotein predicts treatment outcome in chronic hepatitis C patients regardless of HCV genotype. PLoS One. 2008;3(6):e2391. Pubmed Central PMCID: PMC2398780, Epub 2008/06/12. eng.
44. Degasperi E, Valenti L, Aghemo A, et al. Interleukin 28B genotype and insulin resistance in chronic hepatitis C patients. Antivir Ther. 2014;19(8): 747–53. Epub 2014/02/14. eng.
45. Vukovic VR, Baskic D, Mijailovic Z, et al. Association between risk factors, basal viral load, virus genotype and the degree of liver fibrosis with the response to the therapy in patients with chronic hepatitis C virus infection. Vojnosanit Pregl. 2015;72(6):505–9. Epub 2015/08/01. eng.

Permissions

All chapters in this book were first published in GASTROENTEROLOGY, by BioMed Central; hereby published with permission under the Creative Commons Attribution License or equivalent. Every chapter published in this book has been scrutinized by our experts. Their significance has been extensively debated. The topics covered herein carry significant findings which will fuel the growth of the discipline. They may even be implemented as practical applications or may be referred to as a beginning point for another development.

The contributors of this book come from diverse backgrounds, making this book a truly international effort. This book will bring forth new frontiers with its revolutionizing research information and detailed analysis of the nascent developments around the world.

We would like to thank all the contributing authors for lending their expertise to make the book truly unique. They have played a crucial role in the development of this book. Without their invaluable contributions this book wouldn't have been possible. They have made vital efforts to compile up to date information on the varied aspects of this subject to make this book a valuable addition to the collection of many professionals and students.

This book was conceptualized with the vision of imparting up-to-date information and advanced data in this field. To ensure the same, a matchless editorial board was set up. Every individual on the board went through rigorous rounds of assessment to prove their worth. After which they invested a large part of their time researching and compiling the most relevant data for our readers.

The editorial board has been involved in producing this book since its inception. They have spent rigorous hours researching and exploring the diverse topics which have resulted in the successful publishing of this book. They have passed on their knowledge of decades through this book. To expedite this challenging task, the publisher supported the team at every step. A small team of assistant editors was also appointed to further simplify the editing procedure and attain best results for the readers.

Apart from the editorial board, the designing team has also invested a significant amount of their time in understanding the subject and creating the most relevant covers. They scrutinized every image to scout for the most suitable representation of the subject and create an appropriate cover for the book.

The publishing team has been an ardent support to the editorial, designing and production team. Their endless efforts to recruit the best for this project, has resulted in the accomplishment of this book. They are a veteran in the field of academics and their pool of knowledge is as vast as their experience in printing. Their expertise and guidance has proved useful at every step. Their uncompromising quality standards have made this book an exceptional effort. Their encouragement from time to time has been an inspiration for everyone.

The publisher and the editorial board hope that this book will prove to be a valuable piece of knowledge for researchers, students, practitioners and scholars across the globe.

List of Contributors

Hala I. Mohamed, Hamdy A. Mokarib, Zienab M. Saad and Wael M. Abd El Ghany
Faculty of Medicine, Gastroenterology and Endemic Medicine Department, Minya University, Minya, Egypt

Maria Stepanova, Mehmet Sayiner, Leyla de Avila, Zahra Younoszai, Andrei Racila and Zobair M. Younossi
Betty and Guy Beatty Center for Integrated Research, Inova Health System, Claude Moore Health Education and Research Building 3300 Gallows Road, Falls Church, VA 22042, USA

Maria Stepanova
Center for Outcomes Research in Liver Diseases, Washington, DC, USA

Zobair M. Younossi
Center for Liver Diseases, Department of Medicine, Inova Fairfax Hospital, Falls Church, VA, USA

Stefan Bourgeois
Department of Gastroenterology and Hepatology, ZNA Antwerp, Antwerpen, Belgium

Hans Van Vlierberghe
Department of Hepatology and Gastroenterology, Universitair Ziekenhuis Gent, Ghent, Belgium

Christophe Moreno
Liver Unit, CUB Hôpital Erasme, Université Libre de Bruxelles, Brussels, Belgium

Hans Orlent
Department of Gastroenterology and Hepatology, AZ Sint-Jan AV Hospital, Bruges, Belgium

Frederik Nevens
Department of Liver and Biliopancreatic Disorders, University Hospitals KU Leuven, Leuven, Belgium

Keikawus Arastéh
EPIMED/Vivantes-Auguste-Viktoria-Klinikum, Berlin, Germany

Yves Horsmans
Hepato-gastroenterology, Cliniques Universitaires Saint-Luc, Université Catholique de Louvain, Brussels, Belgium

Jörn M. Schattenberg
Department of Medicine, University Medical Center Mainz, Mainz, Germany

Peter Buggisch
IFI, Liver Center Hamburg, Asklepiosklinik St. Georg, Hamburg, Germany

Sven Francque
Department of Gastroenterology and Hepatology, Universitair Ziekenhuis Antwerpen, Antwerp, Belgium

Leen Vijgen and Bert Jacquemyn
Janssen Pharmaceutica NV, Beerse, Belgium

Thomas N. Kakuda
Alios BioPharma Inc, South San Francisco, CA, USA

An Vandebosch, René Verloes and Eva Hoeben
Janssen Research and Development BVBA, Beerse, Belgium

Donghan Luo and Pieter Van Remoortere
Janssen Pharmaceuticals LLC, Titusville, NJ, USA

Yang-Sheng Lin, Shou-Chuan Shih, Horng-Yuan Wang, Chen-Wang Chang and Ming-Jen Chen
Division of Gastroenterology, Department of Internal Medicine, MacKay Memorial Hospital, Taipei Campus, No. 92, Sec

Yang-Sheng Lin, Horng-Yuan Wangn and Ming-Jen Chen
Chungshan North Road, 104 Taipei, Taiwan. MacKay Junior College of Medicine, Nursing, and Management, Taipei, Taiwan

Shou-Chuan Shih, Yang-Sheng Lin and Ching-Chung
MacKay Medical College, New Taipei City, Taiwan

Jian-Hua Lei, Xu Yang, Xin-Qiang Xiao, Zi Chen and Feng Peng
Department of Infectious Diseases, the Second Xiangya Hospital, Central South University, No.139 Middle Renmin Road, Changsha, Hunan 410011, People's Republic of China

Ji Won Park, Sung Eun Kim and Choong Kee Park
Department of Internal Medicine, Hallym University Sacred Heart Hospital of Hallym University Medical Center, 22, Gwanpyeong-ro 170 beon-gil, Dongan-gu, Anyang-si, Gyeonggi-do 14068, Republic of Korea

Ji Won Park
Department of Biomedical Gerontology, Graduate School of Hallym University, 1 Hallymdaehak-gil, Chuncheon-si, Gangwon-do 24252, Republic of Korea

Kyeong Min Kwak
Department of Occupational and Environmental Medicine, Hallym University Sacred Heart Hospital of Hallym University Medical Center, 22, Gwanpyeong-ro 170 beon-gil, Dongan-gu, Anyang-si, Gyeonggi-do 14068, Republic of Korea

Kyeong Min Kwak
Department of Environmental Health, Seoul National University School of Public Health, 1, Gwanak-ro, Gwanak-gu, Seoul 08826, Republic of Korea

Hyoung Su Kim and Myoung Kuk Jang
Department of Internal Medicine, Kangdong Sacred Heart Hospital of Hallym University Medical Center, 18, Cheonho-daero 173-gil, Gangdong-gu, Seoul 05355, Republic of Korea

Dong Joon Kim and Ki Tae Suk
Department of Internal Medicine, Chuncheon Sacred Heart Hospital of Hallym University Medical Center, 77, Sakju-ro, Chuncheon-si, Gangwon-do 24253, Republic of Korea

Sang Hoon Park and Myung Seok Lee
Department of Internal Medicine, Kangnam Sacred Heart Hospital of Hallym University Medical Center, 1, Singil-ro, Yeongdeungpo-gu, Seoul 07441, Republic of Korea

Weihui Sun, Lei Ma, Anhua Hao, Bo Zhao, Lin Zhou and Fengzhu Li
Department of Hepatology, Chengyang People's Hospital of Qingdao, Qingdao 266109, Shandong Province, China

Shangfei Zhao and Mingquan Song
Department of Gastroenterology, The Affiliated Hospital of Qingdao University, Qingdao 266011, Shandong Province, China

Hongqin Xu, Wenli Kong, Lei Liu, Xiumei Chi, Xiaomei Wang, Ruihong Wu, Xiuzhu Gao, Huan Wang, Yue Qi, Yu Pan and Junqi Niu
Department of Hepatology, First Hospital of Jilin University, Jilin University, Changchun 130021, China

Junqi Niu
Ministry of Education Key Laboratory of Zoonosis, Changchun 130061, China

Hongqin Xu, Xiumei Chi, Xiaomei Wang, Ruihong Wu and Xiuzhu Gao
Jilin Province Key Laboratory of Infectious Diseases, Laboratory of Molecular Virology, Changchun 130061, China

Limei Qu
Department of Pathology, First Hospital of Jilin University, Jilin University, Changchun 130021, China

Ming-Shyan Lin
Department of Cardiology, Department of Internal Medicine, Chang Gung Memorial Hospital, Yunlin, Taiwan

Tien-Hsing Chen
Department of Cardiology, Department of Internal Medicine, Chang Gung Memorial Hospital, Chang Gung University College of Medicine, Keelung, Taiwan

Wey-Yil Lin and Chi-Hung Liu
Stroke Center and Department of Neurology, Chang Gung Memorial Hospital, Linkou Medical Center, Chang Gung University College of Medicine, Taoyuan, Taiwan

Yung-Yu Hsieh
Department of Hepato-Gastroenterology, Chang Gung Memorial Hospital, Chiayi, Taiwan

Wen-Nan Chiu
Department of Hepato-Gastroenterology, Chang Gung Memorial Hospital, Yunlin, Taiwan

Chih-Hsiang Chang
Department of Nephrology, Kidney research center, Chang Gung Memorial Hospital, Chang Gung University, College of medicine, Taoyuan, Taiwan

Mei-Yen Chen
College of Nursing, Chang Gung University of Science and Technology (CGUST), Taoyuan, Taiwan

Mei-Yen Chen
Department of Nursing, Chang Gung University, Taoyuan, Taiwan

Chang-Min Chung and Yu-Sheng Lin
School of Traditional Chinese Medicine, College of Medicine, Chang Gung University, Taoyuan County, Taiwan

Chang-Min Chung and Yu-Sheng Lin
Department of Cardiology, Chiayi Chang Gung Memorial Hospital, 6, Sec. West Chai-Pu Road, Pu-TZ City, Chai Yi Hsien 61363, Taiwan

Yan Xu, Xu Wang, Zhenhua Liu, Changyu Zhou, Wenqian Qi, Jian Jiao, Fan Yu, Honghua Guo, Ping Zhao and Jiangbin Wang
Department of Gastroenterology, China–Japan Union Hospital, Jilin University, Changchun, Jilin Province 130033, China

Faisal M. Sanai and Khalid AlSwat
Liver Disease Research Center, King Saud University, Riyadh, Saudi Arabia

Khalid I. Bzeizi
Department of Gastroenterology, Prince Sultan Military Medical City, Riyadh, Saudi Arabia

Mohammed A. Babatin
Division of Gastroenterology, Department of Medicine, King Fahad Hospital, Jeddah, Saudi Arabia

Hamad Al-Ashgar
Division of Gastroenterology, Department of Medicine, King Faisal Specialist Hospital and Research Center, Riyadh, Saudi Arabia

Hadeel AlMana
Department of Pathology, King Faisal Specialist Hospital and Research Center, Riyadh, Saudi Arabia

Khaled S. Alsaad
Department of Pathology, King Abdulaziz Medical City, Riyadh, Saudi Arabia

Abdulrahman Aljumah and Ibrahim H. AlTraif
Hepatobiliary Sciences and Liver Transplantation, King Abdulaziz Medical City, Riyadh, Saudi Arabia

Taha Farah, Khalid Albeladi, Faisal Batwa, Yaser Dahlan and Faisal M. Sanai
Gastroenterology Unit, Department of Medicine, King Abdulaziz Medical City, Jeddah 21423, Saudi Arabia

Abdulrahman Aljumah and Ibrahim H. AlTraif
King Saud bin Abdulaziz University for Health Sciences, Riyadh, Saudi Arabia

Bahaa E. Kailani
Gastroenterology Unit, Department of Medicine, King Fahad Armed Forces Hospital, Jeddah, Saudi Arabia

Hugo Perazzo, Valdilea Gonçalves Veloso and Rodolfo Castro
Fundação Oswaldo Cruz, FIOCRUZ, Instituto Nacional de Infectologia Evandro Chagas, INI, Laboratório de Pesquisa Clínica em DST e AIDS, LAPCLIN-AIDS, Rio de Janeiro, Brazil

Marcelino Jose Jorge, Alexandre Monken Avellar and Patrícia Santos Silva
Fundação Oswaldo Cruz, FIOCRUZ, Instituto Nacional de Infectologia Evandro Chagas, INI, Laboratório de Pesquisa em Economia das Organizações de Saúde, LAPECOS, Rio de Janeiro, Brazil

Julio Castro Silva
Fundação Oswaldo Cruz, FIOCRUZ, Instituto Nacional de Infectologia Evandro Chagas, INI, Plataforma de Pesquisa Clínica, Rio de Janeiro, Brazil

Carmen Romero
Fundação Oswaldo Cruz, FIOCRUZ, Centro de Desenvolvimento Tecnológico em Saúde, CDTS, Rio de Janeiro, Brazil

Ruben Mujica-Mota, Rob Anderson and Chris Hyde
University of Exeter Medical School, UEMS, Evidence Synthesis and Modelling for Health Improvement, ESMI, Exeter, UK

Rodolfo Castro
Universidade Federal do Estado do Rio de Janeiro, UNIRIO, Instituto de Saúde Coletiva, ISC, Rio de Janeiro, Brazil

Mary Ellen Dias Barbosa and Ana Luiza Zaninotto
Division of Psychology, Clinics Hospital, University of Sao Paulo School of Medicine, Avenida Dr. Eneas Carvalho de Aguiar, 255, São Paulo 05403-900, Brazil

Mario Guimarães Pessoa, Cláudia Pinto Marques Souza de Oliveira, Flair José Carrilho, Alberto Queiroz Farias, Mary Ellen Dias Barbosa and Daniel Ferraz de Campos Mazo
Division of Clinical Gastroenterology and Hepatology, Clinics Hospital, Department of Gastroenterology, University of São Paulo School of Medicine, Avenida Dr. Eneas Carvalho de Aguiar, 255, sala 9159, São Paulo 05403-900, Brazil

Daniel Ferraz de Campos Mazo
Division of Gastroenterology, School of Medical Sciences, University of Campinas, Rua Carlos Chagas, 420, Campinas 13083-878, Brazil

Mary Ellen Dias Barbosa
Departmen of Gastroenterology, University of Sao Paulo School of Medicine, Av. Dr. Enéas de Carvalho Aguiar n° 255, São Paulo 05403-000, Brazil

Chien-Yuan Chen, Feng-Ming Tien, Shang-Yi Huang, Wen-Chien Chou, Ming Yao, Jih-Luh Tang and Hwei-Fang Tien
Division of Hematology, Department of Internal Medicine, National Taiwan University Hospital, Taipei, Taiwan

Wang-Huei Sheng and Aristine Cheng
Division of Infectious Disease, Department of Internal Medicine, National Taiwan University Hospital, 7 Chung-Shan South Road, Taipei 10002, Taiwan

Wen-Chien Chou
Department of Laboratory Medicine, National Taiwan University Hospital, Taipei, Taiwan

Jih-Luh Tang
Tai-Cheng Stem Cell Therapy Center, National Taiwan University Hospital, Taipei, Taiwan

Rie Harada, Masako Kimura, Yasushi Sato, Tatsuya Taniguchi, Tetsu Tomonari, Takahiro Tanaka, Hironori Tanaka, Naoki Muguruma and Tetsuji Takayama
Department of Gastroenterology and Oncology, Tokushima University Graduate School of Biomedical Sciences, 3-18-15, Kuramoto-cho, Tokushima 770-8503, Japan

Hirohiko Shinomiya
Department of Gastroenterology, Yoshinogawa Medical Center, Yoshinogawa, Tokushima 776-8511, Japan

Hirohito Honda
Department of Internal Medicine, Tokushima Health Screening Center, 1-10-3, Kuramoto-cho, Tokushima 770-0042, Japan

Issei Imoto
Department of Human Genetics, Tokushima University Graduate School of Biomedical Sciences, 3-18-15, Kuramoto-cho, Tokushima 770-8503, Japan

Masahiro Sogabe and Toshiya Okahisa
Department of General Medicine and Community Health Science, Tokushima University Graduate School of Biomedical Sciences, 3-18-15, Kuramoto-cho, Tokushima 770-8503, Japan

Rita Moretti, Paola Caruso and Matteo Dal Ben
Neurology Clinic, Department of Medical, Surgical, and Health Sciences, University of Trieste, 34100 Trieste, Italy

Silvia Gazzin, Claudio Tiribelli and Matteo Dal Ben
Italian Liver Foundation, Centro Studi Fegato, AREA Science Park, Bldg. Q, Ss 14, km 163.5, 34149 Trieste, Italy

Surbhi Jain, Sierra McCloud, Wei Song and Jamin D. Steffen
JBS Science, Inc., Doylestown, PA 18902, USA

Ying-Hsiu Su, Yih-Ping Su and Tai-Jung Lee
The Baruch S. Blumberg Institute, Doylestown, PA 18902, USA

Ruixia Xue
The Second Hospital of Yuncheng, Yuncheng, Shanxi Province 044000, China

Shu-Chuan Lin and Chi-Tan Hu
Buddhist Tzu Chi General Hospital and Tzu Chi University, 707, Sec. 3, Chung-Yang Rd, Hualien 970, Taiwan, R.O.C

Selena Y. Lin and Wei Song
U-Screen Dx Inc., Doylestown, PA 18902, USA

Jamin D. Steffen
Hepron Molecular Lab, Inc., Doylestown, PA 18902, USA

Yue Ying, Yue-Kai Hu, Jia-Lin Jin, Ji-Ming Zhang, Wen-Hong Zhang and Yu-Xian Huang
Department of Infectious Diseases, Huashan Hospital Affiliated to Fudan University, 12, Middle Wulumuqi Road, Shanghai 200040, China

Xiuqing Pang, Xinhua Li, Zhishuo Mo, Jing Huang, Hong Deng, Ziying Lei, Xingrong Zheng Dongying Xie and Zhiliang Gao
Department of Infectious Diseases, Third Affiliated Hospital of Sun-Yat-SenUniversity, GuangZhou, China
GuangDong Provincial Key Laboratory of Liver Disease, Third Affiliated Hospital of Sun-Yat-Sen University, GuangZhou, China

Zhiying Feng
Department of Pathology, Third Affiliated Hospital of Sun-Yat-Sen University, GuangZhou, China

Dongying Xie and Zhiliang Gao
GuangZhou, China

Henry H. Nguyen, Abdullah Khathlan, Marvin J. Fritzler and Mark G. Swain
Division of Gastroenterology and Hepatology, University of Calgary Liver Unit, Calgary, Canada

Marvin J. Fritzler
University of Calgary, Calgary, AB, Canada

Mark G. Swain
Teaching Research and Wellness Centre, 3280 Hospital Drive NW, Calgary, AB T2N 4N1, Canada

Wenhui Li, Li Jia, Xin Zhao and Xiaoyuan Wu
Department of Infectious Disease, Children's Hospital of Hebei Province, 133 South Jianhua Street, Shijiazhuang 050031, Hebei, China

Hongxia Tang
Department of Neurology, Children's Hospital of Hebei Province, 133 South Jianhua Street, Shijiazhuang 050031, Hebei, China

Fangyuan Gao, Xiaoshu Li, Yuxin Li, Qun Zhang, Yao Liu, Huimin Liu and Xianbo Wang
Center of Integrative Medicine, Beijing Ditan Hospital, Capital Medical University, Beijing, China

Gang Wan
Statistics Room, Beijing Ditan Hospital, Capital Medical University, Beijing, China

Hai Li
Department of Gastroenterology, Ren Ji Hospital, School of Medicine, Shanghai Jiao Tong University, Shanghai, China

Majid Mahmood
Department of Zoology, The University of Poonch, Rawalakot, Azad Jammu and Kashmir 12350, Pakistan
Department of Zoology, Pir Mehr Ali Shah Arid Agriculture University, Rawalpindi 46300, Pakistan

Muhammad Asim Anwar
Department of General Medicine, Pakistan Atomic Energy Commission (PAEC) General Hospital, Islamabad 44000, Pakistan

Azra Khanum
Barani Institute of Management Sciences (BIMS), Rawalpindi 46300, Pakistan

Nasib Zaman
Center for Biotechnology and Microbiology, University of Swat, Swat 19130, Pakistan

Abida Raza
Diagnostic Department, Nuclear Medicine, Oncology and Radiotherapy Institute (NORI), Islamabad 44000, Pakistan

Nattiya Kapol and Surasit Lochid-amnuay
Department of Community Pharmacy, Faculty of Pharmacy, Silpakorn University, Nakhon Pathom, Thailand73000

Yot Teerawattananon
Health Intervention and Technology Assessment Program (HITAP), Ministry of Public Health, Nonthaburi, Thailand

Naruhiko Nagata, Tatehiro Kagawa, Shunji Hirose, Yoshitaka Arase, Kota Tsuruya, Kazuya Anzai, Koichi Shiraishi and Tetsuya Mine
Division of Gastroenterology and Hepatology, Department of Internal Medicine, Tokai University School of Medicine, Shimokasuya 143, Isehara 259-1193, Japan

M. O. El-Derany, N. M. Hamdy and H. O. El-Mesallamy
Biochemistry Department, Faculty of Pharmacy, Ain Shams University, Cairo, Egypt

N. L. Al-Ansari
Endemic Medicine Department and Hepatology Unit, Faculty of Medicine, Ain Shams University, Cairo, Egypt

Index

www.ingramcontent.com/pod-product-compliance
Lightning Source LLC
LaVergne TN
LVHW080702210926
848485LV00003B/408